CASE STUDIES

Stahl's Essential Psychopharmacology

Volume 3

CASE STUDIES Stahl's Essential
Psychopharmacology

Volume 3

Edited by

Takesha Cooper

*Director of the Psychiatry Residency Training Program,
University of California, Riverside, CA, USA*

Gerald Maguire

Chair, University of California, Riverside, CA, USA

Stephen M. Stahl

*Adjunct Professor of Psychiatry,
University of California San Diego, CA, USA*

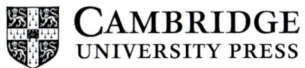
CAMBRIDGE
UNIVERSITY PRESS

CAMBRIDGE
UNIVERSITY PRESS

University Printing House, Cambridge CB2 8BS, United Kingdom

One Liberty Plaza, 20th Floor, New York, NY 10006, USA

477 Williamstown Road, Port Melbourne, VIC 3207, Australia

314–321, 3rd Floor, Plot 3, Splendor Forum, Jasola District Centre,
New Delhi – 110025, India

103 Penang Road, #05–06/07, Visioncrest Commercial, Singapore 238467

Cambridge University Press is part of the University of Cambridge.

It furthers the University's mission by disseminating knowledge in the pursuit of
education, learning, and research at the highest international levels of excellence.

www.cambridge.org
Information on this title: www.cambridge.org/9781009012898
DOI: 10.1017/9781009026499

First published 2022

Printed in the United Kingdom by TJ Books Limited, Padstow Cornwall

A catalogue record for this publication is available from the British Library.

ISBN 978-1-009-01289-8 Paperback

Cambridge University Press has no responsibility for the persistence or accuracy of
URLs for external or third-party internet websites referred to in this publication
and does not guarantee that any content on such websites is, or will remain,
accurate or appropriate.

Every effort has been made in preparing this book to provide accurate and
up-to-date information that is in accord with accepted standards and practice
at the time of publication. Although case histories are drawn from actual cases,
every effort has been made to disguise the identities of the individuals involved.
Nevertheless, the authors, editors, and publishers can make no warranties that the
information contained herein is totally free from error, not least because clinical
standards are constantly changing through research and regulation. The authors,
editors, and publishers therefore disclaim all liability for direct or consequential
damages resulting from the use of material contained in this book. Readers
are strongly advised to pay careful attention to information provided by the
manufacturer of any drugs or equipment that they plan to use.

Contents

Introduction

Following on from the success of the second volume of *Case Studies* in 2016, we are very pleased to present a third collection of new clinical cases. This third collection of cases is the result of a special project of the Department of Psychiatry and Neuroscience of the University of California, Riverside, where all three editors are faculty members. Each case is taken from the clinical practices of the department and each is written by a team comprising a medical student or resident/fellow in psychiatry paired with a faculty member in the UCR psychiatry and neuroscience department. This volume of cases thus showcases not only the clinical practice in our department, but the teamwork of faculty and trainees to produce a scholarly and educational book to enrich and inform our colleagues who treat mental illness. *Stahl's Essential Psychopharmacology* started in 1996 as a textbook (currently in its fourth edition) on how psychotropic medications work. It expanded to a companion Prescriber's Guide in 2005 (currently in its fifth edition) on how to prescribe psychotropic medications. In 2008, a website was added (**stahlonline.cambridge.org**) with both of these books available online in combination with several more, including an *Illustrated* series of books covering specialty topics in psychopharmacology. The *Case Studies* shows how to apply the concepts presented in these previous books to real patients in a clinical practice setting.

Why a case book? For practitioners, it is necessary to know the science and application of psychopharmacology – namely, both the mechanism of action of psychotropic medications and the evidence-based data on how to prescribe them – but this is not sufficient to become a master clinician. Many patients are beyond the data and are excluded from randomized controlled trials. Thus, a true clinical expert also needs to develop the art of psychopharmacology: namely, how to listen, educate, destigmatize, mix psychotherapy with medications, and use intuition to select and combine medications. The art of psychopharmacology is especially important when confronting the frequent situations where there is no evidence on which to base a clinical decision.

What do you do when there is no evidence? The short answer is to combine the science with the art of psychopharmacology. The best way to learn this is probably by seeing individual patients. Here we hope you will join us and peer over our shoulders to observe 34 complex cases from our own clinical practice. Each case is anonymized in identifying details, but incorporates real case outcomes that are not fictionalized. Sometimes more than one case is combined into a single case. Hopefully, you will recognize many of these patients as similar to those you have seen in your own practice (although they will not be exactly the same patient, as the identifying historical details are changed here to comply with disclosure standards, and many patients can look very much like many other patients you know, which is why you may find this teaching approach effective for your clinical practice).

We have presented cases from our clinical practice for many years online (e.g. in the master psychopharmacology program of the Neuroscience Education Institute (NEI) at neiglobal.com) and in live courses (especially at the annual NEI Psychopharmacology Congress). Over the years, we have been fortunate to have many young psychiatrists from our universities, and indeed from all over the world, sit in on our practices to observe these cases, and now we attempt to bring this information to you in the form of a third case book.

The cases are presented in a novel written format in order to follow consultations over time, with different categories of information designated by different background colors and explanatory icons. For those of you familiar with *The Prescriber's Guide*, this layout will be recognizable. Included in the case book, however, are many unique sections as well; for example, presenting what was on the author's mind at various points during the management of the case, and also questions along the way for you to ask yourself in order to develop an action plan. There is a pretest, asked again at the end as a posttest, for those who wish to gain CME credits (go to **neiglobal.com** to answer these questions and obtain credits). Additionally, these cases incorporate ideas from the recent changes in maintenance of certification standards by the American Board of Psychiatry and Neurology for those of you interested in recertification in psychiatry. Thus, there is a section on Performance in Practice (called here "Confessions of a psychopharmacologist"). There is a short section at the end of several cases looking back and seeing what could have been done better in retrospect. Another section of most cases is a short psychopharmacology lesson or tutorial, called the "Two-minute tutorial," with background information, tables, and figures from literature relevant to the case in hand. Medications are listed by their generic and brand names for ease of learning. Indexes are included at the back of the book for your convenience. Lists of icons and abbreviations are provided in the front of the book. Finally, this third collection updates the reader on the newest psychotropic medications and their uses, and adopts the language of *DSM-V*.

The case-based approach is how this book attempts to complement "evidence-based prescribing" from other books in the *Essential Psychopharmacology* series, plus the literature, with "prescribing-based evidence" derived from empiric experience. It is certainly important to know the data from randomized controlled trials, but after knowing all this information, case-based clinical experience supplements those data. The old saying that applies here is that wisdom is what you learn *after* you know it all; and so, too, for studying cases after seeing the data.

A note of caution: we are not so naïve as to think that there are not potential pitfalls to the centuries-old tradition of case-based teaching. Thus, we think it is a good idea to point some of them out here in order to try to avoid these traps. Do not ignore the "law of small numbers" by basing broad predictions on narrow samples or even a single case.

Do not ignore the fact that if something is easy to recall, particularly when associated with a significant emotional event, we tend to think it happens more often than it does.

Do not forget the recency effect, namely, the tendency to think that something that has just been observed happens more often than it does.

According to editorialists[1], when moving away from evidence-based medicine to case-based medicine, it is also important to avoid:
- Eloquence or elegance-based medicine
- Vehemence-based medicine
- Providence-based medicine
- Diffidence-based medicine
- Nervousness-based medicine
- Confidence-based medicine

We have been counseled by colleagues and trainees that perhaps the most important pitfall for us to try to avoid in this book is "eminence-based medicine," and to remember specifically that:
- Radiance of gray hair is not proportional to an understanding of the facts
- Eloquence, smoothness of the tongue, and sartorial elegance cannot change reality
- Qualifications and past accomplishments do not signify a privileged access to the truth
- Experts almost always have conflicts of interest
- Clinical acumen is not measured in frequent flier miles

Thus, it is with all humility as practicing psychiatrists that we invite you to walk a mile in our shoes; experience the fascination, the disappointments, the thrills, and the learnings that result from observing cases in the real world.

Takesha Cooper, MD

Gerald Maguire, MD

Stephen M. Stahl, MD, PhD

[1] Isaccs D and Fitzgerald D. Seven alternatives to evidence based medicine. *British Medical Journal 1999; 319:1618.*

Contributors

Dennis Alters, MD, DLFAPA
Angharad Ames, MD
Roberto Castaños, MD
Karen Clarey, MD, Psychiatry Resident
Takesha Cooper, MD, MS, Psychiatry Residency Program Director and Associate
Clinical Professor
Evagelos Coskinas, MD, PhD
Courtney DiNicola, BS, MS
Lawrence Faziola, Associate Professor of Clinical Psychiatry
Carl Feinstein, MD
Christopher G. Fichtner, MS, MD, Clinical Professor and Vice Chair for Administration,
Department of Psychiatry and Neuroscience, University of California, Riverside
School of Medicine
Kayla L. Fisher, MD, MBA
Erin Fletcher, MD, MPH
Karla P. Furlong, MD
Sarah Grace, MD
Douglas Grover, MD
Niraj Gupta, MD
Catherine Ha, Medical Student (MS), UCR School of Medicine
Nekisa Haghighat, MD, MPH
Charity Hall, Medical Student (MS), UCR School of Medicine
Carla Hammond, MD, Assistant Clinical Professor, Department of Psychiatry, UC
Riverside School of Medicine
Peter Hauser, MD, LBVA
Dale Hoang, MD, UCR
Ijeoma Ijeaku, MD, MPH, FAPA
Michael T. Ingram, Jr., MS, MD
Eduardo Javier, MD
Brenda Jensen, MD, University of California, Riverside School of Medicine
Sana Johnson-Quijada, MD
Samer Kamal, MD
Justine Ku, MSIII
Lauren Kurz, PMHNP, MSN
Troy Kurz, MD
Niya Larios, BS
Richard J. Lee, MD, UCR Child and Adolescent Psychiatry Training Program Director
Arthur Leitzke, MD

Casey Lester, MD
Matt Jason V. Llamas, BS
Kathleen Lopez, MD
Alex J. Mageno, MD
Gerald Maguire, MD, DFAPA
Ruqayyah Malik, MD
Stephen Maurer, MD
Louis May, MD
Austin Nguy, BA
Alexander Thanh Nguyen, MD MPH, Assistant Clinical Professor, UCR Psychiatry, Long Beach VA Healthcare System
Diem Nguyen, MD, University of California, Riverside School of Medicine
Edgar Ortega, MD
Monish Parmar, MD DABPN
Yatna Patel, BS, UCR MS3
Joshua Poole, MD
Nishant Prakash, BS
Harika Reddy, MD
Madeline Saavedra, MD
Martin Sahakyan, MD
Michael Seigler, MD
Kevin Simonson, MD
Saloni Singh, MD, Resident Physician, Department of Psychiatry, UC Riverside School of Medicine
Sireena Sy, MD, UCR Psychiatry PGY2
Michelle Tom, MD
Alexander H. Truong, MD
Kevin Truong, MD
Joshua Valverde, MD
Alfonso Vera
Darian Vernon, MD
Phuong Vo, BS, MS
Joseph Wong, MS IV
Stephanie Wong, Medical Student
Jami Woods, MD
Joseph Yasmeh, BS
Margaret Yau, MS3
Bo Ram Yoo, MS
Lawrence Yu, MD

List of icons

	Pre- and posttest self-assessment question; question
	Patient evaluation on intake; patient evaluation on initial visit
	Psychiatric history
	Social and personal history
	Medical history
	Family history
	Medication history
	Current medications

	Psychotherapy history; psychotherapy moment
	Mechanism of action moment
	Attending physician's mental notes
	Further investigation
	Case outcome; use of outcome measures
	Case debrief
	Take-home points
	Performance in practice: confessions of a psychopharmacologist
	Tips and pearls
	Two-minute tutorial

Abbreviations

5-HT	serotonin	CBC	complete blood count
AACAP	American Academy of Child and Adolescent Psychiatry	CBT	cognitive behavioral therapy
AAP	American Academy of Pediatrics	CIWA-Ar	Clinical Institute Withdrawal Assessment of Alcohol, Revised
ACE	adverse childhood event	CNS	central nervous system
ADHD	attention-deficit/hyperactivity disorder	COVID-19	coronavirus disease 2019
AF	atrial fibrillation	CPS	Child Protective Services
AIMS	Abnormal Involuntary Movement Scale	CT	computed tomography
ALT	alanine amino transferase	CYP1A2	cytochrome P450 1A2
		CYP2D6	cytochrome P450 2D6
AMPA	α-amino-3-hydroxy-5-methyl-4-isoxazolepropionic acid	DA	dopamine
		DSM-4-TR	*Diagnostic and Statistical Manual of Mental Disorders*, 4th edn., text revision
ANC	absolute neutrophil count		
ANCA	anti-neutrophil cytoplasmic antibody	DSM-4/DSM-5	*Diagnostic and Statistical Manual of Mental Disorders*, 4th/5th edn.
ASD	autism spectrum disorder	ECG	electrocardiogram
ASQ	Ages and Stages Questionnaire	ECT	electroconvulsive therapy
AST	aspartate amino transferase	EEG	electroencephalogram
		EPS	extrapyramidal symptoms
AWS	alcohol withdrawal syndrome	ER	extended-release
BDNF	brain-derived neurotrophic factor	FAST	Functional Adaptation and Skills Training
BDZ	benzodiazepine	FDA	US Food and Drug Administration
BED	binge eating disorder		
BMI	body mass index	fMRI	functional magnetic resonance imaging
BMP	basic metabolic panel		
BPD	brief psychotic disorder	GABA	γ-aminobutyric acid
bpm	beats/min	GAD	generalized anxiety disorder
BUN	blood urea nitrogen		

G-CSF	granulocyte colony-stimulating factor	MoCA	Montreal Cognitive Assessment
GnRH	gonadotropin-releasing hormone	MOR	μ-opioid receptor
		MRI	magnetic resonance imaging
GSK3	glycogen synthase kinase 3	mTOR	mammalian target of rapamycin
HAM-D	Hamilton Depression Rating Scale	NDRI	norepinephrine-dopamine reuptake inhibitor
HbA1c	hemoglobin A1c		
HDL	high-density lipoprotein	NE	norepinephrine
HIV	human immunodeficiency virus	NMDA	N-methyl-D-aspartate
HPA	hypothalamic–pituitary–adrenal	NMS	neuroleptic malignant syndrome
ID	intellectual disability	NPSLE	neuropsychiatric systemic lupus erythematosus
IDD	intellectual developmental disorder		
IEP	Individualized Education Plan	OCD	obsessive–compulsive disorder
IM	intramuscular	ODT	oral disintegrating tablet
IMD	institution for mental diseases	OROS	osmotic-controlled release oral delivery system
IPT	interpersonal psychotherapy	PARS	Pediatric Anxiety Rating Scale
IR	immediate-release		
IV	intravenous	PAWSS	Prediction of Alcohol Withdrawal Severity Scale
KOR	κ-opioid receptor		
LAI	long-acting injectable		
LDL	low-density lipoprotein	PCP	primary care physician
LPS	Lanterman–Petris–Short	PEDS	Parent's Evaluation of Developmental Status
MAO	monoamine oxidase		
MAOI	monoamine oxidase inhibitor	PET-CT	positron emission tomography/computed tomography
MASC	Multidimensional Anxiety Scale for Children	PO	by mouth
MDD	major depressive disorder	PTSD	posttraumatic stress disorder
MDE	major depressive episode	QTc	corrected QT interval
		REM	rapid eye movement
MERS	Middle East respiratory syndrome	RVR	rapid ventricular response
MMSE	mini-mental state examination	SAD	seasonal affective disorder

SARS	severe acute respiratory syndrome	TBS	Therapeutic Behavioral Services
SCA	spinocerebellar ataxia	TCA	tricyclic antidepressant
SCARED	Screen for Child Anxiety and Related Emotional Disorders	TR	time-release
		TSH	thyroid-stimulating hormone
SCAS	Spence Children's Anxiety Scale	UDS	urine drug screen
		VEGF	vascular endothelial growth factor
SCL-90-R	Symptom Checklist-90-Revised	VLPFC	ventrolateral prefrontal cortex
SLD	specific learning disorder		
SLE	systemic lupus erythematosus	VMAT2	vesicular monoamine transporter-2
SNRI	serotonin-norepinephrine reuptake inhibitor	WISC	Wechsler Intelligence Scale for Children
SSRI	selective serotonin reuptake inhibitor	WPATH	World Professional Association for Transgender Health
T3	triiodothyronine		
T4	thyroxine	XL	extended-release
TBI	traumatic brain injury	XR	extended-release

Case 1: Wearing down a diagnosis

The Question: What are the similarities and differences between anxiety and autism spectrum disorder (ASD) in children? How does it affect treatment and prognosis?

The Psychopharmacological Dilemma: Does this patient have an anxiety disorder, which can be treated effectively with a simple regimen that has a good prognosis, or does she have an ASD, which would require a more extensive regimen and possible lifelong treatment?

Karen Clarey, Stephanie Wong, and Takesha Cooper

Pretest self-assessment question (answer at the end of the case)

Which evidence-based treatment is recommended for severe anxiety in the pediatric population?

A. Low-dose benzodiazepines as needed for anxiety attacks
B. Selective serotonin reuptake inhibitor (SSRI) alone
C. Cognitive behavioral therapy (CBT) alone
D. Combination of SSRI with low-dose benzodiazepines as needed
E. Combination of SSRI with CBT

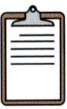

Patient evaluation on intake

- A 7-year-old female with prior diagnoses of unspecified anxiety, obsessive–compulsive disorder (OCD), and Asperger's disorder who is brought in by her mother for treatment and clarification of her previous diagnoses

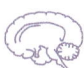

Psychiatric history

- The patient has been anxious for 3–4 years; she was first diagnosed 2 years prior to the initial visit
  - She worries that her neighbors will hurt others, that her dog is hiding under her bed and will bite her, that she will contaminate others when she is ill, that she will get words wrong while reading, etc.
  - She is afraid of the dark and cannot go to the restroom or walk down the hallway alone
- She has panic attacks with hyperventilation leading to syncope
- She has struggled with sleep since birth
  - She is anxious and activated at sleep time
  - Ultimately, she cannot fall asleep unless making physical contact with her mother
- She demonstrates some compulsive behaviors
  - She arranges or rewrites excessively until things are "just right"

- – She throws papers away if mistakes are made or erases the paper until small holes appear
- – She lines toys up
- – She insists on changing clothes when mildly dirty
- – Chips cannot touch the sandwich on a plate, otherwise she will throw a tantrum
- She is hypersensitive to sensory stimuli
  - – She complains to teacher when class is too loud, which leads to switch in classroom
  - – She does not like tags on shirts and must wear soft clothing
  - – She prefers soft food such as mashed potatoes or cooked carrots

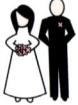

Social and personal history

- She attends elementary school (2nd grade), has a 1st grade reading level, and has no special education
- She lives with three sisters, a cousin, and her mother
- Her parents divorced when she was 3 years old
- Her parents have joint legal custody; her mother has physical custody and her father sees her one weekend a month
- She has a normal developmental history

Medical history

- She has astigmatism and wears glasses
- There is no history of head injury, loss of consciousness, seizures, or cardiac problems

Family history

- Mother and father have a history of depression treated with paroxetine (Paxil)
- Maternal side
  - – Depression with substance use disorder in aunt and uncle (heroin and methamphetamine, respectively)
  - – Bipolar disorder in aunt and uncle
  - – Thyroid disorder in grandfather and cousin
- Paternal side
  - – Anxiety in grandmother
  - – Substance use disorder in grandfather (substance unknown)

Medication history

- Clonidine (Catapres) 0.1 mg at bedtime for insomnia
- Previously used melatonin, dose unknown, but was not effective

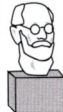

Psychotherapy history
- There is no psychotherapy history to report

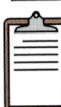

Patient evaluation on initial visit
- The patient has reported symptoms of anxiety pertaining to various aspects of her life – school, family, safety, and health
- She appears restless with baseline anxious affect worsened when challenged to do something she is uncomfortable with (e.g. she bangs her head on a book when struggling to read)
- She is preoccupied with structure and is rigid and inflexible in her routine
- She is obsessive about organization of objects, writing, and self
- She shows hypersensitivity to various sensory stimuli with poor coping
- It is reported that patient has had poor sleep due to overactivation since she was an infant
- There is no history of psychotherapy or special education
- She is compliant with clonidine (Catapres) for sleep with little improvement; no other medication trials
- The provider decided to start sertraline (Zoloft) 12.5 mg daily for anxiety
- Continue clonidine 0.1 mg at bedtime for insomnia

Question
Does this choice of medication make sense?
- Yes
- No

Attending physician's mental notes: initial evaluation
- The child exhibits constant worry, restlessness, and somatic symptoms, and thus best meets the criteria for generalized anxiety disorder (GAD). It is reasonable to rule out OCD
- Autism is not likely given that social emotional reciprocity is intact, she is able to maintain peer friendships, plays imaginatively, uses and understands non-verbal gestures appropriately, and has good eye contact consistently
- The overlap between symptoms of autism spectrum disorder (ASD) and anxiety includes repetitive motor movements (lining toys up, rocking), insistence on sameness/inflexibility, and fixated interests, yet given her lack of impairment socially, the above symptoms are better explained by GAD
- She would benefit from CBT and an SSRI

Case outcome: first interim follow-up visit at 4 weeks

- The patient still has anxiety-driven outbursts but these are less intense and less frequent
- She is still sleeping in her mother's bed
- She is open to more clothing options
- Her teacher reported an improvement in reading
- She has good medication adherence
- She denies side effects
- Therapy is pending due to insurance issues
- She continues with clonidine (Catapres) 0.1 mg at bedtime for insomnia

Question

What would be your next step?

- Increase sertraline (Zoloft) to 25 mg
- Maintain sertraline dose and wait for a further response

Attending physician's mental notes: first interim follow-up visit at 4 weeks

- The child is on a very low dose of sertraline (Zoloft) with continued significant symptoms of anxiety; thus, a dose increase is indicated. The mother is agreeable to increasing sertraline to 25 mg daily for further improvement of symptoms
- She would benefit from CBT, but the insurance is pending
- Psychoeducation provided on anxiety and how thoughts impact feelings and behaviors
- Also practiced abdominal breathing with the patient and parent, with homework to practice for 1–2 minutes each day

Case outcome: interim follow-up visit at 9 months

- Sertraline (Zoloft) has been steadily increased and she has been taking 100 mg daily for about 1 month
- The patient still has some anxiety, but described it as mild and only occurring with reasonable triggers
- She is still sleeping in her mother's bed
- She has received various awards in school, including reading awards
- The patient was reading at pre-K level 1 year ago and is now at 3rd grade level
- Overall, the most improvement seen since the initial evaluation
- The therapy referral is still in progress
- Continue sertraline at 100 mg for now; continue clonidine (Catapres) 0.1 mg at bedtime for sleep
- The mother reports the primary care physician (PCP) also started diphenhydramine (Benadryl) 25 mg at bedtime for sleep

Question

Is diphenhydramine (Benadryl) a reasonable choice for insomnia in children?

- Yes, for a short-term daily use
- Yes, for long-term daily use
- Yes, but only as needed
- No

Attending physician's mental notes: first interim follow-up visit at 9 months

- The patient is tolerating sertraline (Zoloft) well with significant improvements in functioning from prior to medication
- As therapy referral is still pending, the parent is working with the child using a structured CBT manual, which appears to help
- Addition of diphenhydramine (Benadryl) by the PCP is helping, and the parent wishes to continue
- Diphenhydramine is a reasonable short-term option for pediatric insomnia. An alternative would be increasing dose of clonidine (Catapres) or initiating melatonin (Table 1.1)
- Will consider taper off of clonidine to avoid polypharmacy if sleep improves alone with diphenhydramine

Table 1.1 Sleep medications used in the pediatric population

Medication class	Examples	Take-home point
Non-prescription medications		
Antihistamine	Diphenhydramine, hydroxyzine, chlorpheniramine	Short-term use in younger children, especially those with atopy
Melatonin	Several over-the-counter preparations available	Best for circadian rhythm phase delay or sleep-onset insomnia
Prescribed medication		
Benzodiazepine	Lorazepam, temazepam, etc.	Limit use in children as can be habit forming. Anxiolytic properties can be useful short term (<1 week)
Non-benzodiazepine receptor agonists	Zaleplon, zolpidem, eszopiclone	Sleep-related behavioral side effects limit utility in pediatric population
Off-label medication		
Antidepressants	Atypical antidepressants: trazodone, mirtazapine Sedating SSRIs: fluvoxamine, citalopram Tricyclic antidepressants: imipramine, amitriptyline	Most useful with comorbid mood/anxiety disorders
α-Agonists	Clonidine, guanfacine	Often used for pediatric insomnia. Generally safe and effective despite little data to support their use. Can lead to hypotension

Case outcome: interim follow-up visit at 2.5 years

- The patient has been followed every 1–2 months
- Sertraline (Zoloft) has been gradually increased and is now at 150 mg; she has been on this dose for about 1 year and 8 months
- Clonidine (Catapres) was tapered off and discontinued approximately 1 year ago, as it was no longer helping with sleep
- She is still taking diphenhydramine (Benadryl) at bedtime for sleep as of 3 months earlier, and was sleeping alone in her own bed most nights; however, recently anxiety due to sleeping alone has returned
- The patient began therapy 1.5 years ago and went for approximately 8 months; however, her mother felt it was ineffective and quit
- She is more adventurous in her choice of clothing and foods
- She has more restlessness and irritability
- She has more complaints about loud noises to the point of leaving the classroom in the middle of lessons
- Bullying at school might explain the spike in anxiety

Question

What would you do next?

Attending physician's mental notes: interim follow-up visit at 2.5 years

- There has been exacerbation of symptoms with continued impairing anxiety
- Her mother is agreeable to raising sertraline (Zoloft) to 175 mg due to the spike in anxiety and resulting poor sleep
- In order to augment the increased SSRI dose, she is encouraged to return for booster CBT sessions
- The parent will talk with the school about bullying and assist the patient with coping skills

Case outcome: interim follow-up visit at 3.5 years

- 1 year ago, the patient began a sertraline (Zoloft) taper due to ongoing improvement in anxiety symptoms
- It was tapered by decrements of 25–50 mg every 1–2 months; she is currently on 25 mg daily
- The patient has not returned for therapy
- She has been sleeping in her own bed with no problems for 3 months
- Her sensory issues have diminished and she is enjoying different textures, food, and environments
- She is functioning well both at home and at school

- The patient was challenged to have a playdate at a friend's house to challenge her anxiety and this was successful
- She continues to use diphenhydramine (Benadryl) for sleep

Question

What would you do next?

Attending physician's mental notes: interim follow-up visit at 3.5 years

- The patient has responded well to sertraline (Zoloft) over the past 3.5 years from titration to 175 mg to gradual taper completely off medication
- Although the patient would have benefited from consistent CBT from a trained provider, this was not available in the locale. Nonetheless, the patient and parent were able to implement some CBT techniques and the parent's willingness to work with the patient on a manualized treatment, while not ideal, was helpful
- After more than 3 years of treatment, the patient has gained confidence in her ability to manage her anxiety and use her cognitive skills to reduce thinking errors, and has increased willingness to face her fears

Case debrief

- Our patient was initially diagnosed with unspecified anxiety, OCD, and Asperger's disorder by multiple physicians
  - A proper diagnosis guides proper treatment. Adequate treatment was not started in this case due to an unclear diagnosis. Also, patients with multiple diagnoses often experience polypharmacy, and thus diagnostic clarity is key
  - The patient was started on clonidine (Catapres) to target sleep problems and this was likely to address other behaviors, such as outbursts. If sleep problems were secondary to the underlying anxiety disorder, it is possible the sertraline (Zoloft) alone would have resolved the sleep difficulties
- After a full history review of all symptoms, the patient appeared to more closely fit into a diagnosis of GAD
  - The treatment became more simplified and targeted, and there was hope for remission of her symptoms
- The SSRI sertraline, which is FDA approved for OCD in children, is widely used off label for GAD in children. It has been shown to reduce somatic symptoms of anxiety in children with GAD,

including a reduction in the Hamilton Anxiety Rating Scale in a double-blind, placebo-controlled trial of children aged 5–17 years

- CBT was recommended but, unfortunately, access was limited
- Sertraline, along with clonidine for sleep, was used and slowly titrated to alleviate symptoms
- There were frequent follow-ups at 1–2-month intervals, and the patient began to show significant improvement in her symptoms
- Diphenhydramine (Benadryl) was initiated by her PCP for further augmentation for insomnia
  - Due to the risk of unnecessary polypharmacy, clonidine was eventually discontinued
- There were instances of deterioration, which were effectively managed by increasing the dose of sertraline
  - A benefit of sertraline is the wide dosage range, which was essential in this case
- At her peak dose, the patient improved quickly and tolerated a slow taper to ultimately completely discontinue medication and achieve symptom remission

Take-home points

- Anxiety disorders and ASD have multiple overlapping symptoms, which can make diagnosis difficult
- Distinguishing between the two can be done by assessing all symptoms exhibited by the child and obtaining a thorough history to find key symptoms missing for a certain diagnosis
  - In this case, persistent deficits in social impairment and communication that are classic in ASD were missing
  - Objective assessments such as the Autism Diagnostic Observation Scale are often used to make an ASD diagnosis, but are not widely available
- It is also important to assess the underlying motivation for symptoms
  - For example, refusal to separate from the caregiver, as in our patient, can be seen both in anxiety disorders and ASD
  - In anxiety, the refusal to separate is driven by fear of what might occur to the caregiver or to the patient if they are separated
  - In autism, refusal to separate is more likely a result of unwillingness to change routine without any overt "fear" involved
- The correct diagnosis leads to proper treatment, better understanding of the disorder by caregivers, and a decrease in overmedication/undermedication in children

- SSRI/serotonin-norepinephrine reuptake inhibitor (SNRI) in combination with CBT is the gold standard for treatment of GAD in children
  - They may benefit from the addition of other medications to target symptoms not addressed by an SSRI alone, such as insomnia
- To taper sertraline (Zoloft), reduce by 25–50 mg weekly to avoid discontinuation symptoms
- If the patient does respond to sertraline, a trial of another SSRI would be recommended. After failure of two SSRIs, an SNRI would be indicated
  - Duloxetine (Cymbalta) is FDA approved in children with GAD
- Benzodiazepines have a limited role in pediatric anxiety but can cautiously be used transiently while waiting for an SSRI to begin working
- Clinical trials have found mixed results for tricyclic antidepressants in pediatric anxiety disorder. Side effects limit their usefulness in this population

Performance in practice: confessions of a psychopharmacologist

What could have been done better here?

- As mentioned previously, CBT is an important part in the treatment of pediatric GAD. For mild to moderate GAD, CBT alone is preferred but for severe GAD, a combination approach is indicated
- CBT offers tools such as cognitive reframing and self-monitoring to help patients gain control over their symptoms
- CBT access to this patient was very limited and could have hindered her eventual remission
- While some elements of CBT were presented to the patient during psychiatric follow-ups and at home, she would have benefited from increased access to CBT done in a structured and focused setting
- Earlier and longer access may have led to earlier control of her symptoms and thus decreased the need for psychopharmacological management

What are possible action items for improvement in practice?

- Become familiar with cognitive behavioral principles to teach your patients during their medication follow-up visits or, better yet, become a CBT-trained provider to avoid split treatment
- Research and better understand the pediatric options for sleep, including sleep hygiene and other behavioral interventions in addition to medication options

Tips and pearls

- Diagnosis guides treatment, and thus it is imperative to perform a thorough assessment to ensure you are treating the proper condition
- For children, it is generally recommended to start low and go slow with medication
- Children often require the full doses used in adults due to more rapid drug metabolism at younger ages
- When medicines are indicated for pediatric anxiety, SSRIs are first line
- The goal of treatment with sertraline (Zoloft) is complete remission of current symptoms and prevention of future relapses
- The more anxious the patient appears, the lower the starting dose of sertraline should be and the slower the titration upward
  - This is due to possible activating effects of the medication when first started
- If sertraline seems to wear off before the end of the day, sometimes giving it twice per day can help
- Sertraline must be tapered to avoid withdrawal effects
- It is important to taper clonidine (Catapres) to prevent rebound hypertension that may occur with abrupt discontinuation, especially in children who are more sensitive to the hypertensive effects
- Remember to warn parents and children of the black box warning for all SSRIs warning of increased risk of suicidal ideation and behavior

Two-minute tutorial

Recognition and management of pediatric anxiety disorders

- Anxiety disorders are one of the most common psychiatric conditions seen in the pediatric population
- Screening for the presence and severity of anxiety symptoms along with comorbid psychiatric and medical conditions is recommended when evaluating all pediatric patients
- Recognition and management of these disorders is critical in preventing the development of other psychiatric disorders, such as depression and substance use disorders in adulthood
- Various brain structures have been implicated in anxiety disorders
  - The amygdala plays a prominent role in an individual's fear response
    - Hyperactivity of this structure is seen in functional magnetic resonance imaging (fMRI) studies in anxiety disorders

- The ventrolateral prefrontal cortex (VLPFC) regulates activity in the amygdala
  - ○ Increased VLPFC activity is seen in patients with anxiety disorders and there is an inverse relationship between VLPFC activity and the severity of anxiety
- The cingulate cortex plays a role in emotional regulation
  - ○ Overactivity of this structure and increased glutamatergic activity is found in anxiety disorders
- Several treatment methods involving psychological and psychopharmacological therapies have been effective in the management of pediatric anxiety disorders
  - A personalized approach is recommended to achieve optimal outcomes

Clinical pearls should include the following:

- Utilize any of the following screening measures when evaluating pediatric patients with suspected anxiety disorders:
  - Multidimensional Anxiety Scale for Children (MASC)
  - Screen for Child Anxiety and Related Emotional Disorders (SCARED)
  - Spence Children's Anxiety Scale (SCAS)
  - Pediatric Anxiety Rating Scale (PARS)
  - Social Anxiety Scale, the Social Worries Questionnaire, and the social phobia subscale of SCARED, in patients suspected of having social phobia or social anxiety
- Pay careful attention to symptoms such as crying that may be mistaken as disobedience
  - Such symptoms can be signs of a child trying to avoid situations that cause anxiety
- Consider the combination of CBT and SSRIs when treating patients with anxiety disorders
  - Suggested SSRIs include: fluoxetine (Prozac), sertraline (Zoloft), fluvoxamine (Luvox), and paroxetine (Paxil)
    - ○ Watch for side effects such as nausea/vomiting, headaches, abdominal pain, appetite changes, or sleep disturbances
  - Other forms of therapy that can be used include mindfulness-based psychotherapies and psychodynamic psychotherapy
- Treatment response can be predicted by the following factors, and the presence of any of the following can be associated with poorer outcomes:
  - Family history of anxiety, especially in a first-degree relative
  - Older age at diagnosis
  - More severe anxiety at baseline
  - Limited social support

Posttest self-assessment question and answer

Which evidence-based treatment is recommended for severe anxiety in the pediatric population?

A. Low-dose benzodiazepines as needed for anxiety attacks
B. SSRI alone
C. CBT alone
D. Combination of SSRI with low-dose benzodiazepines as needed
E. Combination of SSRI with CBT

Answer: E

References

1. Guyer, AE, Masten, CL, Pine, DS. Neurobiology of pediatric anxiety disorders. In: Vasa, RA, Roy, AK, eds. *Pediatric Anxiety Disorders: A Clinical Guide*. New York, NY: Humana Press, 2013; pp. 23–46.
2. Kerns CM, Rump K, Worley J, et al. The differential diagnosis of anxiety disorders in cognitively-able youth with autism. *Cogn Behav Pract* 2016; 23:530–47. https://doi.org/10.1016/j.cbpra.2015.11.004
3. Mobach L, Gould K, Husdon JL. Comorbidity in childhood anxiety disorders. In: Compton SN, Villabø MA, Kristensen H, eds. *Pediatric Anxiety Disorders*. Cambridge: Elsevier/Academic Press, 2019; pp. 277–98.
4. Rynn MA, Siqueland L, Rickels K. Placebo-controlled trial of sertraline in the treatment of children with generalized anxiety disorder. *Am J Psychiatry* 2001; 158:2008–14. https://doi.org/10.1176/appi.ajp.158.12.2008
5. Sateia, MJ, Buysse, DJ, Krystal, AD, et al. Clinical practice guideline for the pharmacologic treatment of chronic insomnia in adults: an American Academy of Sleep Medicine Clinical Practice Guideline. *J Clin Sleep Med* 2017; 13:307–49. https://doi.org/10.5664/jcsm.6470
6. Stahl SM. *Stahl's Essential Psychopharmacology: Prescriber's Guide*, 6th edn. Cambridge, UK: Cambridge University Press, 2017.
7. Stahl SM *Stahl's Essential Psychopharmacology: Prescribers Guide – Children and Adolescents*. New York, NY: Cambridge University Press, 2019.
8. Wehry, AM, Beesdo-Baum, K, Hennelly, MM, et al. Assessment and treatment of anxiety disorders in children and adolescents. *Curr Psychiatry Rep* 2015; 17:591. https://doi.org/10.1007/s11920-015-0591-z
9. White, SW, Lerner, MD, Mcleod, BD, et al. Anxiety in youth with and without autism spectrum disorder: examination of factorial equivalence. *Behav Ther* 2015; 46:40–53. https://doi.org/10.1016/j.beth.2014.05.005

Case 2: The woman who couldn't handle her lips smacking any longer

The Question: Is tardive dyskinesia permanent?

The Psychopharmacological Dilemma: Finding various options for treating tardive dyskinesia

Douglas Grover, Michael T. Ingram, Jr., and Christopher G. Fichtner

Pretest self-assessment question (answer at the end of the case)

What are the approved treatments for tardive dyskinesia?

A. Deutetrabenazine (Austedo)
B. Propranolol (Inderal)
C. Olanzapine (Zyprexa)
D. Diphenhydramine (Benadryl)
E. Aripiprazole (Abilify)
F. Valbenazine (Ingrezza)

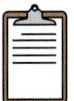

Patient evaluation on intake

- A 50-year-old female with the chief complaint of persistent lip smacking

Psychiatric history

- The patient has diagnoses of schizoaffective disorder depressed type and posttraumatic stress disorder
- As a child, she experienced physical abuse by her stepfather and mother and sexual abuse by her aunt
- Her first psychotic episode requiring hospitalization was in her early 30s and she has been on various antipsychotic treatment regimens since then
- She has been hospitalized five times for psychosis and once after a suicide attempt by overdosing
- She has been disabled since 2009, receiving social security income due to ongoing and persistent episodes of psychosis and depression with suicidal ideation in addition to other medical comorbidities such as narcolepsy
- Her primary symptoms include command auditory hallucinations, paranoia, racing thoughts, depression, nightmares, and suicidal ideation
- She spends most of her time alone reading her Bible to help drown out the negative hallucinations
- She developed orofacial tardive dyskinesia after a brief trial of haloperidol (Haldol) 5 months ago that continued with treatment of risperidone (Risperdal)

Medication history

- The patient has been on numerous psychotropic medications including antipsychotics, mood stabilizers, benzodiazepines, and antidepressants
- Current medications have improved her hallucinations, delusions, and depressed symptoms

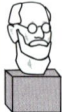

Psychotherapy history

- The patient has had a few attempts with various psychotherapists over the years but does not consistently follow through

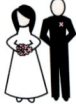

Social and personal history

- The patient never knew her biological father. Starting around 6 years of age, she began to undergo physical abuse by her stepfather and biological mother
- She was sexually abused by an aunt from 9 years of age until her early teenage years
- She dropped out of high school in 10th grade, went to a vocational school and became a teacher's aid
- She was able to work as an aid until becoming completely disabled in 2009 following another hospitalization for psychosis
- She was married for 8 years but divorced. She does not have any biological children. She helped raise three foster children but was not able to adopt them after she and her husband separated
- She was physically abused by her ex-husband
- The patient lives with her biological mother

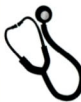

Medical history

- Narcolepsy
- Restless leg syndrome
- Hypothyroidism
- Arthritis/chronic pain

Family history

- Mother with depression
- She does not know about her biological father's family history

Patient evaluation on initial visit

- Severe and persistent tardive dyskinesia involving only her mouth, lip smacking
- An Abnormal Involuntary Movement Scale (AIMS) examination was 7 with regard to facial oral movements, 4 for lip smacking (severe)

and 3 for jaw clenching (moderate). The total AIMS was 18 after adding 11 for global judgments. She has no issues with her teeth and does not wear dentures

- The patient is aware of the involuntary movements, which cause severe distress and embarrassment
- She developed the involuntary movements within the last couple months after a trial of haloperidol (Haldol)
- After haloperidol was discontinued, the involuntary movements persisted with risperidone (Risperdal) treatment
- She denies depression and manic/hypomanic symptoms, and has no current suicidal ideations
- She denies paranoia but has occasional auditory hallucinations that she describes as always in the background but not necessarily distressing

Current medications

- Risperidone (Risperdal) 2 mg twice per day
- Trazodone (Desyrel) 300 mg at bedtime
- Prazosin (Minipress) 5 mg at bedtime
- Lorazepam (Ativan) 1 mg three times per day as needed for anxiety
- Topiramate (Topamax) 125 mg twice per day (for psychotropic-induced weight gain)
- Levothyroxine (Synthroid) 200 µg daily for thyroid
- Omeprazole (Prilosec) 20 mg daily for gastroesophageal reflux disease
- Tramadol (Ultram) 50 mg four times per day as needed for pain
- Mixed amphetamine salts (Adderall) 20 mg three times per day for narcolepsy

Attending physician's mental notes: initial visit

- This patient has tried a variety of antipsychotics in the past and continues to have occasional hallucinations but is currently improved compared with past medication trials
- When she decompensates, she requires prolonged hospitalization for paranoia, command auditory hallucinations, and suicidal ideation
- She developed orofacial tardive dyskinesia with a trial of haloperidol (Haldol) about 5 months ago, and it persists after switching to risperidone (Risperdal)
- The patient is reluctant to try different medications because she currently feels relatively stable

Further investigation

Is there anything else you would especially like to know about this patient? What about further details about the tardive dyskinesia and whether she has tried one of the approved treatments for it?

- The tardive dyskinesia has been persistent for 5 months and it seems to have been worsening over time despite switching from haloperidol (Haldol) to risperidone (Risperdal)
- The involuntary movements only affect her mouth, primarily just lip smacking, which is causing conflict with her mother
- The patient has never tried one of the approved treatments for tardive dyskinesia

Case outcome: first interim follow-up visit at week 2

- The patient continued to take risperidone (Risperdal) 2 mg twice per day due to good benefit of psychosis and mood
- She was started on valbenazine (Ingrezza) 40 mg daily with a partial response of involuntary orofacial movements. Subjectively, the patient had a 50% improvement
- Valbenazine was increased to 80 mg daily

Case outcome: second interim follow-up visit at week 6

- The patient no longer displays any involuntary movements in the office and reports the movements are completely gone at home
- AIMS score has reduced from 18 to 0
- She continues to report very occasional auditory hallucinations but wishes to remain at the current dose of risperidone (Risperdal)

Case outcome: third interim follow-up visit at week 12

- The patient stopped taking valbenazine (Ingrezza) 2 weeks ago because she wanted to see if the tardive dyskinesia was gone without the medication
- During the visit, she again displayed persistent involuntary lip smacking
- The patient wanted to continue treatment with risperidone (Risperdal) as it was still providing benefit with psychosis and mood
- The patient was restarted on valbenazine 40 mg daily for 1 week and then increased back to 80 mg daily

Further investigation

Would you resume treatment with valbenazine (Ingrezza) or change strategy?

- Resume treatment with valbenazine and titrate again to 80 mg daily
- Increase the dose of risperidone (Risperdal) without adding valbenazine
- Increase the dose of risperidone and add valbenazine
- Decrease the dose of risperidone and add valbenazine
- Switch to a different antipsychotic before prescribing valbenazine again or trying deutetrabenazine (Austedo)
- Try to decrease amphetamine which may be exacerbating the movements

Attending physician's mental notes

- The patient appears to have responded to valbenazine (Ingrezza), helping to confirm that this was a case of orofacial tardive dyskinesia
- Increasing the dose of risperidone (Risperdal) may decrease the severity or resolve the involuntary movements briefly, but in time tardive dyskinesia will likely return and perhaps worsen
- Her psychotic and mood symptoms are responding to the current dose of risperidone
- She has been taking antipsychotics for nearly the last 20 years. Is the tardive dyskinesia a culmination of long-term antipsychotic use over that time or was it caused directly by haloperidol (Haldol) and risperidone, or a combination of everything?

Case outcome: fourth interim follow-up visit at week 16

- Although the patient restarted and titrated valbenazine (Ingrezza) back to 80 mg daily where she had previously found complete resolution of tardive dyskinesia, this time it is not providing her with much benefit
- She continues to complain of nearly unrelenting lip smacking, which is clearly visible in the office. Her AIMS score is 6 with regard to oral facial movements, with a total of 17 with global judgments
- The patient desired at this point to try a different antipsychotic as she had never experienced tardive dyskinesia prior to haloperidol (Haldol) and risperidone (Risperdal). The risks of tardive dyskinesia with all antipsychotics were discussed
- The patient was started on aripiprazole (Abilify) 10 mg daily and risperidone was discontinued

Attending physician's mental notes

- Aripiprazole (Abilify) is a partial dopamine agonist with some cases showing improvement of tardive dyskinesia with its use, possibly due to masking of the movements due to the very high-potency partial agonist actions at dopamine D_2 receptors
- She may not experience the same benefits for controlling psychosis with aripiprazole that she found with risperidone (Risperdal)
- It should be noted that all antipsychotics, even aripiprazole, have the risk of developing or worsening tardive dyskinesia

Case outcome: fifth interim follow-up visit week 18

- The patient reports her lip smacking seems to have reduced by about 50%. She still has involuntary movements of her mouth during the visit but they are certainly reduced from 2 weeks ago
- The patient complains of more frequent persecutory auditory hallucinations
- Aripiprazole (Abilify) was increased to 20 mg daily

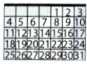

Case outcome: sixth interim follow-up visit at week 22

- The patient reports complete resolution of tardive dyskinesia. Her AIMS score is 0
- She continues to have worsening auditory hallucinations, which are distracting and causing some distress
- She denies command auditory hallucinations and denies suicidal ideations
- Aripiprazole (Abilify) was increased to 30 mg daily

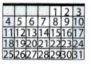

Case outcome: seventh interim follow-up visit at week 26

- The patient continues not to have any involuntary movements
- Her psychotic symptoms have responded to higher doses of aripiprazole (Abilify), but although not subjectively as good as risperidone (Risperdal) in treating auditory hallucinations, the patient is pleased with the absence of lip smacking
- The patient has found other means to help alleviate any persistent auditory hallucinations, such as meditation and reading her Bible

Case debrief

- After 20 years of being treated with antipsychotics, the patient developed tardive dyskinesia after a trial of haloperidol (Haldol), which continued once haloperidol was discontinued and switched to risperidone (Risperdal)

- The patient initially responded to valbenazine (Ingrezza), one of the FDA-approved treatments for tardive dyskinesia. However, she stopped taking it because she thought she was cured. She was restarted on valbenazine a second time but the involuntary movements persisted
- The patient was switched from risperidone to aripiprazole (Abilify) due to some evidence showing improvement of tardive dyskinesia because of its partial agonist on dopamine D_2 receptors rather than full antagonism
- After titrating aripiprazole to the least-effective dose to treat her psychosis, she no longer displayed symptoms of tardive dyskinesia, which has remained stable for a few months

Take-home points

- One of the more severe and debilitating potential side effects of antipsychotics is the development of tardive dyskinesia
- Providers should be aware that the incidence of tardive dyskinesia is greater with typical antipsychotics; however, there is a risk, regardless of whether typical or atypical medications are used
- Not all cases of tardive dyskinesia are "classic". Tardive dyskinesia is characterized by involuntary and abnormal muscle movements, usually by long-term use of neuroleptics, but can also occur rather quickly
- Tardive dyskinesia most often affects the mouth, lips, tongue, and facial muscles, but in some cases may affect the arms, legs, neck, and trunk
- The only FDA-approved treatments for tardive dyskinesia are valbenazine (Ingrezza) and deutetrabenazine (Austedo), which are both vesicular monoamine transporter-2 (VMAT2) inhibitors
- Although the patient is no longer experiencing tardive dyskinesia, it is possible that the high dose of aripiprazole (Abilify) is masking the symptoms rather than providing a long-term cure
- If psychotic symptoms return in the future, the need to either titrate aripiprazole or switch to another antipsychotic may reintroduce involuntary movements
- A trial of deutetrabenazine rather than another trial of valbenazine may be indicated for emergent tardive dyskinesia in the future, as there is more dose flexibility and titration possible with deutetrabenazine and the patient may require a higher degree of VMAT2 inhibition

Performance in practice: confessions of a psychopharmacologist

What could have been done better here?

- Was the differential diagnosis for this being tardive dyskinesia too narrow? Could this have been "rabbit syndrome" of perioral Parkinson's tremor instead?
- Rabbit syndrome is a form of extrapyramidal syndrome that resembles the chewing movements of the mouth and could be resolved by using either higher anticholinergic medications or less potent antipsychotics; however, orofacial exam revealed not the fine, rapid, rhythmic tremor of rabbit syndrome, but irregular lip movements of lower frequency
- Should the patient have been given a trial of deutetrabenazine (Austedo)?

Is there anything else that could be a potential culprit for the involuntary movements?

- The patient is on mixed amphetamine salts (Adderall) for narcolepsy, which act directly on dopamine by inhibiting its reuptake and increasing its release. Although more likely with illicit amphetamines due to the neurotoxicity, there is still a possibility with prescribed stimulants that they are exacerbating her tardive dyskinesia movements

What are the chances that this patient may have ongoing tardive dyskinesia in the future?

- It is likely that this patient may develop symptoms of tardive dyskinesia again in the future. Perhaps the mechanism of aripiprazole (Abilify) is only masking the underlying tardive dyskinesia, which may present more severely in the coming years

What is the mechanism of action of aripiprazole that was thought to play a role in improving this patient's tardive dyskinesia?

- Aripiprazole has a unique mechanism of action as a partial D_2 receptor agonist, a partial 5-HT_{1A} receptor agonist and a 5-HT_{2A} receptor antagonist, and is thought to normalize dopamine upregulation compared with other antipsychotics that cause striatal dopamine receptor hypersensitivity
- It is also thought that activation of the 5-HT_{1A} receptor mediates the release of dopamine in the striatum, decreasing extrapyramidal side effects without affecting the antipsychotic properties within the mesolimbic system

Tips and pearls

What are the risk factors for tardive dyskinesia?

- Advanced age, female gender, alcohol or other substance abuse, pre-existing extrapyramidal symptoms, long-term treatment with antipsychotics particularly high-potency first-generation, severe negative symptoms of schizophrenia, low levels of brain-derived neurotrophic factor (BDNF), and polymorphisms in the enzymes involved with metabolism of the offending drug

How can you diagnose tardive dyskinesia with your eyes closed?

- History taking: has the patient been treated with a dopamine receptor blocking agent such as various antipsychotics, tricyclic antidepressants, or some antiemetics?
- How long has the patient been treated with these agents? Take into account the age of the patient and the other risk factors as described above
- What happened with the tardive dyskinesia symptoms when there was a dose reduction or discontinuation? It may worsen initially before it improves
- What happened with the tardive dyskinesia symptoms when there was a dose increase? It improves initially but later worsens
- What happened when an anticholinergic agent was added? It would worsen tardive dyskinesia

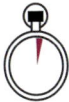

Two-minute tutorial

Tardive dyskinesia

- 5% of patients on typical antipsychotics develop tardive dyskinesia every year, and this may be as high as 25% in elderly patients within the first year of exposure to a typical antipsychotic
- It is usually caused by long-term blockade of D_2 receptors in the nigrostriatal dopamine pathway, which leads to upregulation of these receptors causing the hyperkinetic involuntary motor movements of tardive dyskinesia (Figure 2.1)
- It may be reversible if the offending agent is discontinued early, allowing the dopamine receptors to "reset" themselves
- It most often affects the face (facial grimacing/chewing), lips (smacking, puckering), and tongue (darting/protrusions), but may also affect the neck, arms, and legs with quick jerky movements
- Tardive dyskinesia occurs more often with high-potency typical antipsychotics but is possible with atypical antipsychotics, tricyclic antidepressants, and certain antiemetics

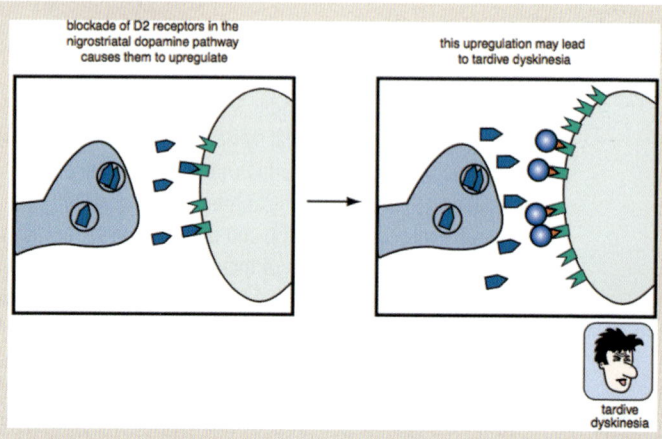

Figure 2.1. Long-term dopamine D_2 receptor antagonism causes upregulation of the D_2 nigrostriatal postsynaptic receptors leading to increased sensitivity and tardive dyskinesia.

Treatments for tardive dyskinesia

- The FDA has approved two treatments: valbenazine (Ingrezza) and deutetrabenazine (Austedo), which are both VMAT-2 inhibitors
- These treatments reduce dopamine availability to the hypersensitive and upregulated postsynaptic D_2 receptors in the motor striatum (Figure 2.2)
- Valbenazine is converted to only one active metabolite, $(+)$-α-dihydrotetrabenazine and is only selective for VMAT2
- Deutetrabenazine is metabolized into four active isomers, two of which act on VMAT2 with a longer half-life, allowing less-frequent dosing
- Other experimental treatments for tardive dyskinesia include donepezil (Aricept), melatonin, vitamins E and B_6, dextromethorphan, clonazepam (Klonopin), propranolol (Inderal), amantadine (Gocovri), and branched-chain amino acids or other antioxidant supplements

AIMS examination

- This is a 12-item clinician-rated scale
- It is completed while the patient is sitting on a firm chair without arm rests
- Ask whether the patient wears dentures and whether they or their teeth are bothering them?
- Ask whether the patient notices any movements in their hands, face, mouth, or feet, and to what extent it bothers them

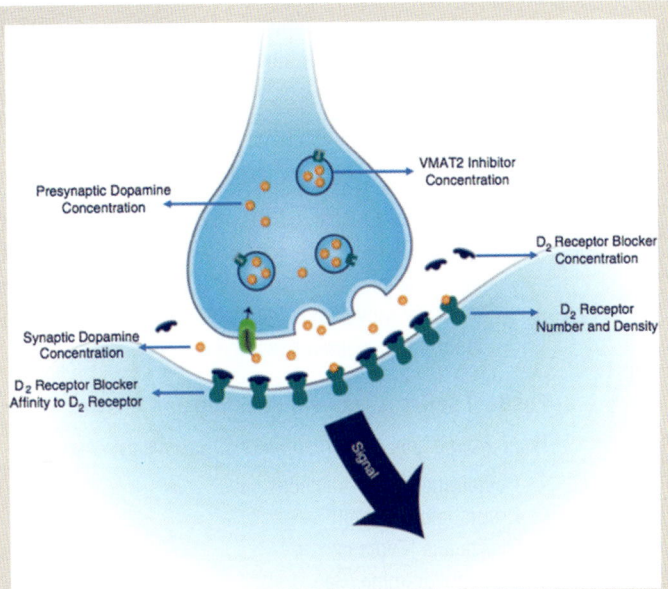

Figure 2.2. The multiple factors that affect the concentration of dopamine within the synaptic cleft including the activity of vesicular monoamine transporter-2 (VMAT2) inhibitors within the presynaptic neuron. VMAT2 inhibition decreases presynaptic dopamine concentration, which results in a downstream effect of reducing synaptic and postsynaptic dopamine levels.

- Observe the patient's movements with their hands on their knees and feet on the ground
- Ask the patient to open their mouth and observe tongue movements; then ask them to protrude their tongue twice
- Have the patient tap each finger with their thumb as fast as possible for 10–15 seconds, one hand at a time
- Flex and extend the patient's arms, one at a time
- Have the patient stand up and observe all their limbs and face again
- Ask the patient to extend both arms out in front with their palms facing down
- Ask the patient to walk a few paces back and forth two times
- Score the procedure: 0 = none, 1 = minimal (may be extreme normal), 2 = mild, 3 = moderate, 4 = severe
  - Muscles of facial expression (eyebrow, forehead, periorbital, cheeks, which includes frowning, blinking, grimacing)
  - Lips and perioral (puckering, smacking, pouting)
  - Jaw (biting, clenching, chewing, mouth opening, lateral movements)
  - Tongue (only increase in movement both in and out of mouth)

- Upper extremities (arms, wrists, hands, fingers, which includes choreic and athetoid movements only, not tremors)
- Lower extremities (legs, knees, ankles, toes, which includes tapping, heel drop, inversion/eversion of foot, lateral movements)
- Trunk (neck, shoulders, hips, which includes rocking, twisting, squirming, pelvic gyrations, diaphragmatic movements)
- Global judgments: severity of abnormal movements (based on highest single score above scored 0–4), incapacitation due to abnormal movements (scored 0–4), and patient's awareness of abnormal movements (scored 0–4))

Posttest self-assessment question and answer

What are the approved treatments for tardive dyskinesia?

A. Deutetrabenazine (Austedo)
B. Propranolol (Inderal)
C. Olanzapine (Zyprexa)
D. Diphenhydramine (Benadryl)
E. Aripiprazole (Abilify)
F. Valbenazine (Ingrezza)

Answer: A and F

References

1. Cornett, EM, Novitch, M, Kaye, AD, et al. Medication-induced tardive dyskinesia: a review and update. *Ochsner J* 2017; 17: 162–74.
2. Kang NR, Kim MD. Tardive dyskinesia: treatment with aripiprazole. *Clin Psychopharmacol Neurosci* 2011; 9:1–8. https://doi.org/10.9758/cpn.2011.9.1.1
3. Kim SW, Lee SY, Kim JM, et al.Resolution of tardive dyskinesia following a switch from long-acting injectable risperidone to aripiprazole. *Clin Psychopharmacol Neurosci* 2008; 6:75–8.
4. Stahl SM. Antipsychotic agents. In: *Stahl's Essential Psychopharmacology: Prescriber's Guide*, 5th edn. New York, NY: Cambridge University Press, 2013; pp. 133–53.
5. Stahl SM. Neuronal traffic signals in tardive dyskinesia: not enough "stop" in the motor striatum. *CNS Spectr* 2017; 22: 427–34. https://doi.org/10.1017/s109285291700061x
6. Stahl SM. (2018). Comparing pharmacologic mechanism of action for the vesicular monoamine transporter 2 (VMAT2) inhibitors valbenazine and deutetrabenazine in treating tardive dyskinesia: does one have advantages over the other? *CNS Spectr*, 23: 239–47. https://doi.org/10.1017/s1092852918001219

Case 3: The depressed bipolar patient on multiple medications

The Question: Can reduction of polypharmacy optimize mood stabilization and reduce risk of subsequent manic or depressive episodes in this patient?

The Psychopharmacological Dilemma: Starting new medications and altering current ones can give rise to new adverse effects

Dale Hoang, Catherine Ha, and Peter Hauser

Pretest self-assessment question (answer at the end of the case)

Which of the following statements is correct regarding treatment for bipolar disorder? (select all that apply)

A. Initial lamotrigine (Lamictal) dosage should be halved in patients on stable dose of valproic acid (Depakote)
B. Patients who develop a severe rash while on lamotrigine should not be rechallenged
C. Antipsychotic medications are the gold standard for maintenance prevention of mania
D. Initial lamotrigine dose should be halved in patients on stable dose of carbamazepine (Equetro)

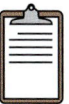

Patient evaluation on intake

- A 52-year-old male with the chief complaint of "evolving depression"
- Evolving depression over 4 weeks despite stable living circumstances, compliance with current psychotropic medications, and no stressors

Psychiatric history

- The patient was diagnosed with bipolar disorder in his early 20s
- He has a 30-year history of frequent decompensation into manic episodes
  - Symptoms include: irritability, grandiose delusions, insomnia resulting in 0–3 hours of sleep per night, pressured speech, racing thoughts, and intrusiveness
- He has had one or more hospitalizations per year in the last 15–20 years
  - Notable medication changes during these hospitalizations including ± thioridazine (Mellaril), perphenazine (Trilafon), olanzapine (Zyprexa), risperidone (Risperdal)
- He has been followed for the last 3 years by intensive case management and day treatment
- Did not admit any prior suicide attempts

Medication history

- Various typical and atypical antipsychotic trials
- Long history of being on mood stabilizers:
  - Lithium for the past 6 years
  - Past valproic acid trial added to lithium for period of 1 year with little benefit
- Antidepressants avoided due to potential mania induction
- Omega-3 supplement as treatment adjunct for bipolar depression
- Verapamil (Veralan) trial as an adjunct medication for mood stabilization
- Trial of carbamazepine (Equetro), a well-established anticonvulsant used for maintenance therapy for bipolar disease
- Trial of lorazepam (Ativan) switched more recently to clonazepam (Klonopin). Benzodiazapines frequently used as targeted, short-term therapy for sleep stabilization and attenuating mania, although it can worsen impulse dysregulation
- Low-dose trial of quetiapine (Seroquel) was tried during an inpatient stay – result of therapy unknown, but most likely as targeted treatment for insomnia

Question

What is your provisional diagnosis?

1. Major depressive episode
2. Schizoaffective disorder
3. Bipolar II disorder
4. Bipolar I disorder, most recent episode mixed
5. Bipolar I disorder, most recent episode depressed

Answer - #5

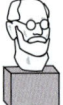

Psychotherapy history

- Unknown other than supportive therapy given with each office visit and intensive care management

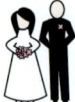

Social and personal history

- The patient is a veteran who is unemployed with 100% service connection and veteran benefits for bipolar disorder
- He graduated college with a degree in education and mathematics
- He has no siblings
- He has never married and has no children
- He lives with a roommate, who is schizophrenic
- He is in a stable relationship of 4 years' duration
- He has a guardian who manages his money
- He reports no substance abuse but he uses various Chinese herbals

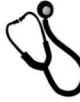

Medical history

- Not reported

Family history

- Mother with alcoholism and chronic tobacco smoker
- Father who is diabetic
- Maternal grandfather who was "mentally ill," possible tertiary syphilis

Patient evaluation on initial visit

- Alarming and apparent depressive symptoms including fatigue, amotivation, insomnia (middle and late), depressed mood, loss of appetite, irritability, anxiety, occasional wishes to be dead and, interestingly, paranoid ideation
- There are no reported or apparent life stressors
- He has good insight into his own symptoms and illness, and motivated for psychopharmacologic treatment
- He is future-orientated with good reasons for living: roommate, positive and hopeful outlook, planned vacation to Hawaii

Medications at time of initial evaluation

- Lithium 900 mg twice per day; last blood level 1.1 mEq/L
- Ziprasidone (Geodon) 80 mg twice per day
- Clonazepam (Klonopin) 1 mg every morning and 1.5 mg every evening
- Risperidone (Risperdal) 1 mg every evening (recently added from last hospitalization)

Questions

In your clinical experience, would you expect a patient such as this one to respond to any medication regimen alone?

- Yes
- No

Answer - No. Multiple episodes of illness on multiple medications

As the consulting psychiatrist, which of the following would be your next step?

- Maximize the dose of lithium
- Begin a selective serotonin reuptake inhibitor (SSRI)
- Discontinue ziprasidone (Geodon) and risperidone (Risperdal) and begin another atypical antipsychotic with better documentation for treating depression, such as cariprazine (Vraylar), lurasidone (Latuda), quetiapine (Seroquel), or olanzapine (Zyprexa)

- Make sure he is taking ziprasidone with food
- Begin Valproic Acid (Depakote)
- Begin lamotrigine (Lamictal)
- None of the above

Attending physician's mental notes: initial visit

- Bipolar disorder is a lifelong condition, with more time depressed than manic
- This patient has a history of more severe manic episodes requiring multiple hospitalizations. Preventing relapse of mania is still the utmost priority
- The patient was previously stabilized on multiple medications. If possible, doses should be optimized and unnecessary/redundant medications should be tapered/discontinued safely
- Depressive episodes within the context of bipolar disorder are challenging to treat
  - Lithium level is within high normal range so increasing lithium dose not recommended and less beneficial for bipolar depression
  - SSRIs while beneficial for treatment of depression. However with an extensive and well-documented history of bipolar disorder and manic episodes, the risk associated with starting an SSRI (inducing a potentially severe manic episode or rapid cycling) are an important consideration
  - Changing antipsychotics at this time is a lower priority
  - As patient is depressed but not a high suicide risk, lamotrigine (Lamictal) can be added and titrated slowly
- If treatment of the evolving depression and continued prevention of mania can be achieved with fewer medications, and there is a reduced likelihood of adverse effects resulting from polypharmacy
- Whenever starting new medications, especially in patients on multiple pre-existing medications, the chance for drug-to-drug interactions increases greatly
  - Safe titration along with close monitoring of adverse effects is of high priority
- The patient has been on a stable dose of benzodiazepines. If possible, long-term use should be discontinued due to potential addiction/dependence
  - If discontinued, it should be tapered gradually due to potential withdrawal from developed dependency
  - However, if benzodiazepines are required to achieve adequate maintenance of the patient's illness, the benefits outweigh the risks in this patient, given his history of multiple psychiatric hospitalizations due to relapse/decompensation

- Lamotrigine (Lamictal) was initiated due to its efficacy in treating acute bipolar depression. It also provides mood stabilization as a maintenance treatment phase of bipolar I disorder
  - Due to need for slow titration lamotrigine may take weeks to improve bipolar depression, weeks to months for mood stabilization, but ultimately may reach complete remission of symptoms
  - If there is an improvement, treatment can continue indefinitely to avoid the recurrence of mania and/or depression
  - When starting lamotrigine, all patients should always be cautioned about possible rash as a side effect and instructed to be evaluated immediately in an emergency or urgent clinic setting should a rash develop
  - Initial montitoring for rash or Stevens–Johnson syndrome is of utmost importance during initial titration of lamotrigine. Development of Stevens–Johnson syndrome would be uncommon after 4 weeks of treatment
  - Remember that valproic acid (e.g. Depakote) increases blood levels of lamotrigine. Initial starting dose of lamotrigine should be halved (i.e. 12.5 mg starting daily dose) if patient on valproic acid prior to starting lamotrigine
  - Conversely carbamazepine (Equetro) decreases blood levels of lamotrigine. If patient on carbamazepine, initial starting dose of lamotrigine can be accelerated
  - Due to its limitation regarding slow titration, lamotrigine is not recommended in the acutely suicidal patient

Case outcome: first interim follow-up visits through initial 3 months

Patient medication changes

Date	Medications	Mood	Concerns
Month 1 (March 2002)	Lithium 1800 mg Lamotrigine 25 mg Ziprasidone 160 mg Risperidone 1 mg Clonazepam 1.0/1.5 mg	Depressed	Insomnia "Paranoid"
Month 2 (April 2002)	Lithium 1800 mg Lamotrigine 75 mg Ziprasidone 160 mg Risperidone discontinued Clonazepam 1.0/0.5/1.5 mg	Depression improved Anxiety	Insomnia "Paranoid"
Month 3 (May 2002)	Lithium 1800 mg Lamotrigine 100 mg Ziprasidone 160 mg Clonazepam 1.0/0.5/1.5 mg	Euthymic Anxiety gone	Insomnia Paranoid thoughts improved Downward nystagmus

Question

Given that the patient is now presenting with downward nystagmus, what change to his medication list would you make?

- 1. Check lithium blood level and decrease the dose of lithium
- 2. Discontinue lamotrigine (Lamictal)
- 3. Discontinue ziprasidone (Geodon)
- 4. Decrease clonazepam (Klonopin)
- 5. Review the chart

Answer - #1

Case outcome: follow-up visits 4 months through 5 months
Patient medication changes

Date	Medications	Mood	Concerns
Month 4 (June 2002)	Lithium 1200 mg Lithium level 0.88 mEq/l Lamotrigine 125 mg Ziprasidone 160 mg Clonazepam 1.0/0.5/1.5 mg	Euthymic	Insomnia Nystagmus improved slightly Patient wishes to discontinue lithium and start carbamazepine or valproic acid
Month 5 (July 2002)	Lithium 1050 mg Lamotrigine 200 mg Ziprasidone 160 mg Clonazepam 1.0/0.5/1.5 mg	Euthymic	Insomnia Nystagmus continues to improve "Paranoid"

Question

Because of the continued insomnia and paranoid ideation, what would be your next step?

- 1. Discontinue lithium
- 2. Discontinue lamotrigine (Lamictal)
- 3. Discontinue ziprasidone (Geodon) and start olanzapine (Zyprexa)
- 4. Discontinue clonazepam (Klonopin)
- 5. Start quetiapine (Seroquel) at night and once benefit shown begin taper discontinue ziprasidone

Case outcome: follow-up visits 6 months through 12 months
Patient medication changes

Date	Medications	Mood	Concerns
Month 6 (August 2002)	Lithium 900 mg Lamotrigine 200 mg Ziprasidone tapered Quetiapine started Clonazepam 1.0/0.5/1.5 mg	Euthymic	Insomnia Nystagmus "Paranoid"
Month 7 (September 2002)	Lithium 600 mg Lamotrigine 200 mg Ziprasidone discontinued Quetiapine 400 mg Clonazepam decreased 1.0/1.5 mg	Euthymic	Insomnia gone Nystagmus Paranoia gone

Date	Medications	Mood	Concerns
Month 8 (October 2002)	Lithium 450 mg Lamotrigine 200 mg Quetiapine 400 mg Clonazepam 0.5/1.5 mg	Euthymic	Nystagmus improved Patient admits mood is now stable
Month 9 (November 2002)	Lithium 300 mg Lamotrigine 200 mg Quetiapine 400 mg Clonazepam 0.5/1.0 mg	Euthymic	Nystagmus still present
Month 10 (December 2002)	Lithium discontinued Lamotrigine 200 mg Quetiapine 400 mg Clonazepam 0.5/0.5 mg	Euthymic	Nystagmus resolved Patient can drive again
Month 12 (February 2003)	Lamotrigine 200 mg Quetiapine 400 mg Clonazepam discontinued	Euthymic	

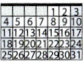

Case summary

- By the end of a rather long (12-months) and gradual process of medication changes/titration, the patient achieved euthymia and had no significant adverse reactions
- Polypharmacy was avoided as the patient improved with dual-therapy lamotrigine (Lamictal) and quetiapine (Seroquel) and was no longer on multiple antipsychotics or benzodiazepines

Take-home points

- Mood stabilization without induction of mania or rapid cycling is the paramount goal in the treatment of bipolar depression
- Standard antidepressants have the potential to destabilize bipolar disorder; however, lithium and lamotrigine (Lamictal) are recommended as first-line treatments
- Currently, there are only four medications currently approved by the FDA to treat bipolar depression: cariprazine (Vraylar), lurasidone (Latuda), olanzapine-fluoxetine (Symbax), and quetiapine (Seroquel)[6]
- While the adverse effects of lithium including hypothyroidism, renal failure, and an increase in peripheral calcium and parathyroid hormone have been well described, lithium can induce downbeating nystagmus and other ocular motor abnormalities such as gaze palsies that may persist despite discontinuation of the medication

Tips and pearls

- To start lamotrigine (Lamictal), take a slow titration approach. Begin with 25 mg daily and increase gradually, with daily dose increases weekly or biweekly from 25 mg to 50 mg to 100 mg and after 4

Table 3.1 Mood stabilizers: evidence from controlled clinical trials

Drug	Depression		Mania	
	Acute	Maintenance	Acute	Maintenance
Divalproex sodium	–	+	++	+
Lamotrigine	++	++	–	–
Lithium	+	+	++	++
Atypicals	+	+	++	++

Quality of evidence/effect size: ++, marked; +, moderate; –, minimal/inadequate evidence.
Modified from Keck and McElroy (2003).

Table 3.2 Medication effects on weight

Increase weight	Neutral	Decrease weight
Olanzapine ↑↑↑	Oxcarbazepine ↔	Topiramate ↓↓
Divalproex sodium ↑↑		Lamotrigine ↓
Lithium ↑↑		Bupropion ↓
Gabapentin ↑		

Modified from Allison et al. (1999).

weeks obtain a blood level. If blood levels permit, the dose can titrate dose up to 200 mg or higher

- Black box warnings
  - Lithium: narrow therapeutic index
  - Divalproex sodium (Depakote): hepatotoxicity, teratogenicity, pancreatitis
  - Carbamazepine (Equetro): aplastic anemia, agranulocytosis
  - Lamotrigine: serious rashes, Stevens–Johnson syndrome
- Consider the need for antipsychotic medications for maintenance therapy in bipolar patients (Table 3.1). Although they might have been required initially to treat acute manic episodes, always factor in the long-term adverse effects, including tardive dyskinesia, hyperglycemia, hyperlipidemia, and weight gain (Table 3.2), especially when on multiple agents

Posttest self-assessment question and answer

Which of the following statements is correct regarding treatment for bipolar disorder?

A. Initial lamotrigine (Lamictal) dosage should be halved in patients on stable dose of valproic acid (Depakote)

B. Patients who develop a severe rash while on lamotrigine should not be rechallenged

C. Antipsychotic medications are the gold standard for maintenance prevention of mania

D. Initial lamotrigine dose should be halved in patients on stable dose of carbamazepine (Equetro)

Answer: A and D

Lithium and valproic acid (Depakote) have strong evidence in head-to-head trials versus antipsychotics for the maintenance of bipolar disorder, specifically preventing mania. Lamotrogine is FDA approved for bipolar depression but can cause severe rashes (e.g. Stevens–Johnson syndrome). Patients should NOT be rechallenged as Stevens–Johnson syndrome can potentially be fatal. Carbamazepine lowers blood levels of lamotrigine; therefore doses should be doubled, not halved. Some studies have shown that calcium-channel blockers can improve outcomes in mania initially unresponsive to lithium monotherapy, but only in conjunction with lithium.

References

1. Allison DB, Mentore JL, Heo M, et al. Antipsychotic-induced weight gain: a comprehensive research synthesis. *Am J Psychiatry* 1999; 156:1686–96. https://doi.org/10.1176/ajp.156.11.1686

2. Biton V, Mirza W, Montouris G, et al. Weight change associated with valproate and lamotrigine monotherapy in patients with epilepsy. *Neurology* 2001; 56:172–7. https://doi.org/10.1212/wnl.56.2.172

3. Bowden CL, Calabrese JR, McElroy SL, et al. A randomized, placebo-controlled 12-month trial of divalproex and lithium in treatment of outpatients with bipolar I disorder. *Arch Gen Psychiatry* 2000; 57:481–9. https://doi.org/10.1001/archpsyc.57.5.481

4. Bozzatello P, Brignolo E, de Grandi E, Bellino S. Supplementation with omega-3 fatty acids in psychiatric disorders: a review of literature data. *J Clin Med* 2016; 5:67. https://doi.org/10.3390/jcm5080067

5. Calabrese JR, Sullivan JR, Bowden CL, et al. Rash in multicenter trials of lamotrigine in mood disorders: clinical relevance and management. *J Clin Psychiatry* 2002; 63:1012–19. https://doi.org/10.4088/jcp.v63n1110

6. Carvalho AF, Firth J, Vieta E. Bipolar disorder. *N Engl J Med* 2020; 383:58–66. https://doi.org/10.1056/NEJMra1906193

7. Chengappa KNR, Rathore D, Levine J, et al. Topiramate as add-on treatment for patients with bipolar mania. *Bipolar Disord* 1999; 1:42–53. https://doi.org/10.1034/j.1399-5618.1999.10111.x

8. Dunner DL. Optimizing lithium treatment. *J Clin Psychiatry* 2000; 61 (Suppl. 9):76–81.

9. Fountoulakis KN, Grunze H, Vieta E, et al. The International College of Neuro-Psychopharmacology (CINP) Treatment Guidelines for Bipolar Disorder in Adults (CINP-BD-2017), Part 3: The Clinical Guidelines. *Int J Neuropsychopharmacol* 2017; 20:180–95. https://doi.org/10.1093/ijnp/pyw109

10. Frye MA, Ketter TA, Kimbrell TA, et al. A placebo-controlled study of lamotrigine and gabapentin monotherapy in refractory mood disorders. *J Clin Psychopharmacol* 2000; 20:607–14. https://doi.org/10.1097/00004714-200012000-00004

11. Gidal BE, Maly MM, Nemire RE, Haley K. Weight gain and gabapentin therapy. *Ann Pharmacother* 1995; 29:1048. https://doi.org/10.1177/106002809502901019

12. Goodwin GM, Consensus Group of the British Association for Psychopharmacology. Evidence-based guidelines for treating bipolar disorder: revised second edition--recommendations from the British Association for Psychopharmacology. *J Psychopharmacol* 2009; 23:346–88. https://doi.org/10.1177/0269881109102919

13. Keck PE Jr, McElroy SL. Redefining mood stabilization *J Affect Disord* 2003; 73:163–9. https://doi.org/10.1016/s0165-0327(01)00355-x

14. Knowles SR, Shapiro LE, Shear NH. Anticonvulsant hypersensitivity syndrome: incidence, prevention and management. *Drug Saf* 1999; 21:489–501. https://doi.org/10.2165/00002018-199921060-00005

15. Mallinger AG, Thase ME, Haskett R, et al. Verapamil augmentation of lithium treatment improves outcome in mania unresponsive to lithium alone: preliminary findings and a discussion of therapeutic mechanisms. *Bipolar Disord* 2008; 10:856–66. https://doi.org/10.1111/j.1399-5618.2008.00636.x

16. McElroy S, Suppes T, Keck PE Jr, et al. Open-label adjunctive topiramate in the treatment of bipolar disorders. *Biol Psychiatry* 2000; 47:1025–33. https://doi.org/10.1016/s0006-3223(99)00316-9

17. Melkersson KI, Hulting A-L, Brismar KE. Elevated levels of insulin, leptin, and blood lipids in olanzapine-treated patients with schizophrenia or related psychoses. *J Clin Psychiatry* 2000; 61:742–9. https://doi.org/10.4088/jcp.v61n1006

18. *Physicians' Desk Reference*, 56th edn. Montvale, NJ: Medical Economics Company, 2002.

19. Rosa AR, Fountoulakis K, Siamouli M, et al. Is anticonvulsant treatment of mania a class effect? Data from randomized clinical trials. *CNS Neurosci Ther* 2011; 17: 167–77. https://doi.org/10.1111/j.1755-5949.2009.00089.x

20. Sanger TM, Grundy SL, Gibson PJ, et al. Long-term olanzapine therapy in the treatment of bipolar I disorder: an open-label continuation phase study. *J Clin Psychiatry* 2001; 62:273–81. https://doi.org/10.4088/jcp.v62n0410

21. Schein F, Manoli P, Cathébras P. Lithium-induced downbeat nystagmus. *Am J Ophthalmol Case Rep* 2017; 7:74–5. https://doi.org/10.1016/j.ajoc.2017.06.012

22. Schlienger RG, Shear NH. Antiepileptic drug hypersensitivity syndrome. *Epilepsia* 1998; 39 (Suppl. 7):S3–7. https://doi.org/10.1111/j.1528-1157.1998.tb01678.x

23. Stahl SM. *Stahl's Essential Psychopharmacology: Prescriber's Guide*, 6th edn. Cambridge, UK: Cambridge University Press, 2017.

24. Tohen M, Sanger TM, McElroy SL, et al. Olanzapine versus placebo in the treatment of acute mania. Olanzapine HGEH Study Group. *Am J Psychiatry* 1999; 156:702–9. https://doi.org/10.1176/ajp.156.5.702

25. Tohen M, Jacobs TG, Grundy SL, et al. for the Olanzapine HGGW Study Group. Efficacy of olanzapine in acute bipolar mania: a double-blind, placebo-controlled study. *Arch Gen Psychiatry* 2000; 57:841–9. https://doi.org/10.1001/archpsyc.57.9.841

26. Young LT, Robb JC, Patelis-Siotis I, et al. Acute treatment of bipolar depression with gabapentin. *Biol Psychiatry* 1997; 42:851–3. https://doi.org/10.1016/s0006-3223(97)00305-3

Case 4: The agitated patient who finally wasn't

The Question: What do you do when a patient is taking appropriate scheduled medications, but is frequently agitated and requiring medication intramuscularly (IM) or as needed on top?

The Psychopharmacological Dilemma: This patient had a significant history of violence and required heavy utilization of emergency IM medications in addition to scheduled medications. How do you balance the safety needs of the patient and staff while still respecting consent, ethical rights, and the risk of serious side effects?

Alex J. Mageno, Nekisa Haghighat, and Arthur Leitzke

Pretest self-assessment question (answer at the end of the case)

What is the expected effective therapeutic range of plasma levels for olanzapine (Zyprexa)?

A. 10–50 ng/ml
B. 20–100 ng/ml
C. 30–150 ng/ml
D. 40–200 ng/ml

Patient evaluation on intake

- A 28-year-old female, who has been dropped off at the psychiatric emergency room by her family, who left without providing further information. The patient reports that "the medication isn't working. I haven't slept in 3 days." On presentation, the patient is hyperverbal, hypersexual and labile, with delusions of grandeur. She requests "the shots in my butt that help me sleep"
- The patient is known to the nursing staff as one who previously caused a physical altercation on the unit, resulting in several injuries among staff and other patients, two of whom ended up in the medical emergency department for further treatment. At 350 lbs (160 kg), the patient is difficult to subdue, particularly when agitated. Tonight, she warns, "If anyone messes with me, I'll mess them up!"

Psychiatric history

- She has a prior diagnosis of "bipolar disorder versus schizophrenia" and has been admitted to the emergency room/hospital several times, most recently about 3 months ago. She also has a history of incarceration, during which she was also admitted to a psychiatric facility

- Per chart review, the patient was most recently admitted to this psychiatric hospital 2 months ago after calling her landlord to tell him that she had a knife and was going to stab someone. She presented in a similar, labile state and required frequent emergency IM medications throughout her admission
- She denies prior suicide attempts but did report prior self-harm by cutting when she was a teenager

Medication history

- Trials of risperidone (Risperdal), divalproex sodium (Depakote), and prazosin (Minipress), as well as the long-acting injectable form of paliperidone (Invega)

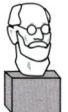

Psychotherapy history

- She has not established care with a therapist or counselor

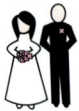

Social and personal history

- The patient is married and lives with her husband and their daughter. She is not employed but receives government disability benefits. She graduated from high school. She has been incarcerated one time
- She reports a history of methamphetamine use but says she is not a regular user and that she last used several years ago. She does admit to drinking alcohol daily and had a "tall one" prior to admission
- She also smokes a pack per day of cigarettes and reports almost daily marijuana use. She last smoked cigarettes and marijuana on the day of admission. She denies other substance use

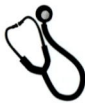

Medical history

- She reports a history of hypertension and hypothyroidism but says she was never on any medications for either problem
- No known drug allergies

Family history

- Mother with bipolar disorder

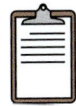

Patient evaluation on initial visit
Vitals and laboratory results on admission

Blood pressure	146/82 mmHg (agitated)
Heart rate	82 bpm
Respiratory rate	19 breaths/min
Temperature	98.9°F
Height	5'5" (165 cm)
Weight	350 lbs (160 kg)
Complete blood count	Within normal limits
Comprehensive metabolic panel	Within normal limits
Lipid profile	Within normal limits
Hemoglobin A1c	5.9%
Thyroid-stimulating hormone	1.2 mIU/l
Urine drug screen	Positive for tetrahydrocannabinol
Blood alcohol level	Not ordered

- The patient is extremely distracted throughout the interview, making her a poor historian. She has a pressured, hyperverbal speech pattern, and extreme distractibility. The patient admits racing thoughts and insomnia. She has not slept in 3 days. Instead of sleeping, she is "writing a book and music" because she is "an author, a songwriter", after which she proceeds to sing a song in demonstration. In the same sentence, she talks about going back to college to become a "probation officer, pediatrician, and career counselor"
- She is very labile throughout the conversation, suddenly crying out "I need the shots in my butt to help me sleep!" and becoming tearful
- The patient acknowledges auditory hallucinations but cannot clearly describe them
- She denies suicidal ideation and specific homicidal ideation but again threatens violence against anyone who "messes" with her
- She denies the use of illicit substances but reports having a "tall beer" prior to coming to the hospital

Current medications
- Risperidone (Risperdal) 3 mg twice per day
- Trazodone (Desyrel) 100 mg for insomnia every night as needed

Questions

The patient states that she takes her medication regularly. Despite her high dose of risperidone (Risperdal) (6 mg per day), she believes the medications are not helping. Would you consider changing her medication regimen at this time?

- Yes
- No

Would you perform any of the following actions next?

- Order a plasma drug level of risperidone and 9-hydroxyrisperidone
- Order pharamacogenomic profile
- Decrease the dose of risperidone
- Start a mood stabilizer
- Switch to a different antipsychotic
- Add a second antipsychotic
- Administer paliperidone long-acting injection (Invega)

Attending physician's mental notes: initial visit

- The patient is presenting with clear features of mania in the absence of amphetamine use, per urine drug screen. These include minimal sleep, emotional lability, flight of ideas, pressured speech, and grandiosity. Given the severity of her symptoms, she will likely require admission
- Olanzapine (Zyprexa) and divalproex sodium (Depakote) have both been shown to be effective in the treatment of acute mania. The patient does not want to start olanzapine because it "hasn't worked" in the past. She has, however, tried divalproex sodium and is agreeable to starting this medication now
- Staff have already alerted you to this patient's history of violence while on the unit. The patient is starting to make vaguely threatening remarks. During previous admissions, she has demonstrated her ability to inflict serious bodily harm and property damage. Maintaining a safe and therapeutic environment is of the utmost importance. It would thus be wise to maintain a low threshold for emergency medications with this patient

Case outcome: hospital day 1

- The patient was calm during processing onto the unit. She was cooperative and tried to rest for the first few hours, but suddenly became agitated in the early morning. Ultimately, she was redirectable and agreed to take oral medications. She briefly calmed down after taking lorazepam (Ativan) 2 mg and olanzapine (Zyprexa) 10 mg PO as an oral disintegrating tablet (ODT)
- Later, the patient became agitated. She began to throw chairs at staff and threatened further violence against anyone who came near her. This time she was not redirectable and required emergency IM medications. She was given haloperidol (Haldol) 5 mg + lorazepam 2 mg + diphenhydramine (Benadryl) 50 mg IM, after which she became calmer

- Around dinner time, the patient suddenly began shouting at another patient, despite seemingly being unprovoked. This time, she was not only non-redirectable, but also attempted to escape from the unit by forcing open the patio door. She was again given emergency haloperidol 10 mg + lorazepam 2 mg + diphenhydramine 50 mg IM, after which she eventually slept
- Approximately 5 hours later – shortly before midnight – the patient woke up and began pounding on the nursing staff's window, demanding to leave and refusing to return to bed. When the on-call physician arrived to evaluate the situation, the patient became even more threatening and required emergency IM medications. This time she was given chlorpromazine (Thorazine) 100 mg IM
- The total antipsychotic load in the first 24 hours was:
  - 10 mg oral olanzapine (Zyprexa) ODT
  - 15 mg haloperidol IM
  - 100 mg chlorpromazine IM

Attending physician's mental notes: end of hospital day 1

- As initially feared, the patient's agitation and tendency toward violence is already proving to be difficult to manage. In less than 1 day, she has tried throwing furniture and forcefully leaving the unit, and continues to spontaneously lash out at patients and staff alike
- Like any emergency department, multiple attending physicians are managing the unit throughout the day and night. In an emergency situation, any physician can and should evaluate the situation and make the decision that is best for the safety of patients and staff alike. That said, the more physicians evaluate and treat the patient, the more likely the patient is to get varying medications at different doses. Additionally, a physician who has never met the patient will not have established a therapeutic rapport, making it unlikely that they will be able to de-escalate the situation without the use of emergency medications
- In this case, the patient is becoming more and more agitated throughout the day and requires increasing doses of emergency IM medications. When the on-call physician arrives on the scene, it is apparent that IM haloperidol (Haldol) has not been effective in keeping the patient calm for long, even at an increased dose. The anticholinergics she is receiving with each IM injection in order to minimize extrapyramidal symptoms are also accumulating. Thus, switching to a different antipsychotic that does not require a concurrent anticholinergic may be a better option – hence the use of chlorpromazine (Thorazine)

- The patient's obesity affects not only the dosage but also the method of administration. Patients with excessive adipose tissue may require longer needles than what is standard for emergency medications in order to allow IM delivery. If the patient was receiving IM medications through a needle of insufficient length, the chances are the medication administered was not adequately absorbed. It could also explain her weak response to the long-acting injectable form of paliperidone (Invega) in the past. In obese patients, a needle of at least 1.5″ should be used

Case outcome: hospital days 2 and 3

- The patient was able to sleep on and off through the night. When she awoke, she was initially cooperative. Her current regimen is divalproex sodium (Depakote) 500 mg twice per day and olanzapine (Zyprexa) ODT 10 mg PO twice per day, which she took as prescribed throughout the day
- The calm was short lived, however, as the patient became agitated immediately before breakfast. She began yelling at other patients, wanting to "fight them" and the responding staff. She also appeared to be responding to auditory hallucinations and ultimately received chlorpromazine (Thorazine) 200 mg IM
- Although she continued to be irritable throughout the day, staff became hopeful when she went for 8 hours without requiring emergency intervention. After lunch, however, she became hostile, agitated, disorganized, and once again threatened to assault staff and other patients. She received haloperidol (Haldol) 10 mg + lorazepam (Ativan) 2 mg + diphenhydramine (Benadryl) 100 mg IM
- 7 hours later, a little after dinner, the patient suddenly punched another patient in the face. She received chlorpromazine 200 mg IM. The patient became calm and apologetic afterwards, although staff noted that she appeared paranoid before finally retiring to bed
- Total antipsychotic load in the second 24 hours:
  - 20 mg oral olanzapine ODT
  - 10 mg haloperidol IM
  - 400 mg chlorpromazine IM
- The next day followed a similar pattern. The patient was compliant with her prescribed medications but would become intermittently and progressively agitated throughout the day. After one instance of agitation in the afternoon, she became somewhat redirectable and agreed to take chlorpromazine 100 mg PO. Her evening dose of olanzapine was doubled to 20 mg ODT, with plans to continue at 20 mg ODT PO twice per day starting with tomorrow morning's

dose. Nevertheless, the patient ended up receiving chlorpromazine 200 mg IM after teaming up with a peer and attempting to start a riot among the patients. She then used the hospital phone to call 911 and threatened the responding operator

- Total antipsychotic load in third 24 hours:
  - 35 mg olanzapine ODT, including additional 5 mg PO received as needed
  - 100 mg oral + 200 mg chlorpromazine IM

Questions

Is there anything about this patient's history that would make you reconsider the starting dose of her olanzapine (Zyprexa)?
Would you have made any adjustments to the route or method of administration of her medications?

Attending physician's mental notes

- In retrospect, a few things about the patient could have clued us into the fact that she would need a higher dose of olanzapine (Zyprexa) than what we started out with, or even the maximum FDA-approved dose of 20 mg
- The patient smokes a pack a day of cigarettes in addition to marijuana. This means that she will likely need a higher starting dose of olanzapine compared with non-smokers. Olanzapine is metabolized mainly by the enzymes cytochrome P450 1A2 (CYP1A2) and UDP-glucuronosyltransferase. Hydrocarbon by-products of smoking are known inducers of these two enzymes, meaning that they kick them into overdrive and cause them to metabolize substrates such as olanzapine at a faster rate.[3] It follows, then, that smokers will have lower plasma levels of olanzapine, indicating that a higher dose is needed to reach therapeutic levels
- Interestingly, caffeine is a prominent competitive inhibitor of CYP1A2 and would therefore have the opposite effect of smoking.[3] In other words, a high caffeine intake will cause CYP1A2 enzymes to metabolize less olanzapine, leading to higher plasma levels and a lower therapeutic range

Case outcome: hospital day 4

- As the third day drew to a close, the on-call physician was called to evaluate the patient a little after midnight. Nursing staff reported that the last IM dose of chlorpromazine (Thorazine) appeared ineffective, as the patient was still exhibiting verbal and motor agitation. She had been pacing around the unit for hours, intermittently punching the walls

- Upon evaluation, the physician noted that the patient was tearful and wanting to talk, although she found it difficult to articulate her feelings. She was no longer threatening staff but appeared frustrated and anxious
- The physician wondered if the patient was experiencing akathisia. She agreed to take lorazepam (Ativan) 4 mg PO. Shortly afterwards, the patient stopped pacing and returned to her room, where she eventually fell asleep. No further incidents were reported during the night
- The next morning, the patient was continued on oral divalproex sodium (Depakote) 500 mg twice per day and olanzapine (Zyprexa) 20 mg ODT twice per day. She also agreed to take chlorpromazine 100 mg PO on three separate occasions throughout the day, as needed for breakthrough symptoms. She did not receive any emergency IM medications on this day

Case outcome: hospital day 5 through discharge

- The patient had no further behavioral emergencies and required no further adjustments to her daily psychopharmacological regimen. Over the next few days, the patient's mood showed signs of stabilizing. She began sleeping through the night, became conversational, and participated in group activities. She was discharged 9 days after admission on divalproex sodium (Depakote) 500 mg twice per day and olanzapine 20 mg ODT twice per day, with plans to follow up on an outpatient basis

Attending physician's mental notes

- The patient's initial days on the unit were marked by extreme agitation and volatility, punctuated by frequent emergency IM medications for sedation. Although the patient would initially become calm or even sedated after doses of IM haloperidol (Haldol) or oral olanzapine (Zyprexa), the effect was always short lived. Within a few hours, the patient would become agitated and require emergency intervention
- Perhaps the patient's morbid obesity could explain these diminished therapeutic effects. Thus, both IM and oral chlorpromazine (Thorazine) was tried, as its high lipid solubility suggests it would have a longer half-life in this patient
- Even with the addition of chlorpromazine, the patient continued to be volatile and threatening. However, when the on-call physician was asked to evaluate her yet again for reported agitation, she presented in a slightly different matter. It would have been easy

for the physician to discount the patient's lashing out at the walls as a sign of further agitation, warranting emergency intervention. However, when taken into consideration with her relentless pacing in the setting of frequent doses of antipsychotics, a different picture begins to emerge. It would not be surprising if the patient is experiencing progressively worsening akathisia or signs of extrapyramidal symptoms – perhaps she is unable to articulate her feelings, and her resulting frustrations are misinterpreted as violent agitation. Thus, the physician foregoes another antipsychotic in favor of a benzodiazepine, with the hopes that treating akathisia may provide the patient with some relief

Case debrief

- When evaluating a patient for agitation, staff and patient safety have to be weighed against the right of the patient to refuse medications. Your clinical judgment should be based on a nuanced understanding of evidence-based medicine and shaped by your own personal experience as a physician
- It is important to reassess patients in person each and every time they are agitated. Your next course of action should be based on the person you see before you and not the person you may have heard about from staff or who you remember seeing a few days earlier
- Granted, collateral and a patient's individual history are important when making an overall diagnosis or treatment plan. However, agitation is an acute state and should be treated as such. Just because a patient required emergency medications yesterday does not mean they need them today or at the first sign of conflict
- You may find the unexpected, such as your previously violent patient is now displaying akathisia or excited catatonia. These states require different, and often much less drastic, therapeutic interventions than violent agitation alone

Take-home points

- Violence associated with psychosis or mania is a commonly encountered problem in the psychiatric hospital setting. Second only to law enforcement, the inpatient psychiatric setting is one of the most violent workplace settings in the USA. Every setting is different, and providers must understand the needs, risks, and resources available in their specific population setting
- Always be on the lookout for side effects of medications that can be causing behavioral issues or agitation. These include constipation or ileus, anticholinergic confusion, orthostatic hypotension, and

akathisia. It is always better to use as few medications as possible at the lowest effective dose

- If available, plasma levels of medications and pharmacogenomic testing can be extremely helpful. Without them, you are dosing in the dark based on population studies that may not apply to the patient in front of you. When documented appropriately, such testing can also help justify to other providers why the patient needs an abnormally high or low dose of a particular medication
- One must consider pharmacokinetics when reviewing this patient. Her lack of response to IM medications may be a mechanical failure related to utilizing a needle with insufficient length to account for the patient's obesity. Social factors, such as smoking cigarettes and marijuana, can also play a biological role in the metabolism and efficacy of medications

Tips and pearls

- Olanzapine (Zyprexa) can be used in some patients with treatment-resistant psychosis or bipolar disorder
- Olanzapine is a preferred augmenting agent in bipolar depression or treatment-resistant unipolar depression
- The immediate-release olanzapine injection is useful when rapid onset of anti-agitation action without drug titration is needed
- Alternative antipsychotics should be considered for patients who have a personal or family history of diabetes mellitus, obesity, and/or dyslipidemia
- Use of plasma antipsychotic and mood stabilizer levels correlate more precisely with relevant receptor occupancies than the standardized, prescribed doses of a medication
- If one can afford an individual approach for each patient, better control of symptoms will likely follow

Mechanism of action moment

Mechanism of action at specific receptors

Dopamine	Robust antagonism at D_2 and D_3 receptors decreases positive psychotic symptoms and contributes to mood stabilization Clinical effects of robust binding at D_4 receptors is unknown
Serotonin	Robust antagonism at $5\text{-}HT_{2A}$ receptors increases dopamine release in the mesocortical, nigrostriatal, and tuberoinfundibular tracts and likely improves frontal lobe functioning, diminishing neurological motor symptoms, and avoiding prolactin elevation, respectively Antagonism at $5\text{-}HT_{2C}$ receptors likely increases carbohydrate craving and may contribute to improved cognitive and affective symptoms
Acetylcholine	Antagonism at M_1–M_5 receptors produces anticholinergic effects including blurred near vision, dry mouth, decreased gastrointestinal motility, and urinary retention

Glutamate	At high plasma concentrations (120–200 ng/ml), allosteric modulation (increase) in glutamate signal transduction may be a major factor in treating psychosis and improving frontal lobe functions including cognition, a reduction in negative symptoms, and improved executive functions
Histamine	Inverse agonism at histamine H_1 receptors produces sedation and weight gain
Epinephrine/ norepinephrine	Antagonism at α_1-adrenergic receptors causes orthostatic hypotension

From Cummings and Stahl (2020).

Plasma concentrations and treatment response

Initial target range	40–120 ng/ml
Range for treatment resistance	120–200 ng/ml (more resistant patients)
Typical time to response	Therapeutic improvement can be seen within 1–2 weeks for aggression, agitation, insomnia Therapeutic improvement can be seen within 3–6 weeks for control of mania and positive psychotic symptoms Therapeutic improvement can be seen within 1–6 weeks
Time course of improvement	If no response by 4 weeks at maximum tolerated dose or in upper therapeutic plasma concentration range (120–200 ng/ml), taper and withdraw therapy or cross-titrate with clozapine

From Cummings and Stahl (2020).

Posttest self-assessment question and answer

What is the expected effective therapeutic range of plasma levels for olanzapine (Zyprexa)?

A. 10–50 ng/ml
B. 20–100 ng/ml
C. 30–150 ng/ml
D. 40–200 ng/ml

Answer: D

In a non-smoking patient, it is reasonably expected that plasma levels below 40 mg will have no effect on target symptoms, whereas there is evidence to suggest that, for most patients, levels above 200 ng/ml will have reached receptor saturation and will likely have no further benefit. To estimate the expected plasma level based on daily dose, multiply the daily dose in milligrams by 2.0 (non-smokers only).

References

1. Baker, RW, Kinon, BJ, Maguire, GA, et al. Effectiveness of rapid initial dose escalation of up to forty milligrams per day of oral olanzapine in acute agitation. *J Clin Psychopharmacol* 2003; 23:342–8. https://doi.org/10.1097/01.jcp.0000085406.08426.a8
2. Cummings M, Stahl SM, eds. *Management of Complex Treatment-resistant Psychotic Disorders*. Cambridge, UK: Cambridge University Press, 2021.

3. de Leon, J. Glucuronidation enzymes, genes and psychiatry. *Int J Neuropsychopharmacol* 2003; 6: 57–72. https://doi.org/10.1017/S1461145703003249

4. Meyer, JM, Cummings, MA, Proctor, G, et al. Psychopharmacology of persistent violence and aggression. *Psychiatr Clin North Am* 2016; 39, 541–56. https://doi.org/10.1016/j.psc.2016.07.012

5. Phillips JP. Workplace violence against health care workers in the United States. *N Engl J Med* 2016; 374:1661–9. https://doi.org/10.1056/NEJMra1501998

6. Schoretsanitis G, Kane JM, Correll CU, et al. (2020). Blood levels to optimize antipsychotic treatment in clinical practice: a joint consensus statement of the American Society of Clinical Psychopharmacology and the Therapeutic Drug Monitoring Task Force of the Arbeitsgemeinschaft für Neuropsychopharmakologie und Pharmakopsychiatrie. *J Clin Psychiatry*, 81: 19cs13169. https://doi.org/10.4088/JCP.19cs13169

Case 5: The George who was not psychotic but anxious and distracted

The Question: How common is psychosis seen in the spectrum of psychiatric comorbidities in DiGeorge syndrome?

The Psychopharmacological Dilemma: Treating anxiety in a patient with a comorbid medical condition, symptoms of mood elevation, and a family history of bipolar disorder

Edgar Ortega, Michael Seigler, and Takesha Cooper

Pretest self-assessment question (answer at the end of the case)

Which anxiolytic acts as a partial agonist, with a strong affinity for the serotonin 5-HT$_{1A}$ receptors, has a weak affinity for the serotonin 5-HT$_2$ receptors, and acts as a weak antagonist of the dopamine D$_2$ autoreceptors?

A. Venlafaxine (Effexor)
B. Vilazodone (Viibryd)
C. Buspirone (BuSpar)
D. Vortioxetine (Trintellix)

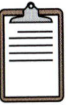

Patient evaluation on intake

- A 16-year-old male accompanied by his mother for initial evaluation
- The mother has been concerned about behavioral disturbances and anxiety, and has concerns for possible psychotic-like symptoms
- The patient was formally diagnosed with DiGeorge syndrome (velocardiofacial syndrome) in 2015

Psychiatric history

- Multiple diagnoses at 5 years: attention-deficit/hyperactivity disorder (ADHD), intellectual disability (ID) and autism spectrum disorder (ASD)

Medication history from age 5 to 15 years

- ADHD was treated in the past with mixed amphetamine salts (Adderall) leading to weight loss and depression
- He was switched to atomoxetine (Strattera) with only partial effectiveness
- Aripiprazole (Abilify) was added to atomoxetine due to behavioral issues, impulsivity, and concerns for some bizarre hallucinations
- Atomoxetine was eventually discontinued due to continuous weight loss and "mood swings"

- He remained on aripiprazole, and guanfacine extended-release (ER) (Intuniv) was added for ADHD and impulsivity. Melatonin was added as a sleep aid
- Aripiprazole was discontinued due to increased anxiety and restlessness, possibly akathisia

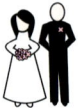

Social and personal history

- Developmental history: full term, forceps birth, walked at 11 months, language delayed at around 2 years of age, toilet trained at 2 years. He is sensitive to touch, loud music, and bright lights
- He lives at home with his mother, two siblings, and stepfather (no frequent contact with biological father)
- He attends 11th grade, has an Individualized Education Plan (IEP) and Regional Center services, and receives special education (classes for emotionally disturbed) for impulsive behaviors in the setting of cognitive impairment
- He has had over 20 school suspensions for fighting

Medical history

- DiGeorge Syndrome (velocardiofacial syndrome), diagnosed in 2015 as a teenager after extensive treatment by pediatricians and specialists
- He was previously thought to have Beals syndrome due to facial features and structural hand deformities

Family history

- Father's side: multiple family members with schizophrenia or bipolar disorder
- Mother's side: uncle with ADHD

Current medications

- Guanfacine ER (Intuniv) 4 mg at bedtime for ADHD
- Melatonin 6 mg at bedtime

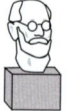

Psychotherapy history

- The patient has never received individual therapy. His mother was advised to participate in Therapeutic Behavioral Services (TBS)
- TBS is a short-term intensive program aimed at reducing challenging behaviors that are placing a youth at risk of psychiatric hospitalizations or out-of-home placement. The goal of TBS is to reduce challenging behaviors while emphasizing the youth's and

family's strengths and abilities. Services are provided at the time and place the behaviors occur, typically in the home

- Plans are individualized and should include the behavioral problems that need to be changed, including responsibilities for the patient, coach, and family members/caregivers/guardian. Needs will determine the frequency and length of treatment, with a gradual taper in frequency as the patient improves

Attending physician's mental notes: initial evaluation

- The patient presents with prior diagnoses and current chief complaints:
  - Behavioral issues have worsened over the last 1.5 years (being told "no" is a big stressor, aggression at school and home, fighting, profanity)
  - Suspected psychotic symptoms: when having to go to bed alone in his room, he reports seeing a green light and says he sees bad spirts in his bedroom. This improves when he is able to sleep with a sibling. However, reality testing is intact and he recognizes these disturbances are not real
  - Mood symptoms: depressed or irritable, decreased interest/ pleasure, worthlessness, guilt, insomnia, inability to concentrate. However, at times he presents with elevated mood: he feels on top of the world, has many goals, and tried to open a window believing he could fly. Duration is a few hours
  - Anxiety symptoms: excessive anxiety/worry, distressing dreams, restlessness, feeling on edge, irritable, and acts out behaviorally when anxious. Overreacts when triggered "to the next level beyond what is considered a normal response" according to the parent. He elopes from class when in stressful situations
  - Hyperactivity, impulsivity, and inattention. The symptoms presented before 7 years of age: difficulty staying quiet and still, fidgety, interrupts others, talks excessively, difficulty with sustaining attention, easily distracted, avoids detailed tasks, carelessness

Question

Based on your clinical experience, is monotherapy with an α-agonist for ADHD a good alternative in controlling ADHD symptoms in the context of anxiety symptoms?

- Yes
- No
- Sometimes

Attending physician's mental notes: initial evaluation (continued)

- The patient presents with symptoms from multiple domains (mood, anxiety, rule out psychotic, disruptive behavior) with a family history of mental illness (schizophrenia and bipolar), and a diagnosis of DiGeorge syndrome increases the predisposed risk of developing psychotic symptoms
- However, at this time he is not exhibiting auditory/visual hallucinations or paranoia
- Behavioral outbursts seem to be related to the patient's anxiety and fear (fight/flight response)
- He has restlessness, worries about the future, irritability, and sleep disturbance, and admits perceptual disturbances only when anxious
- The patient has cognitive impairments but makes an effort to focus and does not appear to be easily distracted or exhibiting significant attention deficit and hyperactivity symptoms at this time, possibly because guanfacine ER (Intuniv) is addressing the ADHD symptoms well

Question

What would be your next step?

- Raise guanfacine ER (Intuniv) to 6 mg daily
- Augment with clonidine (Catapres) to better target impulsivity, hyperactivity, and other ADHD symptoms
- Start a selective serotonin reuptake inhibitor (SSRI), a first-line medication for generalized anxiety disorder (GAD), despite the risk of triggering mania
- Start a medication that is an agonist of the 5-HT$_{1A}$ receptor
- Continue with the current regimen and wait to restart TBS
- Restart treatment with a different antipsychotic such as risperidone (Risperdal) for behavioral issues

Further investigation

Is there anything else you would especially like to know about the patient?

- What is DiGeorge syndrome and what are the implications regarding its psychiatric comorbidities?
  - A syndrome caused by the heterogeneous chromosomal deletion of 22q11.2
  - There are several disorders that fall under the umbrella of 22q11.2 deletion syndromes

- DiGeorge syndrome is characterized by the classic triad of cardiac abnormalities, hypoplastic thymus, and hypocalcemia
- Psychiatric comorbidities are commonly seen in 9–60% of children with the chromosomal 22q11.2 deletion. The most common comorbidities are anxiety disorders, ADHD and ASD
- Emotional dysfunction, inhibition, and attention disorders are among the symptoms seen in these patients
- Up to 75% present with moderate developmental delay
- Up to one-third of adolescents with DiGeorge syndrome develop schizophrenia-like psychosis
- The risk of developing psychosis appears to be as high as 25 times that of the general population
- The average age of onset of psychosis in DiGeorge syndrome is reported as 19–26 years

Attending physician's mental notes: initial evaluation (continued)

- The patient's symptoms are subthreshold for a bipolar or psychotic illness; what appears most impairing is anxiety, which manifests as irritability and acting-out behavior
  - GAD due to general medical condition
  - ADHD
  - Neurocognitive disorder due to another medical condition, with behavioral disturbance (DiGeorge syndrome)
  - Rule out ASD and unspecified schizophrenia spectrum and other psychotic disorder
- To address anxiety given the concern for activation (symptoms of mood elevation and family history of bipolar disorder)
  - Defer first-line SSRIs due to history of manic-like symptoms and strong family history of bipolar disorder
  - Start buspirone (BuSpar) 5 mg twice per day for 2 weeks and titrate to 10 mg twice per day to target anxiety
  - Change melatonin to melatonin time release (TR) 3 mg at bedtime to help with sleep maintenance
  - Continue guanfacine ER (Intuniv) 4 mg at bedtime for ADHD as this is working well
- Other therapeutic interventions that are being considered
  - Parent support to ensure IEP meets the patient's needs
  - Additional services by the Regional Center, the local agency providing a milieu of services to people with intellectual disabilities
  - The mother is considering TBS, an intensive, one-to-one behavioral therapy available for children and adolescents with serious emotional disturbances

Case outcome: first interim follow-up visit at 4 weeks

- The patient is tolerating buspirone (BuSpar) well
- He is sleeping better in his new room and is "less paranoid"
- He attends school regularly, with only one minor incident
- TBS is beginning soon with home support and on-the-spot guidance
- He is now on buspirone 10 mg twice per day; continue as is. Continue guanfacine ER (Intuniv) 4 mg PO at bedtime, and melatonin TR 3 mg PO at bedtime

Attending physician's mental notes: interim follow-up visit at 3 months

- The patient has difficulty controlling behaviors and impulses, and has eloped from the classroom during stressful situations
  - These reactions and behaviors seemed to be related to his anxiety: fight or flight kicks in
  - Other symptoms include restlessness, excessive worry about the future, irritability, and sleep disturbances
  - No psychotic symptoms were noted
- Will benefit from continuing treatment targeting his anxiety and moderate ADHD symptoms. Based on the above, medication changes as it follows
  - Increase buspirone (BuSpar) to 15 mg PO twice per day
  - Add diphenhydramine (Benadryl) 25–50 mg PO at bedtime as needed for sleep
  - Continue guanfacine ER (Intuniv) 4 mg PO at bedtime and TBS

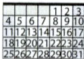

Case outcome: interim follow-up visit at 5 months

- The patient came to his appointment with his mother, who believes he is more mature and is doing better overall. He is taking his medications as indicated without side effects
- He is participating in TBS therapy and has learned new coping skills
- Current medication:
  - Guanfacine ER (Intuniv) 4 mg at bedtime
  - Diphenhydramine (Benadryl) 50 mg at bedtime
  - Buspirone (BuSpar) 15 mg twice per day
- He is irritable with his stepfather when he gives him a direction, and this causes anxiety
- He still feels anxious and wants to increase the medicine
- He is not having suicidal ideations, homicidal ideations, or auditory or visual hallucinations except for seeing "some flashing lights"

Question

What would you do next?

- Continue to titrate buspirone (BuSpar) to better target his residual anxiety
- Consider adding a benzodiazepine to better treat the patient's anxiety
- Augment with clonidine (Catapres) to better target impulsivity, hyperactivity, and other ADHD symptoms
- Consider adding a mood stabilizer of an atypical antipsychotic to target behavioral issues

Attending physician's mental notes: interim follow-up visit at 5 months

- He has difficulty in controlling behaviors and impulse, and would elope from the classroom during stressful situations
  - These reactions and behaviors seemed to be related to his anxiety
  - Other symptoms include restlessness, worrying about the future, irritability, and sleep disturbances
- Although he has cognitive impairments, he makes effort to focus and does not appear to be easily distracted or to exhibit other significant signs of ADHD at this time
- He will benefit from continuing treatment targeting his anxiety and moderate ADHD symptoms
- Based on the above, his medication changes as follows
  - Increase buspirone (BuSpar) 15 mg to PO three times a day
  - Continue diphenhydramine (Benadryl) 25–50 mg PO at bedtime as needed
  - Continue guanfacine ER (Intuniv) 4 mg PO at bedtime
  - Continue TBS

Case outcome: interim follow-up visit at 15 months

- The patient is now almost 18 years old and was seen for his 15-month follow-up visit with his mother. He is medication adherent, without adverse reactions
- He reports he is doing well, and the mother has no concerns
  - He is sleeping well now on diphenhydramine (Benadryl)
  - He remains euthymic, with no depression or anxiety
  - He has no suicidal ideations, homicidal ideations, or auditory or visual hallucinations

- He has no behavioral issues at school and is doing well academically
- Continue medications. He is stable at school. Both mother and patient agree on his discharge to the adult clinic due to private insurance and turning 18 years old in a month

Attending physician's mental notes: interim follow-up visit at 15 months

- The patient is a 17-year-old male with DiGeorge syndrome with multiple prior diagnoses, but with primary symptoms of anxiety, ADHD, and cognitive delay
- He has improved at controlling his behaviors and impulses with medication and intensive in-home therapy
  - Prior reactions and behaviors seemed to be related to his anxiety, which can manifest as behavioral outbursts given the fight or flight response, and in cognitively delayed persons can seem like paranoia. His ADHD has responded well to guanfacine ER (Intuniv)
- He is currently stable and ready for transitioning to adult care

Case debrief

- Psychiatric comorbidities are commonly seen in 9–60% of children with chromosome 22q11.2 deletion syndromes such as DiGeorge syndrome. Emotional dysfunction, inhibition, and attention disorders are among the most common
- The diagnosis of 22q11.2 deletion syndrome can be made by a chromosomal microarray. A genetics consultation is recommended
- Up to 75% of patients with 22q11.2 syndromes present with moderate developmental delay
- Up to one-third of adolescents with DiGeorge syndrome develop schizophrenia-like psychosis
- In addition, about 25% of children with anxiety have comorbid ADHD, and it can be difficult to distinguish which disorder is responsible for the symptom when there is symptom overlap. For example, a symptom of anxiety disorders is feeling restless, which can mimic hyperactivity in a child with ADHD. Additionally, both ADHD and anxiety disorders share difficulty concentrating as a core symptom
- In our case, the patient has DiGeorge syndrome, which is known to have multiple comorbidities accompanying the illness. His original presentation of psychotic-like symptoms was most likely a manifestation of his anxiety and illusions, also potentially

complicated by his intellectual disability. Psychotic symptoms would not have resolved with his medication regimen
- Anxiety symptoms were well controlled with buspirone (BuSpar) and ADHD symptoms were well treated with guanfacine ER (Intuniv) at 4 mg daily, the maximal dose recommended for treatment of ADHD
- In addition to this, guanfacine, a second-line ADHD medicine with some anxiolytic properties, may have played a role as an adjunct in controlling anxiety in addition to relieving ADHD symptoms
- Guanfacine as monotherapy for ADHD has been found to be more effective for children under 12 years of age, although older children can experience symptom relief
- The addition of TBS, with better behavioral control with buspirone (BuSpar) and guanfacine, helped the patient in achieving further long-term symptomatic control

Take-home points

- Comorbid anxiety, when severe, can present like psychosis, especially in the setting of intellectual disability
    - It is important to clarify diagnoses to treat the underlying disorders and achieve symptom remission
- DiGeorge syndrome is known to have multiple psychiatric comorbidities accompanying the illness
    - It can be difficult to distinguish which disorder is responsible when symptoms of anxiety and ADHD overlap
- Buspirone (BuSpar), a second-line medication for anxiety disorders, can be a good alternative in cases where SSRIs are either ineffective or there may be risks associated with bipolar disorder
- Guanfacine ER (Intuniv), a second-line ADHD medicine with some anxiolytic properties, may have played a role as an adjunct in controlling anxiety in addition to relieving ADHD symptoms

Performance in practice: confessions of a psychopharmacologist

What could have been done better here?

- Maintain a low threshold for treating psychosis and severe behavioral issues with mood stabilizers or antipsychotics as there is high risk in DiGeorge syndrome for psychosis
- Focus on clarifying the diagnosis to best treat the patient's anxiety and ADHD symptoms. While we aim to avoid polypharmacy, it is often necessary to use different medications to treat different disorders

Tips and pearls

- In cases such as this, clarifying the diagnosis is imperative for choosing the most effective treatment as well as its execution. However, while this is acknowledged by many practicing clinicians, it can be difficult to tease apart the intricacies of a diagnosis when multiple symptoms overlap. Collateral history from caregivers becomes vital in determining the final diagnosis
- Another strategy that is used clinically is the use of rating scales to help rule in or out specific diagnosis. For example, the Vanderbilt scale is used as a standardized screening tool by both teachers and caregivers to help determine the possibility of a child having ADHD
- The impact that having a clear diagnosis (anxiety, not psychotic disorder) can have on a patient can be immense, as in this patient's case, where it allowed him to avoid medication with antipsychotics, which potentially would have led to side effects such as metabolic syndrome and sedation

Two-minute tutorial

- Buspirone (BuSpar) is FDA approved for short- and long-term treatment of GAD
- Buspirone works at the serotonin 5-HT$_{1A}$ receptor as a partial agonist, has a weak affinity for the 5-HT$_2$ receptors, and is a weak antagonist of the D$_2$ autoreceptors
- The time of onset is similar to that of the common antidepressants; its use may be limited in acute anxiety, and it is used commonly as augmentation for SSRIs in GAD
- Although there is no comprehensive evidence for its efficacy as monotherapy, based on clinical evidence it may be a good alternative for patients who have failed SSRIs, have intolerable side effects, or are at risk for developing mania when used for GAD

Posttest self-assessment question and answer

Which anxiolytic acts as a partial agonist, with a strong affinity for the serotonin 5-HT$_{1A}$ receptors, has a weak affinity for the serotonin 5-HT$_2$ receptors, and acts as a weak antagonist of the dopamine D$_2$ autoreceptors?

A. Venlafaxine (Effexor)
B. Vilazodone (Viibryd)
C. Buspirone (BuSpar)
D. Vortioxetine (Trintellix)
Answer: C

Buspirone's mechanism of action involves the 5-HT_{1A} receptors (strong, partial agonist) where it is believed to produce its most significant clinical effects, and also acts on 5-HT_2 and D_2 receptors. Venlafaxine is an FDA-approved serotonin-norepinephrine reuptake inhibitor (SNRI) for GAD that acts on reuptake inhibition of serotonin and norepinephrine, and at higher doses, weak inhibition of the reuptake of dopamine. Vilazodone has its effect as an SSRI with the added partial agonism of 5-HT_{1A} receptors (buspirone's main mechanism of action). Vortioxetine has SSRI effects with partial agonism for 5-HT_{1A} receptors and antagonism of 5-HT_{1B}, $5\text{-HT}_{1D,}$ 5-HT_3, and 5-HT_7 receptors.

Case 6: The man who saw enemies everywhere

The Question: What treatment options are left when nearly all treatments have been exhausted and ineffective?

The Psychopharmacological Dilemma: Treating symptoms recalcitrant to even the most robust treatment strategies

Joshua Poole and Stephen Maurer

Pretest self-assessment question (answer at the end of the case)

Which of the following pharmacological treatments is not used in the management of acute aggression?

A. Haloperidol (Haldol) 2–10 mg intramuscularly (IM) or PO
B. Lorazepam (Ativan) 1–2 mg IM or PO
C. Olanzapine (Zyprexa) 5–10 mg IM or PO
D. Lithium 300–600 mg PO
E. Diphenhydramine (Benadryl) 25–50 mg IM or PO
F Ketamine (Ketalar) 4–6 mg IM

Psychiatric history

- The patient is a male in his early 30s who is currently receiving long-term care for schizoaffective disorder
- The patient is a generally poor historian who provides consistent/ useful information sparingly over long periods of time but is generally limited due to disorganization
- Outside records and collateral information suggest that the patient had seen a psychiatrist before long-term treatment in his adolescence but there is no evidence of medication or therapy
- The patient apparently suffered from both visual and auditory hallucinations during his teenage years (approximately age 14)
- The patient has a history of self-harming behaviors such as hitting, scratching, and biting himself (the patient even went so far as to bite off his fingernail)
- The patient has had no prior suicide attempts

Substance use history

- The patient reports that he started using cannabis nearly daily at age 13 with no apparent psychotic symptoms at that time
- The patient reports that he started drinking alcohol at age 19 and would often drink a 24 pack of beer every other day. He reports that when he first stopped drinking during his incarceration he got "the shakes"

- The patient began smoking crack cocaine at age 17 and used it daily as his drug of choice. This was consistent until he was incarcerated. He denies any psychotic symptoms from use of this substance
- The patient denies any use of hallucinogenic substances in his past
- There is suspicion that the patient was exposed to methamphetamine for roughly 1 week at age 16 but he is unable to confirm this information
- The patient began smoking cigarettes at age 27 and smoked four packs per week

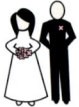

Social and personal history

- The patient was in the juvenile corrections system at age 16 for various drug- and violence-related crimes
- He has also been to jail as an adult, and outside reports indicate that he engaged in seemingly random acts of violence there
- The patient denies any history of physical or sexual abuse as a child
- He denies any intellectual disability or special education, but records of connection to a center for intellectually disabled adolescents make this doubtful
- The patient reports that he was expelled from school for indecent exposure
- The patient did not graduate high school and has worked in food service
- He reports that he was married for a few months once and that he has one child
- There is no evidence of a family history of mental or significant physical illness

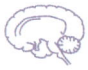

Psychiatric history (continued): a history of violence

- The patient was engaged in multiple fights while growing up in a type of "fight club". This may have been related to his activity in a gang
- The patient engaged in seemingly random acts of violence while in jail. However, it was later explained that the patient would engage in violence to pre-empt bullying and violence against him
- The patient had to be moved from rooms and units while in long-term care for his exceedingly violent attacks on both patients and staff (including several hospitalizations of staff)
- When questioned, the patient often reported delusional and persecutory reasons for attacking others including explaining that he was suffering from visual hallucinations where he saw whoever was talking to him as "standing on [his] mother's head"

- He would experience auditory hallucinations of solicitations to fight
- The patient's violence was so consistent and extreme that he required a constant 2:1 watch and had to perform his activities of daily living at staggered times compared with his peers
- However, it was noted that the patient would often hold back when attacking people, withdrawing his total strength

Question

Based on the information provided above, what would you think is the etiology of this patient's psychiatric symptoms?

- Intellectual disability
- Substance abuse from an early age
- Primary psychotic disorder
- Possible traumatic brain injuries (TBIs) from a long history of physical altercations
- Undiscovered family history of psychiatric illness

Further investigation

What would you do to manage an acutely aggressive patient? How about a patient that is consistently aggressive despite your intervention?

- Currently, most physicians will begin management of aggression by attempting verbal de-escalation. Failing this, many patients can be calmed down by placing them in temporary seclusion with the hope that taking them out of their environment might alleviate environmental causes of agitation. If a physician has concerns that a patient is an immediate harm to themselves or others, temporary restraints should be considered. During this process, the physician should be considering other reversible causes of agitation and potential pharmacological interventions
- Common pharmacological interventions include oral formulations of benzodiazepines, antipsychotics (typical antipsychotics are preferred to atypical antipsychotics), or antihistamines. However, as is frequent in the acutely agitated patient, IM formulations are often required
- Many physicians will consider the potential causes of acute agitation to tailor their medication choice. For instance, if you suspect that a patient is delirious or agitated from alcohol withdrawal, a benzodiazepine would be a wise choice. Another

example can be found in the agitation arising from psychostimulant use or overuse. As these drugs can have psychotomimetic properties, it is reasonable to consider an antipsychotic for acute treatment

- As with any treatment, the benefits must be weighed against the costs. IM formulations of antipsychotics can produce a very rapid D_2 receptor blockade, but in the antipsychotic-naïve patient or medication-sensitive patient, this can often lead to QT prolongation, acute dystonic reactions (e.g. laryngospasm, torticollis, rigidity), or even neuroleptic malignant syndrome. While there is no indication for prophylactic use of either benzodiazepines or antihistamines to treat acute dystonic reactions, there is often a helpful bonus of using these medications in combination with an antipsychotic. What is more, if a patient develops difficulty breathing following an IM formulation of an antipsychotic, an IM version of an antihistamine such as diphenhydramine (Benadryl) can potentially treat both conditions

- Long-standing aggression is a more challenging option. As with acute aggression, it is worth dedicating considerable time to identifying reversible causes of agitation as there are few FDA-approved treatments for aggression, let alone long-term treatments

Attending physician's mental notes: initial evaluation

- The patient was not able to engage in interview in any substantial way due to disorganization
- The patient made reference to both auditory and visual hallucinations, mostly relating to his family
- He was otherwise pleasant during interview
- The patient's complicated history with a panoply of potential etiologies will make a straightforward treatment strategy difficult
- He has likely already had numerous trials of medications if he has had psychotic symptoms since he was young and is now in a long-term care facility
- Outside-the-box thinking will be required to address his symptoms and will likely require off-label considerations

Medication history

- The patient has had past trials of haloperidol (Haldol), haloperidol decanoate (Haldol Decanoate), risperidone (Risperdal), olanzapine (Zyprexa), aripiprazole (Abilify), lithium, valproic acid (Depakote), amantadine (Gocovri), benztropine (Cogentin), diphenhydramine (Benadryl), clonazepam (Klonopin), lorazepam (Ativan), and sertraline (Zoloft) during previous admissions to long-term care

- The patient underwent 36 sessions of electroconvulsive therapy (ECT) in the hopes of mitigating his auditory hallucinations
- The patient's most recent regimen was:
  - Clozapine (Clozaril) 900 mg PO at bedtime, 50 mg in the morning
  - Haloperidol decanoate 300 mg IM twice per month
  - Lithium carbonate 1500 mg PO at bedtime
  - Lamotrigine (Lamictal) at 100 mg PO twice per day
  - Mirtazapine (Remeron) 7.5 mg in the evening
  - Lorazepam 0.5 mg four times per day

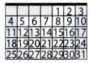

Case outcome: initial evaluation

- The patient's affect became brighter and his cognition improved following several rounds of ECT. However, his violent outbursts also increased dramatically
- He still demonstrated remarkable resistance to treatment and had consistent auditory and visual hallucinations, even while on two antipsychotics, a mood stabilizer, lithium, an atypical antidepressant, and a benzodiazepine
- He continued to experience command auditory hallucinations telling him that others wanted to fight him
- The patient continued to see visual hallucinations of people standing on his mother's head
- Violent outbursts and attacks (or attempted attacks) were still occurring most days of the week

Attending physician's mental notes: interim analysis

- What we know so far:
  - The patient has been experiencing auditory and visual hallucinations since his early teens
  - He has a history of polysubstance abuse beginning at an early age
  - He may have experienced multiple TBIs from fights during his adolescence
  - He may have a history of intellectual disability
- The patient's psychotic features have been resistant to multiple treatments including both first- and second-generation antipsychotics
- His violence seems to be related to the delusion that others want to fight him and the visual hallucination that someone is standing on his mother's head, prompting him to feel that he needs to defend her

- The antipsychotics used so far have provided some relief from auditory hallucinations but appear to have had no effect on the frequency or duration of his visual hallucinations and minimal effect on his disorganization

Questions

Which of the following pathways is most implicated in visual hallucinations?[3]

- Hyperactivity in dopaminergic neurons in the mesolimbic pathway
- Hypoactivity in dopaminergic neurons in the substantia nigra
- Hyperactivity of serotonergic neurons in the cerebral cortex
- Hypoactivity of glutamatergic neurons in the visual cortex

Which of the following is the mechanism of action of pimavanserin (Nuplazid)?

- Full antagonist at the D_2 receptor in the mesolimbic pathway
- Full antagonist at the 5-HT_{1A} receptor in the cerebral cortex
- Partial agonist at the D_2 receptor in the visual cortex
- Inverse agonist at the 5-HT_{2A} receptor in the cerebral cortex

Attending physician's mental notes (continued)

- The patient's violence and psychotic features are related to one another but have, so far, been resistant to combinatorial approaches and last-line-of-defense strategies
- A novel therapeutic intervention was required, and several factors were precluding the feasibility of psychotherapeutic interventions such as cognitive behavioral therapy or psychoanalysis: namely, the patient was too disorganized to participate in these modalities to great effect. Additionally, the patient's violence urged a more immediate response
- Pimavanserin (Nuplazid) carries an FDA indication only for psychosis in Parkinson's dementia. However, it has shown some efficacy as a potential augmentation strategy in schizophrenia[1]
- Pimavanserin was chosen for its properties as a 5-HT_{2A} receptor inverse agonist and antagonist, sparing any D_2 receptor interaction. Furthermore, pimavanserin is known to be effective in treating the psychosis associated with Parkinson's disease, which is characterized more by visual hallucinations than auditory hallucinations
- It is theorized that the pathophysiology for Parkinson's disease psychosis is related not only to the loss of dopaminergic neurons in the substantia nigra but also to the loss of serotonergic neurons in the dorsal striatum. This loss of serotonergic neurons results in

an upregulation of serotonin receptors on neurons in the cerebral cortex, particularly layer V pyramidal neurons in the visual cortex. Additionally, these highly sensitized serotonergic neurons project back to the mesolimbic dopamine tracts, increasing the risk for auditory hallucinations and delusions

- The theorized mechanism of action of pimavanserin involves addressing the upregulation of 5-HT$_{2A}$ receptors in the cerebral cortex by acting as an inverse agonist/antagonist at these receptors and reinstating a balance of serotonin receptors[2]
- As the patient's violent outbursts seem to be at least partially related to offensive visual perceptual disturbances, perhaps a reduction of these through this novel mechanism would provide relief
- Although an off-label use, prescribing pimavanserin in this instance may be justified, given the recalcitrant nature of this patient's psychosis

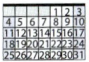

Case outcome: multiple interim follow-ups through month 3

- The patient was started on pimavanserin (Nuplazid) 34 mg per day with no additional changes to his medication regimen
- Over the course of several weeks, the patient was noted to have greater clarity of thought and to be more organized in conversation
- The patient reported that his visual hallucinations have all but disappeared
- Finally, the patient's violent outbursts were dramatically reduced such that he was only gesturing or engaging in violent behaviors on a scale of one to two times per week

Case debrief

- The patient had a convoluted psychiatric history complicated by substance abuse, suggested intellectual disability, and TBIs
- The patient repeatedly participated in violent behaviors that appeared to be linked to his psychotic phenomena
- He was resistant to many first-line treatments for psychosis and mood lability
- He underwent ECT to improve his energy and affect, but ultimately this had a paradoxical effect with regard to violence
- The patient ultimately responded positively to pimavanserin (Nuplazid), used off label to treat his visual hallucinations

Take-home points

- Some patients have extraordinarily complex etiologies to severe psychiatric illness that are often resistant to first-line treatments

- Violence is a difficult and multifactorial issue, particularly with patients in inpatient or custodial care facilities. A thorough investigation of reversible causes should be conducted to treat aggression
- Aggression associated with psychotic illness can be managed effectively through the use of antipsychotic medications, but resistant cases may require higher doses or combinatorial strategies
- Particularly resistant cases like this one may benefit from pharmacological options with an alternative mechanism of action, independent of dopamine blockade at mesolimbic dopamine neurons
- Pimavanserin (Nuplazid) acts as an inverse agonist/antagonist at the 5-HT_{2A} receptors located on glutamatergic neurons in the cortex. When these neurons are excessively stimulated, especially in the visual cortex, they can lead to visual hallucinations. Pimavanserin has the distinct advantage of counteracting this effect without manipulating dopamine receptors directly

Performance in practice: confessions of a psychopharmacologist

- Did we truly consider all possible causes of his psychotic symptoms?
  - The patient's visual hallucinations are atypical for standard schizophrenia and raise questions about psychosis secondary to another medical illness
  - Was the patient's history of potential head trauma from fighting thoroughly evaluated? The sequelae of TBIs are multifaceted and non-specific but may offer some more information about a patient's mood lability and psychotic features
  - Was this patient ever evaluated for more obscure causes of aggression such as a cryptic genetic illness that was not caught at a younger age or perhaps an early presentation of a dementia-related syndrome?
  - What imaging could have been done to offer a more up-close look at the patient's brain for clues?
  - Further work could have been done to contact family to garner collateral information about the patient's family and birth history
- ECT was a good idea for the patient's negative symptoms and it is somewhat unexpected that the patient became more disinhibited and violent as a result of this. This is an important consideration to keep in mind with ECT moving forward

Posttest self-assessment question and answer

Which of the following pharmacological treatments is not used in the management of acute aggression?

A. Haloperidol (Haldol) 2–10 mg IM or PO
B. Lorazepam (Ativan) 1–2 mg IM or PO
C. Olanzapine (Zyprexa) 5–10 mg IM or PO
D. Lithium 300–600 mg PO
E. Diphenhydramine (Benadryl) 25–50 mg IM or PO
F. Ketamine (Ketalar) 4–6 mg IM

Answer: D

Lithium does not have an IM formulation, making its use limited to voluntary administration. Moreover, lithium can take anywhere from 1 to 3 weeks to provide effective mood stabilization; acute agitation requires a medication that can reach effective doses in the bloodstream within 30 minutes to 1 hour. Finally, initiating lithium should be done after kidney and thyroid function have been evaluated and there is little time to do this in the setting of acute agitation.

References

1. Abbas A, Roth BL. Pimavanserin tartrate: a 5-HT2A inverse agonist with potential for treating various neuropsychiatric disorders. *Expert Opin Pharmacother* 2008; 9:3251–9. https://doi.org/10.1517/14656560802532707

2. Stahl SM. Mechanism of action of pimavanserin in Parkinson's disease psychosis: targeting serotonin 5HT2A and 5HT2 C receptors. *CNS Spectr* 2016; 21:271–5. https://doi.org/10.1017/S1092852916000407

3. Stahl, S. Beyond the dopamine hypothesis of schizophrenia to three neural networks of psychosis: Dopamine, serotonin, and glutamate. *CNS Spectr* 2018; 23:187–91. https://doi.org/10.1017/S1092852918001013

Case 7: The young woman with psychosis complicated by substance use and a history of traumatic brain injury

The Question: How do you determine whether psychosis is a primary or secondary illness?

The Psychopharmacological Dilemma: Does treatment depend upon whether psychosis is due to a primary psychiatric illness?

Harika Reddy, Austin Nguy, and Sana Johnson-Quijada

Pretest self-assessment question (answer at the end of the case)

Which of the following statements is false regarding diagnosing a patient with a primary psychiatric illness?

A. A thorough history must include medical and pertinent social history, especially focusing on childhood upbringing and interpersonal trauma

B. Basic laboratory tests including complete blood count (CBC), basic metabolic panel (BMP), and urine drug screen (UDS) must be ordered to rule out secondary causes of psychosis

C. If the patient has a previous psychiatric diagnosis, no further evaluation is necessary

D. A family history of psychiatric illness increases the probability of a primary psychiatric illness

Patient evaluation on intake

- A 20-year-old female presenting with symptoms of psychosis, admitted on an involuntary hold for psychiatric evaluation and treatment. The patient was exhibiting disorganized behavior, responding to internal stimuli, and disrobing in front of patients and staff

Psychiatric history

- Previous diagnoses: schizophrenia, schizoaffective disorder, bipolar disorder with psychosis, unspecified mood disorder, posttraumatic stress disorder, substance use disorder (including methamphetamine, marijuana, alcohol, and cocaine), and amphetamine-induced psychotic disorder
- Previous medication trials included several antidepressants, second-generation antipsychotics, mood stabilizers, prazosin (Minipress), and benzodiazepines
- The patient has utilized mental health and substance use services for 10 years

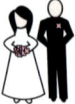

Social and personal history

- The patient suffered physical and emotional abuse in childhood
- She is a victim of sex trafficking
- She is homeless
- She has poor social support
- She is a high-school graduate
- She last worked briefly 3 years prior to admission
- She is supporting herself through supplemental security income

Medical history

- The patient has a history of traumatic brain injury (TBI) as teenager
- She has a congenital eye disorder

Family history

- The patient has a family history of substance use, primarily methamphetamine
- Both parents are homeless

Attending physician's mental notes: initial evaluation

- The patient exhibited little insight into her illness, denying any mental health history but endorsing marijuana, methamphetamine, and cocaine use. She was unable to engage in a meaningful interview due to psychosis
- Mental status examination: she was mildly unkempt, distracted, had irrelevant and tangential speech and grandiose delusions, appeared internally preoccupied, and denied suicidal/homicidal ideation

Questions

What is the differential diagnosis for psychosis?

- Primary psychiatric diagnosis (it is important to note that a primary psychiatric diagnosis is a diagnosis of exclusion)
  - Schizophrenia
  - Bipolar disorder: manic or depressed episode
  - Schizoaffective disorder
  - Severe depressive episode with psychotic features
  - Delusional disorder
  - Posttraumatic stress disorder
  - Obsessive–compulsive disorder
  - Schizotypal or paranoid personality disorder
  - Autism spectrum disorder
  - Attention-deficit/hyperactivity disorder
- Secondary to substance use

- Secondary to a medical condition
  - Delirium
    - Hypo/hyperglycemia
    - Hypoxia
    - Medication interactions or withdrawal
    - Sepsis
    - Serum electrolyte or metabolic abnormalities
    - Sleep deprivation
  - Chronic disturbance in mental condition
    - Autoimmune
    - Endocrine
    - Genetic
    - Neurological
    - Nutritional
    - Oncological
    - Pharmacological

Besides taking a detailed history, what diagnostic tools would be helpful?

- UDS
- CBC
- BMP
- Liver function tests
- Pregnancy test
- May consider calcium, thyroid hormones, and cortisol
- May consider electrophysiological and radiological imaging

Attending physician's mental notes: workup results

- The patient's UDS was positive for amphetamines
- A pregnancy test, urinalysis, hepatic panel, CBC, BMP, alcohol level, thyroid-stimulating hormone, rapid plasma reagin, lipid panel, and hemoglobin A1c (HbA1c) were unremarkable
- The patient was evaluated by an internist and an acute medical process was considered unlikely

Questions

What specific differential diagnosis should now be considered?

- Primary psychiatric illness
- Psychosis secondary to substance use given the patient's positive amphetamine result on UDS as well as a history of several other substances
- Psychosis secondary to TBI

What is the relationship between psychosis and TBI?

- Psychotic syndromes occur more frequently in individuals who have had a TBI than in the general population (Table 7.1). In a Danish study in 2013, individuals with TBI (including concussions) were four times more likely to develop a mental illness. People who had a TBI were 65% more likely to develop schizophrenia, 59% more likely to develop depression, and 28% more likely to develop bipolar disorder

Table 7.1 Risk factors for psychosis following TBI

Family history of psychosis

Genetic risk for schizophrenia

History of congenital neurological disorder

Pre-TBI history of neurodevelopmental and/or neuropsychiatric problem

TBI during adolescence

Involvement of temporal lobe pathology

Greater cognitive impairment

Greater severity of TBI

Psychoactive substances (e.g. amantadine)

Male gender

Sleep disturbance

Modified from van Reekum and van Reekum (2018).

Individuals with schizophrenia have a higher frequency of prior TBI than individuals with other psychiatric disorders

- Key brain regions include the dorsolateral prefrontal cortex, temporal lobe structures, basal ganglia, thalamus, and cingulate gyrus. These brain regions are commonly injured in patients with TBI, suggesting a possible mechanism underlying the observed link between TBI and psychosis
- The time to onset of psychosis following TBI has been found to vary, with typical onset within the first one or two years after the TBI

Further investigation

Is there anything else you would like to know about this patient?

- What about details regarding the TBI and onset of symptoms?
  - TBI
    - Head injury at age 14
    - Hit on left side of head while playing soccer
    - Vomited after injury and had symptoms of headache, sleepiness, dizziness, nausea, and slow speech
    - Neurological examination was unremarkable; she was transferred to hospital emergency room due to increasing headaches and nausea but it is unclear what occurred after

- ◦ She also documented a head injury at age 19 while under the influence of alcohol
- – Psychosis
  - ◦ She first began utilizing mental health services at age 13
  - ◦ At age 15, there was documented hospitalization for danger to self and she was prescribed a selective serotonin reuptake inhibitor (SSRI) and an antipsychotic at this time; she reported several recent hospitalizations but was unclear on the exact age of the first psychotic episode

Question

What risk factors for psychosis following TBI does this patient have?

- TBI during adolescence
- Pre-TBI history of neuropsychiatric symptoms as the patient was already utilizing medical health services prior to the TBI
- Symptoms of psychosis about 1–2 years after the documented TBI
- Use of psychoactive substances

Attending physician's mental notes: initial evaluation (continued)

- It is difficult to narrow down the differential diagnosis further in this patient as the TBI may have precipitated symptoms of psychosis, and substance use is confounding the picture
- Although the patient has had several psychotic episodes before, she has also had long-standing substance use; therefore substance-induced psychosis cannot be ruled out. However, substance use itself also plays a role in increasing the risk of a primary psychiatric illness

Question

This patient primarily was using cannabis and methamphetamine. What is the relationship between substance use and the risk of psychosis?

- Cannabis use in adolescence appears to confer a twofold risk for schizophrenia or schizophreniform disorder in adulthood
- Psychotic symptoms and syndromes are frequently experienced among individuals who use methamphetamine, with recent estimates of up to approximately 40% of users affected
- Distinguishing primary versus substance-induced psychotic disorders among methamphetamine users requires assessing the temporal relationship of symptoms with methamphetamine use, which at times can be difficult to discern

Attending physician's mental notes: initial evaluation (continued)

- Both TBI and substance abuse themselves can lead to psychotic symptoms but also increase the risk for primary psychotic disorders such as schizophrenia. What other risk factors for schizophrenia/primary psychotic disorder does this patient have?
  - She suffered childhood physical and emotional abuse, and was a victim of sex trafficking
- There have been several population-based studies that suggest childhood trauma as a risk factor for psychosis, appearing in adolescence or adulthood. These studies also suggest that early childhood interventions could help manage the potentially detrimental psychosocial outcome in adulthood. This is particularly the case for the long-term effects of adulthood psychosis and substance use abuse, driven by childhood sex abuse
- There are some promising treatments for childhood trauma that include cognitive behavioral therapy with a focus on trauma-informed practices, particularly diagnosing and treating posttraumatic stress disorder when comorbid with schizophrenia. These therapy techniques target and help to reduce tension, hostility, anger, and suspicion
- Although there is a high correlation between schizophrenia and childhood sex abuse, this may be related to the cluster of other risk factors including a family history of mental illness and social deprivation
  - Her socioeconomic status includes the stressor of homelessness
- According to one hypothesis for schizophrenia called the cumulative risk hypothesis, schizophrenia could be related to accumulated risk factors such as low socioeconomics and demographics. A large European meta-analysis study showed an inverse relationship between objective social status and subjective social status with DSM-4 diagnoses.[5,22] The accumulated risk factors of low socioeconomics can predispose people to diagnosable psychiatric disorders such as schizophrenia
- A lower socioeconomic status is associated with increased smoking of marijuana, especially in those with schizophrenia/schizoaffective disorder. One of the major reasons was using smoking as a way to relax and to cope with the stress and boredom of poverty
- She has a family history of substance use and homelessness
  - Studies have shown that the interaction of gene variants and the external environment predispose family members to similar substance abuse

- There is a higher incidence of psychiatric disorders, including substance abuse, among adolescents whose mother or both parents had a history of homelessness
- This patient's family may even have other unknown/undiagnosed psychiatric illnesses, in addition to substance use, leading to their homelessness. In previous assessments, at least 25% of homeless people had a serious mental illness and 45% had any mental illness

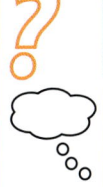

Question

What pharmacotherapy should be considered at this stage?

Attending physician's mental notes: treatment

- The patient seems to be in a psychotic episode and requires acute intervention including an antipsychotic and anxiolytic (e.g. low-dose antipsychotic, benzodiazepine, antihistamine) as needed to stabilize her symptoms. This medication regimen can be helpful for all three differential diagnoses with preference for an atypical antipsychotic for TBI and a favorable side-effect profile
- It is important to consider a patient's preference in selecting a medication to increase medication adherence
- **Hospital course:** the patient consented to aripiprazole (Abilify) and was titrated up to 20 mg daily; this was tolerated well with an improvement in symptoms

Questions

Why is aripiprazole (Abilify) a good choice for this patient?

- It is a second-generation antipsychotic with a more favorable side-effect profile
- It provides a long-acting injectable (LAI) option; it is important to consider adherence for this patient
- There are favorable studies for the use of aripiprazole for TBI. Relative to typical antipsychotic drugs, aripiprazole is a safer alternative for alleviating behavioral disturbances after experimental brain trauma as seen in adult male rats
  - Antipsychotic drugs exhibiting D_2 receptor antagonism impede cognitive recovery after an experimental TBI. A study with risperidone (Risperdal) and haloperidol (Haldol) showed impaired recovery compared to controls with effects lasting up to 3 months[18,24]
  - Aripiprazole is a 5-HT$_{1A}$ receptor agonist
    - 5-HT$_{1A}$ receptor agonists are thought to enhance cognition through enhancing pro-cognitive neurotransmitters including acetylcholine, norepinephrine, and dopamine

- Aripiprazole is a partial D_2 receptor agonist
  - The D_2 receptor agonist bromocriptine (Parlodel) promotes cognitive recovery and also reduces TBI-initiated malondialdehyde in multiple brain regions. Bromocriptine is thought to reduce haloperidol-induced neuronal toxicity by decreasing mitochondrial dysfunction and the production of hydroxyl free radicals. Oxidative stress is considered to be one of many pathophysiological effects induced by TBI that contributes to cognitive dysfunction

Now that the patient has improved, what should be considered?

- It is important to consider a medication that a patient will consent to and is likely to take in the long term. Considering this patient's history of non-compliance, an LAI should be considered

Attending physician's mental notes: treatment prior to discharge

- The patient was administered aripiprazole (Abilify) 882 mg LAI intramuscular (IM) prior to discharge with aripiprazole 21-day PO overlap
- Required doses of risperidone (Risperdal) and hydroxyzine (Vistaril) were prescribed as needed for anxiety/agitation; she also required emergency IM haloperidol-lorazepam-diphenhydramine due to agitated behavior
- At the time of discharge, the patient continued to exhibit some delusions with disorganized thought processes. However, this was attenuated compared with admission and the patient was able to hold a meaningful conversation with the treatment team with decreased paranoia

Case outcome: re-hospitalization: 2 weeks later

- The patient was again admitted on an involuntary hold for attempting to enter other residences and making delusional statements

Question

What factors could have led to re-exacerbation of symptoms?

- Non-compliance of aripiprazole (Abilify) overlap
- Inadequate medication therapy
- Substance use
- Environmental factors such as poor social support or stressors

Case outcome: attending physician's evaluation and treatment on readmission

- The patient had stopped taking aripiprazole (Abilify) PO overlap
- The patient denied recent substance use but refused a UDS, so the role of substance use could not be ruled out in the current presentation
- The patient was restarted on aripiprazole PO overlap for a few days and was given a second dose of aripiprazole LAI when due. As the symptoms of agitation were not adequately controlled requiring IM injections, aripiprazole was increased to 30 mg PO per day

Question

At this point, although the patient's psychosis was better controlled, her mood lability was not adequately controlled. What pharmacotherapy could be considered in adjunct with the current atypical antipsychotic?

- A mood stabilizer would be a reasonable choice

- Valproic acid (Depakote) has been used off label for the management of positive findings of schizophrenia such as impulsivity, agitation, and aggression. A multicenter study showed that treatment with valproic acid in combination with an atypical antipsychotic agent resulted in earlier improvements in a range of psychotic symptoms among acutely hospitalized patients with schizophrenia
  - Valproic acid is typically indicated for bipolar disorder with an unclear mechanism of action. It is known to block voltage-sensitive sodium channels and increase brain concentrations of γ-aminobutyric acid
  - In rat models, administration of chronic valproic acid showed a reduction in protein kinase C (closely associated with bipolar disorder) in the frontal cortex and hippocampus with modulated expression of genes including Bcl-2 (cytoprotective), which may suggest a long-term mood stabilizer use with valproic acid
- There have been some case reports and open-label trials that also include valproic acid in the maintenance of aggression and impulsivity in patients with brain injuries, dementia, and borderline personality disorder
  - Recent mice models have shown promising use of valproic acid as a next-generation tool for TBI. Valproic acid was shown to have an epigenetic modulation ability as a general histone deacetylase inhibitor, which can be used to fight against epigenetic changes following TBI. Mice models showed reduced inflammation and blood–brain barrier dysfunction, attenuated platelet dysfunction, and improved neurological recovery

Attending physician's mental notes: treatment prior to discharge (continued)

- The patient was started on valproic acid (Depakote) 500 mg PO twice per day, which was tolerated well with some improvement in mood lability by discharge
- The patient's aripiprazole (Abilify) PO overlap was discontinued

Case outcome: after discharge

- The patient was out of the hospital for longer this time but was again admitted to the same hospital 3 months later with similar symptoms of paranoia, responding to internal stimuli, and disorganized behavior
- The patient did admit marijuana use at this time, but a UDS was unable to be completed
- The patient was non-compliant with medications and was started on olanzapine (Zyprexa) by a different treatment team prior to discharge

Question

What would you do now?

- Increase the patient's access to mental health services
- Investigate any possible alterations to the patient's living environment
- Refer the patient to therapy
- Continue to consider a second-generation antipsychotic with a mood stabilizer that is effective for the patient with the above points addressed

Case debrief

- This case appears to be a primary psychotic disorder, with several prominent secondary risk factors, notably early-life adversity, mild TBI, and substance abuse
- Many patients with symptoms of psychosis require multiple levels of treatment including psychopharmacology, therapy, and environmental modifications
- Medication adherence is a significant problem in this patient population, given that this patient is of poor socioeconomic status, has poor social support, and is exposed to substance use in her environment. An LAI may be helpful in this situation in reducing hospitalizations but may not be sustainable without further modifications. In this case, the patient was able to be out of hospital for 3 months, which is an improvement from the consecutive

admissions within 2 weeks. Any environmental modifications and increasing access to mental health services by regular follow-up and appointment transportation could be very useful
- This patient has had a lot of trauma in her childhood and adolescence. Therapy should be a strong consideration but may not be feasible for the patient to engage in and follow up with. As such, the patient would benefit from intensive support services
- The patient's significant genetic load and TBI history predisposing to psychosis makes her symptoms more complicated to treat
- Hopefully, the patient can avoid substance abuse while taking antipsychotic medications, as the duration of untreated psychosis can be related to poor outcome
- Over time, psychosis with substance abuse and medication non-compliance is a formula for getting involved in the criminal justice system, and all attempts should be made to try to avoid this outcome

Take-home points
- A primary psychiatric diagnosis is a diagnosis of exclusion
- Substance-induced psychosis and a primary psychiatric diagnosis can be difficult to differentiate, but it is important to consider any temporal relationship of symptoms if known
- A previous history of TBI may predispose the patient to psychosis
- Second-generation antipsychotics, in this case aripiprazole (Abilify), have been shown to be useful for psychosis associated with TBI
- A mood stabilizer may be considered as an adjunct with an antipsychotic when symptoms are not adequately controlled, particularly when symptoms of mood lability are present. Valproic acid (Depakote) would be a reasonable choice
- In addition to adjusting a patient's medication regimen, it is important to take a detailed history to identify other barriers to a successful outcome

Performance in practice: confessions of a psychopharmacologist
What could have been done better here?
- Should aripiprazole lauroxil (Aristada) as an LAI have been considered to eliminate the need for a 21-day overlap?
- Should environmental modifications have been considered more seriously during the first two hospitalizations?
- Should a mood stabilizer or alternative augmentation strategies have been considered earlier?

What are possible action items for improvement in practice?
- Make sure to do a thorough psychiatric, medical, and social history with every patient, as some of the non-psychiatric factors might have been able to be better addressed earlier in treatment
- Consider psychotherapy for a patient with a significant trauma history and environmental stressors
- Consider treatment augmentation early if a patient only partially responds to treatment
- Consider a long-term care facility for this patient if environmental modifications are not able to be made and the patient continues to have repeated hospitalizations

Tips and pearls

- In a patient transitioning to aripiprazole (Abilify) LAI from aripiprazole PO with concern for non-compliance, aripiprazole lauroxil (Aristada) should be considered as only one dose PO is required
- If the patient does get restarted on valproic acid (Depakote) in the future, it would be important to monitor liver function tests and platelet counts regularly during the first few months of treatment and annually thereafter

Posttest self-assessment question and answer

Which of the following statements is false regarding diagnosing a patient with a primary psychiatric illness?

A. A thorough history must include medical and pertinent social history, especially focusing on childhood upbringing and interpersonal trauma
B. Basic laboratory tests including CBC, BMP, and UDS must be ordered to rule out secondary causes of psychosis
C. If the patient has a previous psychiatric diagnosis, no further evaluation is necessary
D. A family history of psychiatric illness increases the probability of a primary psychiatric illness

Answer: C

References

1. Byrne P. Managing the acute psychotic episode. *BMJ* 2007; 334:686–92. https://doi.org/10.1136/bmj.39148.668160.80
2. Casey DE, Daniel DG, Wassef AA, et al. Effect of divalproex combined with olanzapine or risperidone in patients with an acute exacerbation of schizophrenia. *Neuropsychopharmacology* 2003; 28:182–92. https://doi.org/10.1038/sj.npp.1300023

3. Dekker SE, Nikolian VC, Sillesen M, et al. Different resuscitation strategies and novel pharmacologic treatment with valproic acid in traumatic brain injury. *J Neurosci Res* 2017; 96: 711–19. https://doi.org/10.1002/jnr.24125

4. Friedman T, Tin NN. Childhood sexual abuse and the development of schizophrenia. *Postgrad Med J* 2007; 83: 507–8. https://doi.org/10.1136/pgmj.2006.054577

5. Fryers T, Melzer D, Jenkins R, Brugha T. The distribution of the common mental disorders: social inequalities in Europe. *Clin Pract Epidemiol Ment Health* 2005; 1: 14. https://doi.org/10.1186/1745-0179-1-14

6. Glasner-Edwards, S, Mooney LJ. Methamphetamine psychosis: epidemiology and management. *CNS Drugs* 2014; 28:1115–26. https://doi.org/10.1007/s40263-014-0209-8

7. Griswold K, Regno P, Berger R. Recognition and differential diagnosis of psychosis in primary care. *Am Fam Physician* 2015; 91:856–63.

8. Grunze H, Schlösser S, Amann B, Walden J. Anticonvulsant drugs in bipolar disorder. *Dialogues Clin Neurosci* 1999; 1:24–40. https://doi.org/10.31887/DCNS.1999.1.1/hgrunze

9. Hailes HP, Yu R, Danese A, Fazel, S. Long-term outcomes of childhood sexual abuse: an umbrella review. *Lancet Psychiatry* 2019, 6: 830–9. https://doi.org/10.1016/s2215-0366(19)30286-x

10. Henry M, Shivji A, de Sousa T, Cohen R. *The 2015 Annual Homeless Assessment Report (AHAR) to Congress*. 2015. Available from: https://files.hudexchange.info/resources/documents/2015-AHAR-Part-1.pdf

11. Manji HK, Moore GJ, Chen G. Bipolar disorder: leads from the molecular and cellular mechanisms of action of mood stabilisers. *Br J Psychiatry* 2001; 178:s107-19. https://doi.org/10.1192/bjp.178.41.s107

12. McAllister TW. Psychiatric disorders and traumatic brain injury: what is the connection? *Psychiatr Ann* 2010; 40: 533–9. https://doi.org/10.3928/00485713-20101018-04

13. McAllister TW, Ferrell RB. Evaluation and treatment of psychosis after traumatic brain injury. *NeuroRehabilitation* 2002; 17:357–68. https://doi.org/10.3233/nre-2002-17409

14. Meyers JL, Dick DM. Genetic and environmental risk factors for adolescent-onset substance use disorders. *Child Adolesc Psychiatr Clin N Am* 2010; 19:465–77. https://doi.org/10.1016/j.chc.2010.03.013

15. Nilsson SF, Laursen TM, Hjorthøj C, et al. Risk of psychiatric disorders in offspring of parents with a history of homelessness during childhood and adolescence in Denmark: a nationwide, register-based, cohort study. *Lancet Public Health* 2017; 2:E541–50. https://doi.org/10.1016/s2468-2667(17)30210-4

16. Orlovska S, Pedersen MS, Benros ME, et al. Head injury as risk factor for psychiatric disorders: a nationwide register-based follow-up study of 113,906 persons with head injury. *Am J Psychiatry* 2014; 171:463–9. https://doi.org/10.1176/appi.ajp.2013.13020190

17. Peckham E, Bradshaw TJ, Brabyn S, et al. Exploring why people with SMI smoke and why they may want to quit: baseline data from the SCIMITAR RCT. *J Psychiatr Ment Health Nurs* 2015; 23: 282–9. https://doi.org/10.1111/jpm.12241

18. Phelps TI, Bondi CO, Mattiola VV, Kline AE. Relative to typical antipsychotic drugs, aripiprazole is a safer alternative for alleviating behavioral disturbances after experimental brain trauma. *Neurorehabil Neural Repair* 2016; 31: 25–33. https://doi.org/10.1177/1545968316650281

19. Rosenberg G. (2007). The mechanisms of action of valproate in neuropsychiatric disorders: can we see the forest for the trees? *Cell Mol Life Sci* 64: 2090–103. https://doi.org/10.1007/s00018-007-7079-x

20. Schäfer I, Fisher HL (2011). Childhood trauma and psychosis – what is the evidence? *Dialogues Clin Neurosci* 13:360–5. https://doi.org/10.31887/DCNS.2011.13.2/ischaefer

21. Schatzberg, AF, Nemeroff, CB, eds. *Essentials of Clinical Psychopharmacology*. Washington, DC: American Psychiatric Publishing,2013.

22. Scott KM, Al-Hamzawi AO, Andrade LH, et al. Associations between subjective social status and DSM-IV mental disorders. *JAMA Psychiatry* 2014; 71:1400–8. https://doi.org/10.1001/jamapsychiatry.2014.1337

23. Trappler B, Newville H. Trauma healing via cognitive behavior therapy in chronically hospitalized patients. *Psychiatr Q* 2007; 78:317–25. https://doi.org/10.1007/s11126-007-9049-8

24. Umene-Nakano W, Yoshimura R, Okamot, T, et al. Aripiprazole improves various cognitive and behavioral impairments after traumatic brain injury: a case report. *Gen Hosp Psychiatry* 2013: 35; 103. https://doi.org/10.1016/j.genhosppsych.2012.05.002

25. van Reekum R, van Reekum E. Traumatic brain injury and psychosis: clinical considerations. *Psychiatr Times* 2018; 35. Available from https://www.psychiatrictimes.com/view/traumatic-brain-injury-and-psychosis-clinical-considerations (accessed March 26, 2021).

26. Winklbaur B, Ebner N, Sachs G, et al (2006). Substance abuse in patients with schizophrenia. *Dialogues Clin Neurosci* 8:37–43. https://doi.org/10.31887/DCNS.2006.8.1/bwinklbaur

Case 8: The woman with worsening psychosis and a mysterious rash

The Question: What do you do when a psychiatric patient on steroids develops psychosis?

The Psychopharmacological Dilemma: How to address steroid-induced psychiatric disorders

Sireena Sy, Yatna Patel, and Alexander Thanh Nguyen

Pretest self-assessment question (answer at the end of the case)

Which psychiatric adverse effects are most associated with short-term steroid use?

A. Agitation and psychosis
B. Depressive symptoms
C. Euphoria and hypomania
D. Disturbances of cognition

Patient evaluation on intake

- A 52-year-old woman with a history of schizophrenia with the chief complaint of worsening paranoia and delusions for 1 week

Psychiatric history

- The patient has a chronic history of schizophrenia and has been in and out of inpatient hospitals since she was in her 20s
- She is currently on a mental health conservatorship and is living in an institution for mental diseases (IMD)
- She was brought in from her IMD for complaints of increasing restlessness, agitation, and threatening IMD staff for the past week
- She originally presented in the psychiatric emergency room with rambling/pressured speech, paranoia, restlessness, and delusions about being pregnant and that staff wanted to harm her baby and poison her food
- On presentation, she required constant redirection and reorientation secondary to disorganized thought processes
- She was observed sleeping 5–7 hours per night while admitted in the inpatient facility
- There was a reported history of an extremely itchy rash on her torso for the past year that had worsened over the past month, so the patient was recently prescribed oral prednisone 40 mg 3 days prior to admission

- Prednisone was discontinued upon admission. The rash was alleviated to a small degree by diphenhydramine (Benadryl) 25 mg PO twice per day as needed and hydrocortisone cream as needed
- After evaluation by the internal medicine team, the itching was suspected to be scabies and was treated with ivermectin PO and permethrin cream
- The patient showed significant improvement of psychiatric symptoms after 7 days

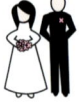

Social and personal history

- The patient had been living at an IMD for the past year after being placed back on Lanterman–Petris–Short (LPS) conservatorship
- She has a history of decompensating when not on mental health conservatorship
- The patient has a sister, but she is not really involved in or aware of the patient's current medical and psychiatric care
- Due to her mental illness, the patient has not been able to independently care for herself since her 30s

Medical history

- Chronic obstructive pulmonary disease, controlled
- Diabetes mellitus, controlled
- Gastroesophageal reflux disease
- Gout
- Overactive bladder
- Chronic constipation
- Vitamin D deficiency

Current medications

- Clozapine (Clozaril) 100 mg PO twice per day
- Aripiprazole (Abilify) 882 mg long-acting injectable every 4 weeks, last administered 2 weeks prior to admission
- Trazodone (Desyrel) 150 mg PO at bedtime
- Paliperidone (Invega) 6 mg PO once per day
- Gabapentin (Neurontin) 600 mg PO three times per day
- Oxybutynin (Ditropan) 5 mg PO four times per day
- Allopurinol (Zyloprim) 100 mg PO once per day
- Vitamin D 2000 units PO once per day
- Metformin (Glucophage) 500 mg PO twice per day
- Senna 8.6 mg PO at bedtime as needed
- Pantoprazole (Protonix) 40 mg PO every morning
- Prednisone 40 mg PO once per day

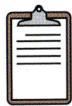

Patient evaluation on intake

- Mental status examination: agitated, uncooperative, labile affect, disorganized and tangential thought processes, paranoid delusions including pseudocyesis
- Vital signs: blood pressure 140/80 mmHg, heart rate 95 bpm, respiration rate 18 breaths/min, O_2 saturation 98% on room air

Attending physician's mental notes: initial evaluation

- There are concerns for polypharmacy with multiple antipsychotics on board, especially with a partial D_2 receptor agonist-antagonist such as aripiprazole (Abilify), which is often associated with akathisia
- Multiple antipsychotics also increase the risk of akathisia, potentially contributing to the patient's initial restlessness and agitation on presentation
- There must also be an assessment for underlying delirium, given the constant need for the patient to be reoriented. It would be important to also rule out any underlying drug/stimulant use that may worsen psychosis
- Steroid-induced psychosis must be considered, as the timing of the steroid treatment for the patient's rash coincides with worsening of the patient's psychotic symptoms

Steroid-induced psychosis versus exacerbation of organic psychosis

- DSM-5 criteria consider steroid-induced psychosis a diagnosis of exclusion, and here the possibility is more of steroid-induced exacerbation of psychosis
- The patient's presenting symptoms and medical history should be carefully reviewed, as psychosis could also be caused by other medical conditions such as:
  - Nervous system conditions (cerebrovascular disease, neoplasms, multiple sclerosis, Alzheimer's disease, Parkinson's disease, Huntington's disease, tertiary syphilis, epilepsy, encephalitis, prion disease, neurosarcoidosis)
  - Endocrine conditions (Cushing's disease, Addison's disease, hyper/hypothyroidism, hyper/hypocalcemia, hypopituitarism)
  - Other conditions (systemic lupus erythematosus and porphyria)
- The diagnosis of steroid-induced psychosis can be made if episodes of psychosis coincide with steroid use and the symptoms cannot be explained by other medical conditions or the use of substances known to induce psychosis[5]
- In most steroid-induced psychosis cases, symptoms tend to occur earlier in the therapeutic course, with the time of onset being

within 1–2 weeks of steroid initiation. Here, our patient's onset of symptoms fits that time frame, and certain laboratory tests could have been ordered to rule out other conditions, such as an autoimmune panel[7]

- Treatment of steroid-induced psychosis involves discontinuation of the offending steroid and supportive therapy. Treatment can also include antipsychotics and other psychotropics, similar to treatment of breakthrough psychosis in a patient with an underlying schizophrenia spectrum disorder. Thus, it can be difficult to distinguish between the two etiologies

Anticholinergic burden

- In looking at the patient's list of medications, oxybutynin (Ditropan) is an anticholinergic medication that exerts antispasmodic effects on smooth muscle, namely, to decrease urinary frequency and urgency for the patient's overactive bladder. This is concerning for the anticholinergic effects of both oxybutynin and concurrent clozapine (Clozaril) treatment, which is also highly anticholinergic, in a patient who presents as disorganized and confused[4]
- As patients age, they are more susceptible to the anticholinergic effects of medications. Special care must be taken in our patient who is now in her fifth decade of life

Delirium

- One can look toward assessing delirium by assessing the patient longitudinally from time of presentation to the subsequent days, focusing particularly on the patient's attention through the Montreal Cognitive Assessment (MoCA) or mini-mental state examination (MMSE) to assess whether their attention was waxing/waning or intact, while ruling out underlying medical causes
- In this patient's case, her confusion and psychosis improved gradually over time and did not have the intermittent episodes of lucidity associated with delirium

Case outcome

- Clozapine (Clozaril) titrated up to 200 mg PO twice per day
- Paliperidone (Invega) discontinued by discharge
- Gabapentin (Neurontin) titrated down to 600 mg PO twice per day in the setting of acute kidney injury

Further investigation

What were the relevant laboratory tests results?

- Complete blood count: significant for mild eosinophilia
- Basic metabolic panel: signs of renal insufficiency were creatinine 1.30 mg/dl, blood urea nitrogen 12 mg/dl, glomerular filtration rate 43 ml/min/1.73 m^2. Most likely secondary to acute kidney injury on chronic kidney disease when compared with the patient's baseline
- Liver function tests: alanine transaminase 50 U/l, aspartate aminotransferase 43 U/l
  - Consider hepatic encephalopathy as a differential diagnosis of acute encephalopathic states; however, this patient's liver function was normal
- Thyroid-stimulating hormone: within normal limits
  - Hyperthyroidism could have been a contributing factor to the patient's acute restlessness and agitation, but her thyroid function was normal
- Clozapine (Clozaril) level: 250 ng/ml
  - This patient was being undertreated with the original clozapine dose. A clozapine, or norclozapine, level is often helpful to assess the medication's efficacy.[2,6] However, the level should not be the only guideline used when treating a patient with clozapine. Be cognizant of clinical efficacy
- Rapid plasma reagin: non-reactive
  - Neurosyphilis can contribute to a presentation of confusion and psychosis
- Human immunodeficiency virus (HIV) antibodies: negative
  - HIV psychosis is a differential diagnosis
- Urinalysis: negative
  - As patients age, urinary tract infections can cause acute delirium
- Urine drug screen: negative
  - Substance use should always be on the differential diagnosis for presentations of acute psychosis

Attending physician's mental notes: follow-up encounter

- As prednisone is metabolized by the liver, it is important to consider any underlying liver disease that may impact the level of corticosteroids in the body. This patient had normal liver function upon presentation
- Evaluating the route of administration would also be helpful as certain steroids received through intravenous (IV) or intramuscular

(IM) injection avoid the first-pass metabolism effects of the liver, as opposed to orally taken steroids

- Orally taken steroids could have lower bioavailability if the liver modifies them into their chemically inactive form. For a similarly administered dose, IV and IM steroids could have higher bioavailability, as these routes avoid the initial modifications through the liver
- Studies have shown that even though dosage is the most important risk factor for corticosteroid-induced adverse psychiatric outcomes, it does not help predict the severity or the duration of the symptoms in patients[3]
- One way to evaluate the risk is to look at the daily dosage of corticosteroids that the patient is receiving. A study carried out by The Boston Collaborative Drug Surveillance Program on patients receiving prednisone therapy showed that patients receiving less than 40 mg per day were at minimal risk for psychiatric disturbances. However, patients receiving 40–80 mg per day of prednisone were at moderate risk, while patients receiving more than 80 mg per day were at high risk[1]
- As different corticosteroids have varying degrees of activity, glucocorticoid-equivalent doses should be considered to evaluate the risk of psychiatric disturbances. Our patient was receiving 40 mg per day of prednisone at the time of the admission, which would put her at a moderate risk. If she was receiving a different steroid medication, prednisone-equivalent doses would have been needed to calculate the risk (Table 8.1)
- For management of acute cases, recommendations are to reduce the corticosteroid dose to as low as can be tolerated by the patient, while still treating the underlying health concern.[7] As our patient was taking prednisone for a suspected scabies rash, it can be completely discontinued as the rash could be managed by ivermectin and permethrin

Table 8.1 Equivalent doses of steroids

Corticosteroid	Glucocorticoid activity	Equivalent dose (mg)	Half-life (h)
Cortisol (hydrocortisone)	1	160	8–12
Cortisone	0.8	200	8–12
Prednisone	**4**	**40**	**18–36**
Prednisolone	4	40	18–36
Methylprednisolone	5	32	18–36
Dexamethasone	25	6.4	36–54

Modified from Warrington & Bostwick (2006).

- If steroids are abruptly withdrawn, patients may experience steroid withdrawal symptoms, such as weakness, fatigue, decreased appetite, weight loss, nausea, vomiting, diarrhea, or abdominal pain. The occurrence of withdrawal symptoms is dependent on the steroid duration and dose of treatment, with higher doses for longer periods of time making patients more susceptible to withdrawal symptoms. In this case, our patient was on prednisone for less than 1 week at a moderate dose of 40 mg per day (Table 8.1). It was considered relatively safe to discontinue immediately

Case outcome (continued)

- With the discontinuation of the oral steroid, the patient's aggression and paranoia gradually improved
- She remained with her baseline chronic delusions but no longer met the criteria for inpatient hospitalization
- This improvement could also be attributed to uptitration of her clozapine (Clozaril) and a careful medication reconciliation leading to reduced polypharmacy
- The patient's mysterious rash was correctly diagnosed as scabies and significantly improved with ivermectin PO and permethrin cream
- The patient was stable enough to be discharged back to her previous IMD

Case debrief

- A 52-year-old woman with a history of schizophrenia presents for worsening agitation and paranoid delusions for the past week in the setting of starting oral prednisone 3 days earlier for a skin rash
- During admission, prednisone was immediately discontinued, the clozapine (Clozaril) dose was increased, and oral paliperidone (Invega) was discontinued
- The patient's psychotic symptoms gradually improved after cessation of the oral steroid
- She eventually returned to her psychiatric baseline and was stable for discharge
- There were several medication-related management issues that could have been improved prior to admission:
  - Avoiding use of steroids, especially for the wrong dermatological indication
  - Avoiding polypharmacy with three antipsychotics, with underdosing of clozapine and use of two other antipsychotics, one which has sufficiently high D_2 receptor-binding affinity (i.e.

aripiprazole (Abilify)) to essentially block the D_2 receptor binding of the other (i.e. paliperidone), with resultant side effects but no additive therapeutic effects

- Avoiding anticholinergics (oxybutynin (Ditropan)) with clozapine, as this can not only exacerbate psychosis and cause delirium and confusion but also cause potentially life-threatening paralytic ileus
- Discontinuing the steroid first rather than concurrently with the increase in clozapine. The patient might have stabilized off the steroid alone and could have been maintained on a lower clozapine dose (the goal is always to use the lowest effective dose). Even though the clozapine level was low, if the patient was stable prior to prednisone then that would be acceptable, as we treat to clinical efficacy and not to the laboratory value

Take-home points

- Consider the initiation of steroids as the potential cause for worsening of psychiatric symptoms, although it is a diagnosis of exclusion (Figure 8.1)

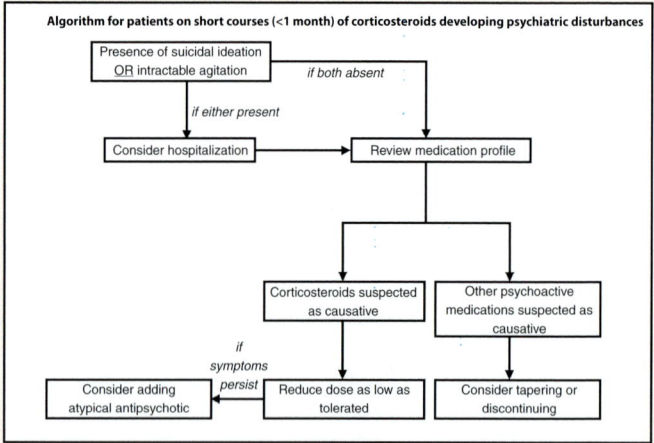

Figure 8.1. Algorithm for treating patients with psychiatric disturbances as a result of short-term corticosteroid use. Modified from Warrington and Bostwick (2006).

- The higher the dose of steroids, the more likely side effects are to occur. Similarly, the longer the duration of treatment, the more likely side effects are to occur[5,7]
- Immediately taper patients off steroids if there is a suspicion of steroid-induced psychosis. Avoid abrupt discontinuation,

if possible, to prevent steroid withdrawal syndrome. Steroid withdrawal syndrome includes symptoms of fatigue, generalized weakness, myalgias, nausea, anorexia, and lightheadedness
- Treatment is typically supportive, but can also include antipsychotics and other psychotropics to manage the agitation, psychosis, depression, hypomania, or disturbances of cognition associated with steroid use
- Polypharmacy is a common issue that providers face daily. When possible, review and consolidate the number of medications that a patient is prescribed and maximize the dose of current medications (i.e. antipsychotics) before adding another medication of the same class
- Be wary of anticholinergics, such as oxybutynin (Ditropan), contributing to a delirium component

Posttest self-assessment question and answer

Which psychiatric adverse effects are most associated with short-term steroid use?

A. Agitation and psychosis
B. Depressive symptoms
C. Euphoria and hypomania
D. Disturbances of cognition

Answer: C

Euphoria and hypomania are the most common psychiatric adverse effects associated with short-term steroid use. Agitation and psychosis are the most easily recognized adverse side effects, despite not being the most common in occurrence.[7] They are what often bring patients to clinical attention. Depressive symptoms are more common with long-term steroid use, specifically, and they may be harder to diagnose. Disturbances in cognition do occur and must be differentiated from frank delirium, which steroids can also induce. However, this does not occur as frequently as symptoms of euphoria and hypomania.

References

1. Boston Collaborative Drug Surveillance Program. Drug-induced convulsions: report from Boston Collaborative Drug Surveillance Program. *Lancet* 1972; 300:677–9. https://doi.org/10.1016/S0140-6736(72)92087-9
2. Ellison JC, Dufresne RL. A review of the clinical utility of serum clozapine and norclozapine levels. *Ment Health Clin* 2015; 5:68–73. https://doi.org/10.9740/mhc.2015.03.068

3. Gagliardi BJP, Muzyk AJ, Holt S. When steroids cause psychosis psychiatric symptoms associated with corticosteroids. *Rheumatologist* October 2010. Available from: https://www.the-rheumatologist.org/article/when-steroids-cause-psychosis/(accessed March 26, 2021).
4. Gulsun M, Pinar M, Sabanci U. Psychotic disorder induced by oxybutynin: presentation of two cases. *Clin Drug Investig* 2006; 25:603–6. https://doi.org/10.2165/00044011-200626100-00007
5. Janes M, Kuster S, Goldson TM, Forjuoh SN (2019). Steroid-induced psychosis. *Proc Bayl Univ Med Cent* 32:614–15. https://doi.org/10.1080/08998280.2019.1629223
6. Meyer JM. *Stahl's Handbooks: The Clozapine Handbook.* Cambridge, UK: Cambridge University Press, 2020.
7. Warrington TP, Bostwick JM. Psychiatric adverse effects of corticosteroids. *Mayo Clinic Proc* 2006; 81:1361–7. https://doi.org/10.4065/81.10.1361

Case 9: The man without a plan

The Question: How to diagnose and treat a patient with a coexisting attention-deficit/hyperactivity disorder (ADHD) and mood symptoms?

The Psychopharmacological Dilemma: Finding an effective medication regimen for a patient previously diagnosed with ADHD and major depressive disorder failing selective serotonin reuptake inhibitors

Alfonso Vera and Gerald Maguire

Pretest self-assessment question (answer at the end of the case)

Which of the following are evidence-based treatments of attention-deficit/hyperactivity disorder (ADHD) in adults?

A. Methylphenidate (Concerta) or amphetamine
B. Atomoxetine (Strattera)
C. Guanfacine (Tenex)
D. Clonidine (Catapres)
E. All of the above

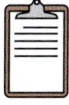

Patient evaluation on intake

- A 64-year-old male presenting with a previous diagnosis of ADHD complaining of "inability to focus and low motivation". He notes stress over his decreased amount of work as a freelance writer
- At the initial consultation, the patient also complained of depressed mood, anhedonia, decreased energy, and decreased concentration. He has a history of poor sleep but this is currently being treated with trazodone (Desyrel)
- The patient notes a good appetite and denies suicidal/ homicidal ideation
- The patient seeks care with this new provider, as he recently moved to the area to live with his father

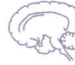

Psychiatric history

- The patient has a childhood diagnosis of ADHD with varied courses of treatment including stimulants and a diagnosis of major depressive disorder (MDD) as an adult with the first episode in his early 30s
- The patient reports failed courses of numerous antidepressant medications including fluoxetine (Prozac), sertraline (Zoloft), and venlafaxine (Effexor). The patient reports lack of efficacy but also experienced sexual dysfunction with each agent
- The patient has no history of psychiatric hospitalizations
- The patient denies a history of hypomanic or manic symptoms

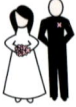

Social and personal history

- The patient is an articulate man who has obtained two graduate-level degrees from prestigious universities
- He is divorced with two children
- He reports that he and his wife divorced due to amicable differences
- He denies any use of alcohol and/or illicit drugs

Medical history

- ADHD
- Diagnosis of MDD
- Hypertension, controlled with diet and exercise
- No surgical history

Family history

- The patient denies any family history of psychiatric diagnoses, but states that he is not close to many of his family members

Current medications

- Trazodone (Desyrel) 100 mg every evening
- Lisdexamfetamine (Vyvanse) 20 mg every morning
- These medications were prescribed by his previous psychiatrist and he presents currently taking these medications

Questions

Based on the patient's presentation and current symptoms, would you consider changing the medication management?

- Yes
- No

If yes, what would you add or discontinue?

- Discontinue trazodone (Desyrel) and add atomoxetine (Strattera)
- Discontinue trazodone and add vortioxetine (Trintellix)
- Increase the dosages of all medications
- Add vortioxetine
- Other

Attending physician's mental notes: initial evaluation

- Given the patient's persistent mood symptoms, poor concentration, failure of numerous antidepressants, and history of antidepressant-induced sexual dysfunction, vortioxetine (Trintellix) at 10 mg/day is started to treat his recurrent MDD

- The recommendation is to treat the patient by manipulating one variable at a time to understand the effects of the added medication
- Therefore, vortioxetine was added and lisdexamfetamine (Vyvanse) and trazodone (Desyrel) continued at the same dosage

Further investigation

Is there anything else you would like to know about this patient?

- Family history
  - The patient gave permission to contact his father who has more knowledge of his family history
- The patient conveys anxiety and worry, stating that this is related to his financial challenges
- He denies sleepless nights, spending sprees, pressured speech, and grandiosity in the past
- He denies adverse reactions to lisdexamfetamine (Vyvanse) and trazodone (Desyrel)
- The patient relates that he did not take the antidepressant medications previously prescribed for long due to their lack of efficacy and the emergence of sexual dysfunction
- The patient feels worthless because he is not working

Case outcome: first interim follow-up at week 2

- The patient follows up with new complaints of increased energy and worsening anxiety
- He now reports restless sleep and the trazodone (Desyrel) is no longer working with sleep-onset insomnia where he sleeps for fewer than 2 hours a night
- The patient relates that he has more energy but feels he cannot relax. He still relates feeling depressed with poor concentration and an inability to focus and start tasks such as his writing
- The patient relates that his diminished interests and pleasure continue. He has no motivation to exercise and relates he is not eating healthily. He is not interacting with his friends and states that his relationship with his father is strained
- The physician was able to speak to the patient's father just prior to the visit. His father relates that his maternal aunt was admitted for years to a psychiatric state hospital with an unknown diagnosis
- On mental status examination, the patient was alert and oriented to person, place, time, and situation. He was cooperative but distracted with pressured speech. His thought process was logical, linear, and goal directed. He related no delusions or hallucinations and denied suicidal or homicidal ideation

Question

What do you now think is the diagnosis for this patient based on his current symptoms?

- Bipolar I disorder
- Bipolar II disorder
- Bipolar depression with mixed features
- MDD
- ADHD presenting with anxiety

Case outcome: first interim follow-up at week 2 (continued)

- The patient was diagnosed with bipolar depression with mixed features based on the mixed features criteria

Attending physician's mental notes: second interim follow-up at weeks 3 and 4

- Vortioxetine (Trintellix) was discontinued due to mixed presentation with increased irritability and agitation
- The patient was initiated on lurasidone (Latuda) 20 mg per day and eventually increased to 40 mg per day after 2 weeks
- The patient was noted to having elevated blood pressure and a past history of hypertension, and was referred to a primary care physician

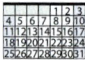

Case outcome: multiple interim follow-ups through week 5

- Upon examination, the patient's hypertension is treated and is normotensive on lisinopril (Zestril) 20 mg per day
- The patient still complains of inattention and difficulty initiating tasks, and his anxiety persists
- His mood is improved and he is sleeping better
- He notes his anxiety to be greater earlier in the day, lessening toward the evening times. The patient relates he still has difficulties in attention and with completing tasks
- The patient was started on atomoxetine (Strattera) for his ADHD, and lisdexamfetamine (Vyvanse) stopped as the stimulant may be exacerbating his anxiety
- He continued on lurasidone (Latuda) 40 mg per day. His sleeping improved and the patient stopped trazodone (Desyrel) 1 week earlier
- An exercise regimen was started to supplement his medication management

Attending physician's mental notes: interim follow-up at week 6

- The patient had improved mood, energy, and sleep
- There was some improvement in attention and focus on atomoxetine (Strattera) 40 mg and then 60 mg per day
- Atomoxetine was increased to 80 mg per day

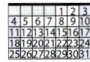

Case outcome: multiple interim follow-ups through weeks 7–10

- The patient has secured employment and is doing well in his writing. He has moved into an apartment separate from his father and has increased self-worth
- His mood is stable on lurasidone (Latuda) 40 mg per day
- His attention is much improved on atomoxetine (Strattera) 80 mg per day
- The patient no longer has anxiety

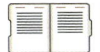

Case debrief

- The patient had a childhood history of previous diagnosis of ADHD and presented with multiple depressive symptoms and difficulty completing tasks
- After the addition of vortioxetine (Trintellix) for his depressed mood, the patient exhibited a mixed presentation with pressured speech, increased energy levels, and insomnia
- The patient's prior lack of response on antidepressants and his reaction to vortioxetine suggest that his initial diagnosis of MDD was incorrect
- In this bipolar patient with coexisting ADHD, the less activating agent atomoxetine (Strattera) did not induce anxiety

Take-home points

- The DSM-5 criteria for manic or hypomanic episode, with mixed features are as follows (Figure 9.1):
  - Full criteria are met for a manic episode or hypomanic episode, and at least three of the following symptoms are present during the majority of days of the current or most recent episode of mania or hypomania
    - Prominent dysphoria or depressed mood as indicated by either subjective report (e.g. feels sad or empty) or observation made by others (e.g. appears tearful)
    - Diminished interest or pleasure in all, or almost all, activities (as indicated by either subjective account or observation made by others)
    - Psychomotor retardation nearly every day (observable by others, not merely subjective feelings of being slowed down)

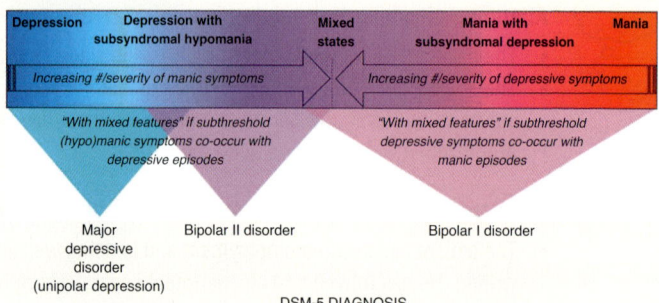

Figure 9.1. Mood disorders spectrum and DSM-5 diagnosis. Mood disorders can be conceptualized as existing along a spectrum that spans from pure unipolar depression with no intra- or inter-episode symptoms of (hypo)mania all the way to threshold-level mania.

- ○ Fatigue or loss of energy
- ○ Feelings of worthlessness or excessive or inappropriate guilt (not merely self-reproach or guilt about being sick)
- ○ Recurrent thoughts of death (not just fear of dying), recurrent suicidal ideation without a specific plan, or a suicide attempt or a specific plan of committing suicide
- – Mixed symptoms are observable by others and represent a change from the person's usual behavior
- – For individuals whose symptoms meet the full episode criteria for both mania and depression simultaneously, the diagnosis should be manic episode, with mixed features, due to marked impairment and clinical severity of full mania
- – The mixed symptoms are not attributable to the physiological effects of a substance (e.g. drug of abuse, medication, or other treatments).

Tips and pearls

- A lack of response or poor tolerability to antidepressant therapy may indicate that the diagnosis of MDD is incorrect. Such patients may actually have bipolar depression. Antidepressant therapy may switch bipolar patients to mixed or manic states
- Treatments for bipolar depression include quetiapine (Seroquel), olanzapine-fluoxetine (Symbax), combination, lurasidone (Latuda) or cariprazine (Vraylar), all of which are approved for this use. Quetiapine has better evidence for treating bipolar II disorder, as the other agents have not been studied in bipolar II disorder. However, lurasidone and cariprazine have better metabolic profiles in comparison with quetiapine or olanzapine-fluoxetine.

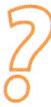

Posttest self-assessment question and answer

Which of the following are evidence-based treatments of ADHD in adults?

A. Methylphenidate (Concerta) or amphetamine
B. Atomoxetine (Strattera)
C. Guanfacine (Tenex)
D. Clonidine (Catapres)
E. All of the above

Answer: E

Methylphenidate or amphetamine is considered the first-line treatment and is used most extensively for its immediate onset of action. Atomoxetine is considered a non-stimulant that inhibits presynaptic norepinephrine reuptake, resulting in increased synaptic norepinephrine and dopamine. Atomoxetine has a decreased abuse profile in comparison with amphetamines. Guanfacine is an α-adrenergic receptor agonist most efficacious in children and adolescents who do not respond to first-line treatments. Clonidine is an α-adrenergic receptor agonist that is most efficacious in children and adolescents; it helps alleviate hyperarousal and agitation but may cause sedation.

References

1. Adler LA, Spencer T, Brown TE, et al. Once-daily atomoxetine for adult attention-deficit/hyperactivity disorder. *J ClinPsychopharmacol* 2009; 29:44–50. https://doi.org/10.1097/jcp.0b013e318192e4a0
2. American Psychiatric Association. *Diagnostic and Statistical Manual of Mental Disorders*, 5th edn. Arlington, VA: American Psychiatric Association, 2013.
3. Berlin RK, Butler PM, Perloff MD. Gabapentin therapy in psychiatric disorders. *Prim Care Companion CNS Disord* 2015; 17:28–32. https://doi.org/10.4088/pcc.15r01821
4. Bymaster FP, Katner JS, Nelson DL, et al. Atomoxetine increases extracellular levels of norepinephrine and dopamine in prefrontal cortex of rats: a potential mechanism for efficacy in attention deficit/hyperactivity disorder. *Neuropsychopharmacology* 2002; 27:699–711. https://doi.org/10.1016/s0893-133x(02)00346-9
5. Clayton AH, Gillespie EH. Bupropion. In: Schatzberg AF, Nemeroff CB, eds. *The American Psychiatric Publishing Textbook of*

Psychopharmacology, 4th edn. Washington, DC: American Psychiatric Publishing, 2009; p. 415.

6. Girard R, Joober R. Treatment of ADHD in patients with bipolar disorder. *J Psychiatry Neurosci* 2017; 42:E11–12. https://doi.org/10.1503/jpn.170097

7. Gitlin MJ. Antidepressants in bipolar depression: an enduring controversy. *Int J Bipolar Disord* 2018; 6:3–6. https://doi.org/10.1186/s40345-018-0133-9

8. Klassen LJ, Katzman MA, Chokka P. Adult ADHD and its comorbidities, with a focus on bipolar disorder. *J Affect Disord* 2010; 124:1–8. https://doi.org/10.1016/j.jad.2009.06.036

9. Li D-J, Tseng P-T, Chen Y-W, et al. Significant treatment effect of bupropion in patients with bipolar disorder but similar phase-shifting rate as other antidepressants: a meta-analysis following the PRISMA guidelines. *Medicine* 2016; 95:e3165. https://doi.org/10.1097/md.0000000000003165

10. Mahableshwarkar AR, Zajecka J, Jacobson W, et al. A randomized, placebo-controlled, active-reference, double-blind, flexible-dose study of the efficacy of vortioxetine on cognitive function in major depressive disorder. *Neuropsychopharmacology* 2015; 40:2025–37. https://doi.org/10.1038/npp.2015.52

11. Marangoni C, de Chiara L, Faedda GL. Bipolar disorder and ADHD: comorbidity and diagnostic distinctions. *Curr Psychiatry Rep*, 2015; 17:1–2. https://doi.org/10.1007/s11920-015-0604-y

12. McIntyre RS, Kennedy SH, Soczynska JK, et al. Attention-deficit/hyperactivity disorder in adults with bipolar disorder or major depressive disorder: results from the International Mood Disorders Collaborative Project. *Prim Care Companion J Clin Psychiatry* 2010; 12: e1–7. https://doi.org/10.4088/pcc.09m00861gry

13. Stahl SM. *Stahl's Essential Psychopharmacology: Prescriber's Guide*, 6th edn. Cambridge, UK: Cambridge University Press, 2017.

14. Stahl SM, Morrissette DA, Faedda G, et al. Guidelines for the recognition and management of mixed depression. *CNS Spectr* 2017; 22:203–19. https://doi.org/10.1017/s1092852917000165

15. Thase ME. Effects of venlafaxine on blood pressure. *J Clin Psychiatry* 1998; 59: 502–8. https://doi.org/10.4088/jcp.v59n1002

16. Tzellos TG, Papazisis G, Toulis KA, et al. A2δ ligands gabapentin and pregabalin: future implications in daily clinical practice. *Hippokratia* 2010; 14:71–5.

17. Wilens TE, Morrison NR, Prince J. An update on the pharmacotherapy of attention-deficit/hyperactivity disorder in adults. *Expert Rev Neurother* 2011; 11:1443–65. https://doi.org/10.1586/ern.11.137

PATIENT FILE

Case 10: The anxious depressed woman who couldn't sit still

The Question: How can you distinguish between bipolar disorder with mixed features and major depressive disorder with mixed features? Is it necessary to differentiate between the two?

The Psychopharmacological Dilemma: Finding an effective regimen for recurrent, anxious depression while minimizing akathisia

Nekisa Haghighat, Charity Hall, Dennis Alters, and Gerald Maguire

Pretest self-assessment question (answer at the end of the case)

What is the first-line treatment of depression with mixed features?

A. Dual therapy with a mood stabilizer plus an atypical antipsychotic
B. Dual therapy with an antidepressant plus an atypical antipsychotic
C. Monotherapy with an antidepressant
D. Monotherapy with an atypical antipsychotic
E. Electroconvulsive therapy

Patient evaluation on intake

- A 62-year-old woman with the chief complaints of anxiety and difficulty sleeping

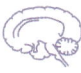

Psychiatric history

- The patient has had intermittent episodes of depression since early adulthood. Typically, her episodes start with feelings of anxiety followed by weeks of anhedonia, listlessness, difficulty getting out bed or caring for herself, loss of appetite, and poor concentration. Ten years ago, she received inpatient psychiatric treatment for a particularly severe episode. At the time, the patient was experiencing multiple psychosocial stressors including her daughter leaving for college and unresolved feelings of abandonment stemming from her mother's death in childhood, as well as a significant loss of income and her family home
- In addition to intensive cognitive behavioral therapy, the patient was started on psychopharmacological therapy. She eventually responded to a combination of venlafaxine (Effexor) XR 150 mg per day and clonazepam (Klonopin) 0.25 mg per day
- During her hospital stay, the patient appeared to make significant improvements. As her overtly depressed symptoms diminished, her affect became brighter and she appeared more energetic, motivated, and talkative. In retrospect, the patient's husband notes that she appeared "manicky" upon discharge. In addition to the abovementioned changes in mood, the patient also exhibited

103

restlessness and impulsive behavior, although the husband acknowledges that these traits may just be part of her baseline personality
- When questioned further about these details, the patient recalls long stretches of time in her 20s and 30s during which she felt similarly hyperactive, with racing thoughts and poor concentration. She denies any periods of excessive spending or risky behavior during these periods
- The patient followed up with a psychiatrist as an outpatient, who ultimately tapered her off all psychotropic medications

Patient evaluation on intake
- Today, the patient is seeing a new psychiatrist. She reports that she has been feeling increasingly anxious over the past few weeks and has had difficulty falling asleep
- Her husband reports that the patient has been very tearful, withdrawn, and anxious at home. Both the patient and her husband worry that she is returning to her previous state of depression, because her emotions and behaviors echo the early stages of her last episode of depression
- On mental status examination, the patient appears restless, anxious, and easily distracted

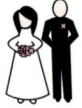

Social and personal history
- The patient's mother died of breast cancer when she was 8 years old
- She and her husband, a clinical psychologist, have been married for 40 years and have two children together
- She likes to be social with her friends and family
- She has no history of drug or tobacco use
- She drinks one to two glasses of wine socially, every few days

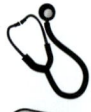

Medical history
- She has essential hypertension, which is well controlled

Current medications
- Amlodipine (Norvasc) 5 mg per day for essential hypertension

Questions
Based on just what you have been told so far about this patient's history and current symptoms, would you consider her period of

hyperactivity following her depressed episode to be indicative of hypomania?

- Yes
- No

Would you restart her previous psychotropic regimen or consider a mood-stabilizing agent?

- Yes, restart her venlafaxine (Effexor) but not her clonazepam (Klonopin)
- Yes, restart her venlafaxine and her clonazepam
- No, start her on a mood-stabilizing agent

Attending physician's mental notes: initial evaluation

- The patient has a history of depression that was triggered by psychosocial factors. The fact that she responded well to venlafaxine XR (Effexor) supports this diagnosis
- However, the patient began to exhibit some hyperactivity and hypomanic tendencies as her depression subsided. Perhaps this is indicative of a subsyndromal hypomania
- One of the major changes introduced by DSM-5 was the addition of the "mixed features" specifier, which can be applied to episodes of major depression, hypomania, or mania. A "major depressive episode (MDE) with mixed features" refers to an episode that is predominantly depressive in nature but is accompanied by a "whiff" of mania (three or more symptoms of mania). Our patient's current presentation is most consistent with this diagnosis, which ultimately changes our approach to treatment
- There are currently no FDA-approved treatments for MDE or major depressive disorder (MDD) with mixed features. Nevertheless, current literature based on studies of mixed depression can help guide us
- In general, the use of antidepressant monotherapy is strongly discouraged in patients with mixed depression. Antidepressants may not only be ineffective but also have the potential to destabilize mood in patients with mixed depression or bipolar disorders. In fact, this may be what happened with this patient during her aforementioned psychiatric hospitalizations, when she began showing hyperactivity and restlessness after being treated with venlafaxine XR (Effexor)
- Atypical antipsychotics, in contrast, have shown to be somewhat effective in the treatment of mixed depression.[1] Originally, lurasidone (Latuda) was considered in this patient. However, her insurance company – like many others – does not cover lurasidone

unless the patient has failed several other medication trials. The risks and benefits of other atypical antipsychotics were discussed with the patient. Ultimately, she agreed to start aripiprazole (Abilify) 5 mg per day, with instructions to uptitrate to 10 mg per day over the next few days

- The patient also has a long history of insomnia, which she attributes to anxious thoughts that prevent her from going to sleep. Her difficulty sleeping may be addressed by treating the underlying anxiety. If it continues, we may consider a sedating atypical antipsychotic, such as asenapine (Saphris) or quetiapine (Seroquel), in the future

Further investigation

Aside from depressed symptoms, which of the following are the three most common symptoms in mixed depression?

- Risky behavior
- Psychomotor agitation
- Elevated mood
- Racing thoughts/flight of ideas
- Irritability

Figure 10.1 shows the most common and least common mania-like symptoms that are seen in depression with mixed features. Note that several of these are not included in DSM-5.

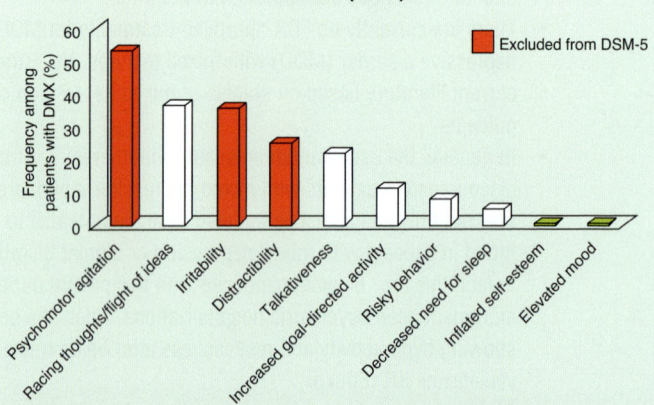

Figure 10.1. Symptoms of depression with mixed features. From Takeshima and Oka (2015).

Case outcome: first interim follow-up at week 4

- Unbeknown to this treating psychiatrist, the patient decided to visit another psychiatrist located closer to her home for her follow-up. Without consultation, this new provider discontinued the patient's aripiprazole (Abilify) and started her on sertraline (Zoloft) 25 mg per day
- After 5 days, the patient started experiencing racing thoughts, anxiety, restlessness, and increased difficulty sleeping. She also reported passive, fleeting suicidal ideation without any intent or plan. She then contacted this treating psychiatrist, who recommended that she discontinue the sertraline and resume aripiprazole at 10 mg per day
- Today, she reports she is doing better and tolerating the aripiprazole well. She still feels overwhelming anxiety but denies suicidal ideation or racing thoughts. She continues to have difficulty sleeping, which she attributes to her anxious thoughts
- A psychiatric pharmacogenomic test was ordered during this visit

Attending physician's mental notes: first interim follow-up at week 4

- The patient's initial response to aripiprazole (Abilify) indicates that we were on the right track with using an agent that potentially targets mixed states. However, her poor response to a selective serotonin reuptake inhibitor (SSRI) – namely hyperactivity and suicidal ideation – are a cause for concern and warrant immediate discontinuation of sertraline (Zoloft)
- The patient has an interesting pattern of responses to antidepressant monotherapy. In the past, treatment with the serotonin-norepinephrine reuptake inhibitor (SNRI) venlafaxine XR (Effexor) appeared to improve her depressed symptoms, although it may have triggered a subsyndromal hypomania. In response to an SSRI, however, she appears to have been flipped into full-blown mania
- Perhaps a psychiatric pharmacogenomic profile may provide insights into which medications may be tolerable and effective. It could also provide information for neurobiologically plausible hypotheses for selection of future therapeutic agents

Case outcome: second interim follow-up at week 5

- A week later, the patient reports that her previously overwhelming feelings of anxiety are now less pronounced and occur less frequently. However, she also reports increasing restlessness, hyperactivity, and difficulty concentrating. In the office, she is easily distracted and continuously fidgets in her chair

- The patient's pharmacogenomic profile is reviewed. Of note, she carries several interesting gene variances, most notably in the *MTHFR*, *SLC6A4*, *CYP2B6*, and *CYP2C19* genes.

Attending physician's mental notes: second interim follow-up at week 5

- The patient's pharmacogenomic profile reveals that she carries a polymorphism in the *MTHFR* gene that limits her ability to convert folic acid into L-methylfolate (Deplin), a key step in the production of serotonin, dopamine, and norepinephrine. As she cannot convert folic acid to L-methylfolate, the patient is prescribed supplementation with L-methylfolate in the hopes of addressing this possible neurotransmitter deficiency

- The pharmacogenomic profile further reveals that the patient is heterozygous for the short/long promoter polymorphism of the serotonin transporter gene *SLC6A4*. The short form of the allele is reported to be associated with decreased expression of the serotonin transporter compared with the long form. Because the patient has one short allele, she has a reduced number of serotonin transporters compared with a person who is homozygous for the long allele. Thus, she may have a decreased likelihood of response to medications that selectively target serotonin reuptake, such as SSRIs like sertraline (Zoloft)

- Furthermore, the pharmacogenomic profile shows that the patient has particular variants in the *CYP2B6* and *CYP2C19* genes encoding the enzymes cytochrome P450 2B6 and cytochrome P450 2C19, respectively, resulting in reduced activity of both enzymes. Sertraline is metabolized, and thus cleared, by the CYP2B6 and CYP2C19 enzymes. Individuals with this phenotype are thought to be intermediate metabolizers of sertraline, meaning that they would metabolize, and thus clear, sertraline at a slower rate than individuals with the normal metabolizer phenotype. Thus, this patient is likely sensitive to even the lowest dose of sertraline. This may explain her dramatic response to sertraline, which appears to have triggered an episode of full-blown mania

Case outcome: third interim follow-up at week 6

- As aripiprazole (Abilify) is uptitrated over the next few days, the patient reports that her anxiety and insomnia appear to be improving. However, she continues to experience hyperactivity and restlessness. In the office, her speech appears somewhat rapid and pressured. The patient also reports continued difficulty falling asleep at night

Attending physician's mental notes: third interim follow-up at week 6

- Although an antipsychotic appears to be improving the patient's anxiety, the accompanying restlessness, hyperactivity, and pressured speech is problematic, as these signs may herald impending mood instability. This "whiff" of mania aligns with a diagnosis of MDD with mixed features but should still be treated like a manic or hypomanic episode
- The patient is thus started on lamotrigine (Lamictal) 25 mg per day, with plans for gradual uptitration over the coming weeks. It is important to start low and go slow with lamotrigine due to the risk of Stevens–Johnson syndrome. At the same time, aripiprazole (Abilify) is gradually discontinued and replaced with nightly quetiapine (Seroquel), uptitrated to 200 mg per night, with the hopes that its sedating properties will help alleviate the patient's insomnia

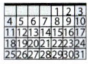

Case outcome: fourth interim follow-up at week 8

- Two weeks later, the patient reports that both her anxiety and sleep have continued to improve. However, she now reports feeling "low", somewhat depressed, and a bit slow; at times, these feelings end up making her feel anxious again. She also admits some passive suicidal ideation but denies intent or plan. Her mental status examination echoes these sentiments: she no longer appears restless or particularly anxious but does seem to exhibit a depressed mood with noticeably slowed movements

Attending physician's mental notes: fourth interim follow-up at week 8

- The patient now appears to have entered a depressed state with concurrent feelings of anxiety, further tipping the scales toward a diagnosis of MDD with mixed features
- In accordance with the patient's pharmacogenomic profile and her history of a positive response to SNRIs, she is started on venlafaxine XR (Effexor) 37.5 mg per day with plans to uptitrate to at least 150 mg per day. This is because at lower doses venlafaxine predominantly targets serotonin reuptake. It is not until higher doses of at least 150 mg that the effect on norepinephrine reuptake becomes apparent. As the patient's serotonin transporters are thought to be essentially ineffective, we want to make sure that we are targeting norepinephrine reuptake in this patient

Question

What adverse effect of venlafaxine (Effexor) should you be wary of in this patient, particularly in light of her medical history?

- Withdrawal syndrome
- Serotonin syndrome
- Hypertension
- Suicidality

Attending physician's mental notes: fourth interim follow-up at week 8 (continued)

- As noted above, the patient's history of essential hypertension indicates that titration of venlafaxine XR (Effexor) should be performed slowly, with particular attention to blood pressure along the way. Thus, her outpatient prescription of amlodipine (Norvasc) is increased from 5 mg to 10 mg per day, and the patient is instructed to carefully monitor her blood pressure at home. Her primary care physician agrees with this course of action
- Meanwhile, lamotrigine (Lamictal) is increased to 25 mg twice per day and the patient is continued on her current dose of quetiapine (Seroquel)

Case outcome: fifth through seventh interim follow-ups through weeks 9–14

- As venlafaxine XR (Effexor) and lamotrigine (Lamictal) are gradually increased over the next few visits, the patient reports that her mood feels more stable overall. Although she still continues to struggle with simultaneous feelings of depression and anxiety, they feel less extreme and overwhelming. Her husband agrees that she appears less hyperactive but notes that she is still far from her baseline. She continues to be socially withdrawn, easily distractible, and has difficulty engaging with the rest of the family or organizing her day
- In person, the patient continues to appear somewhat restless. She denies overt suicidal ideation but admits that she would not particularly care if she were to not wake up the next day

Attending physician's mental notes: fifth through seventh interim follow-ups through weeks 9–14

- On the one hand, the patient has shown some improvement on lamotrigine (Lamictal) and quetiapine (Seroquel). By her own account, her depression and anxiety have become less severe, although both feelings persist simultaneously. On the other hand, merely stabilizing her mood is not our goal. She is simply not herself, as her husband notes, and likely continues to be experiencing a state of mixed depression

- The treating psychiatrist now feels that there is enough evidence that the patient has failed several trials of medications, including combinations of venlafaxine XR (Effexor), sertraline (Zoloft), aripiprazole (Abilify), quetiapine, and lamotrigine. It may be time to visit the original idea of lurasidone (Latuda), an idea that the patient's insurance agrees to authorize now that she has exhausted her alternatives
- Thus, the patient is transitioned to 20 mg lurasidone with food every evening for 1 week and then increased to 40 mg where she is maintained

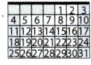

Case outcome: subsequent interim follow-ups

- Once the patient is started on lurasidone (Latuda), she fairly quickly begins to show noticeable improvements in her mood and energy, especially during the second week at 40 mg. With each subsequent visit, the patient reports decreasing feelings of depression, anxiety, and insomnia. She reports improved mental clarity since transitioning to lurasidone
- The patient's husband happily reports that she has started socializing again with her friends and family, is able to focus on the tasks at hand, and remains energized throughout the day
- The patient begins to emphatically deny suicidal ideation. She now looks forward to welcoming a new grandchild in the near future for whom she has started making plans that she admits she never thought she would be making this time last year

Case debrief

- Ten years ago, the patient had a single major depressive episode that was treated to apparent remission with a combination of an SNRI and a long-acting benzodiazepine, venlafaxine XR (Effexor) and clonazepam (Klonopin)
- At the time, there was some concern that she was exhibiting hypomanic symptoms as she recovered from her depressive episode, although her distractibility, hyperactivity, and restlessness could also be attributed to undiagnosed attention deficit hyperactivity disorder or personality traits
- The patient showed signs of an apparent mixed state: depression with concurrent anxiety and restlessness. She was also concerned that her feelings of anxiety might herald a recurrent depressive episode

- After showing a drastic and possibly manic response to an SSRI started by a different provider, the patient was trialed on different classes of psychotropics. She showed a minimal response to monotherapy with an atypical antipsychotic such as aripiprazole (Abilify), along with symptoms of hyperactivity and restlessness concerning for further mood symptoms
- A pharmacogenomic profile guided us against agents that rely solely on serotonin transporter and to avoid/adjust medications based on metabolism profile. Thus, a high dose of venlafaxine XR was used to target the patient's depressive symptoms along with lamotrigine (Lamictal) for mood stabilization and quetiapine (Seroquel) for residual insomnia and anxiety
- Although the patient showed some improvement on this regimen, both she and her family still felt that she was not herself. She continued to exhibit symptoms of both depression and anxiety, albeit milder than before. The decision was made to transition to lurasidone (Latuda) as monotherapy for treatment of MDD with mixed features. Although this idea was considered in the beginning, the health system in the USA, with restrictions mandated by health insurance companies based solely on financial considerations, often puts barriers against patients receiving medications with what would otherwise be considered first-line treatment
- Ultimately, the patient was able to receive lurasidone once she failed a number of other alternatives. She shows remarkable improvement on monotherapy with this treatment, further supporting the diagnosis of MDD with mixed features

Posttest self-assessment question and answer

What is the first-line treatment of depression with mixed features?

A. Dual therapy with a mood stabilizer plus an atypical antipsychotic
B. Dual therapy with an antidepressant plus an atypical antipsychotic
C. Monotherapy with an antidepressant
D. Monotherapy with an atypical antipsychotic
E. Electroconvulsive therapy

Answer: D

Although there are currently no FDA or European Medicines Agency (EMA)-approved medications for the treatment of mixed depression, current evidence supports the use of monotherapy with an atypical antipsychotic such as lurasidone (Latuda), asenapine (Saphris), quetiapine(Seroquel), aripiprazole (Abilify), or ziprasidone (Geodon) as the first-line approach for the acute pharmacological treatment of depression with mixed features. Second-line treatment includes monotherapy with lamotrigine (Lamictal), valproate, lithium, cariprazine (Vraylar), or olanzapine (Zyprexa), or dual therapy with lithium/lamotrigine/valproate plus an atypical antipsychotic, lithium plus valproate, lithium/valproate plus lamotrigine, or olanzapine-fluoxetine (Symbyax).

However, monotherapy with an antidepressant, including SSRIs and SNRIs, is strongly discouraged due to the risk of eliciting an affective switch, in other words, inducing a manic episode. If an antidepressant is to be used, it should be paired with a mood-stabilizing agent and should thus parallel the treatment of bipolar disorder.

References

1. Stahl, SM. Venlaxafine. In: *Stahl's Essential Psychopharmacology: The Prescriber's Guide*, 7th edn. Cambridge, UK: Cambridge University Press, 2020; pp. 841–6.
2. Stahl SM, Morrissette DA. Does a "whiff" of mania in a major depressive episode shift treatment from a classical antidepressant to an atypical/second-generation antipsychotic? *Bipolar Disord* 2017; 19:595–6. https://doi.org/10.1111/bdi.12542
3. Takeshima M, Oka T. DSM-5-defined 'mixed features' and Benazzi's mixed depression: which is practically useful to discriminate bipolar disorder from unipolar depression in patients with depression? *Psychiatry Clin Neurosci* 2015; 69:109–16. https://doi.org/10.1111/pcn.12213
4. Yuce-Artun N, Baskak B, Ozel-Kizil ET, et al. Influence of CYP2B6 and CYP2C19 polymorphisms on sertraline metabolism in major depression patients. *Int J Clin Pharm* 2016; 38:388–94. https://doi.org/10.1007/s11096-016-0259-8

Case 11: The man who thinks it's the end of the world

The Question: Can a pandemic trigger dormant psychiatric symptoms?

The Psychopharmacological Dilemma: If some element of psychosis is personality driven, will the patient benefit from medication therapy or psychotherapy to alleviate symptoms?

Erin Fletcher, Evagelos Coskinas, and Phuong Vo

Pretest self-assessment question (answer at the end of the case)

Which of the following are approved treatments for brief psychotic disorder (BPD)?

A. Haloperidol (Haldol)
B. Risperidone (Risperdal)
C. Olanzapine (Zyprexa)
D. Psychotherapy
E. All of the above

Patient evaluation on intake

- A 39-year-old male who believes that coronavirus disease 2019 (COVID-19) will lead to the end of the world
- He raced his vehicle on the highway at 100 mph, crashed into the center divide, self-extricated, and ran into traffic after he and his wife were both recently diagnosed with flu
- He and his wife both tested negative for COVID-19

Psychiatric history

- The patient was doing well until he became stressed with household and family issues after a shelter-in-place order issued due the COVID-19 pandemic
- He remains gainfully employed despite business closures due to COVID-19 concerns and appears stressed about working from home
- He has no history of mental illness
- He was admitted to the inpatient unit on an involuntarily hold for danger to self after crashing his vehicle and running down the freeway due to visual and auditory hallucinations of Satan chasing him
- He believed TV news covering the COVID-19 pandemic were messages sent to him specifically warning him of the end of the world

- The initial psychiatric interview revealed poor sleep and decreased appetite, and ruminating thoughts about his previous hallucinations. He was cooperative, with anxious, dysphoric affect but not depressed
- When asked about psychotic symptoms, the patient perseverated on thoughts of purgatory, the end of days, and heaven and hell. He denied current psychosis but appeared anxious, dysphoric, and internally preoccupied
- A review of psychiatric systems revealed no formal obsessive–compulsive disorder diagnosed; however, he reports ruminating thoughts regarding somatic symptoms when he becomes ill
- There is no evidence of schizophrenia or mania but he meets some criteria for depression
- There is no history of past hospitalizations
- There have been no suicide attempts

Medical history

- None

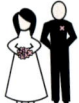

Social and personal history

- The patient lives with his wife and four children
- He graduated from high school and is employed as an electrician supervisor
- He denies current legal issues or past military service
- Alcohol use is occasional, with one or two drinks at social gatherings
- He denies illicit drug use
- A urine drug screen was negative for illicit substances and his ethanol level was negative

Family history

- His mother had possible depression or bipolar disorder. He cannot recollect if she took medication
- No family history of schizophrenia
- His sister has multiple sclerosis

Current medications

- On admission, he was started on olanzapine (Zyprexa) 5 mg per day

Questions

Based on this patient's history and the available evidence, what do you consider his diagnosis to be?

- Brief psychosis
- Adjustment disorder
- Major depressive disorder with psychotic features
- Schizophrenia, late onset

What would your next treatment likely be?

- Increase the olanzapine (Zyprexa) to alleviate psychosis
- Better delineate his diagnosis
- Consider adding a selective serotonin reuptake inhibitor (SSRI), as sometimes this can alleviate depressive psychosis

Attending physician's mental notes: initial evaluation

- This patient is psychotic; it was thought by other providers to be possible delirium or brain trauma due to the car accident
- He is not guarded. It is unclear if this was missed, perhaps as he presents as normal to others, is married with children, is employed, and is of older age. He does not seem schizophrenic to others
- These symptoms may have occurred over several years and this is a case of late-onset schizophrenia
- It will need to be determined whether he is psychotic when euthymic suggesting schizophrenia or if he recovers fully suggesting a brief psychosis
- The patient also presents with a subsyndromal depression and anxiety, which is mild at best
- Substance-induced psychosis will need to be ruled out, although his history suggests no drug abuse
- Medically induced psychosis will need to be ruled out as he is a bit older with regard to developing a psychotic disorder
- He was started on olanzapine (Zyprexa) 5 mg per day

Further investigation

Is there anything else you would especially like to know about this patient?

- Is there a history of PTSD?
  - He denies past symptoms of PTSD
  - There is no history of military service
  - There is no history of physical or mental trauma

Question

Could there be any other cause of his psychotic symptoms?

- Radiological imaging reveals no brain abnormalities
- He had an elevated white cell count of 19×10^9 cells/l upon admission but this quickly normalized over 24 hours. It was likely a stress reaction from the car accident

Attending physician's mental notes: initial evaluation (continued)

- He continues to be psychotic but is improving; his thought process is more linear
- His medical workup is negative
- Brain imaging shows he has no masses, lesions or trauma
- A urine drug screen is negative

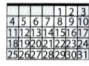

Case outcome: first interim follow-up at 1 week

- The patient is titrated slowly on olanzapine (Zyprexa) without issue, and left on 15 mg per day
- This is effective in treating his positive symptoms
- The hallucinations resolve
- He feels better: he is less tense, has better sleep, and is less ruminative

Attending physician's mental notes: first interim follow-up at 1 week

- The patient now recalls his recent psychotic behavior and hallucinations with disbelief
- His bouts of rumination and hyperawareness seem to be driven by novelty in new social situations and tasks, which may very well be a personality trait, as a response to anxiety, but differentially do not seem to fit generalized anxiety disorder
- He seems to have had a brief psychotic episode
- He also has minor depression and minor anxiety symptoms along with disorder but does not meet full DMS-5 categorical diagnosis

Question

How long would you treat this patient with his antipsychotic?

A. After remission of psychosis, treat for 6 months and then discontinue
B. After remission of psychosis, treat for 1 year and then discontinue
C. After remission of psychosis, treat for 5 years and then discontinue
D. After remission of psychosis, treat indefinitely unless side effects occur
E. As he does not meet categorical obsessive–compulsive disorder, refer for psychotherapy to address his long-term dynamic issues, anxiety, and depression symptoms

Attending physician's mental notes: follow-up at 1 month

- The patient is doing well
- His psychosis has resolved, and he is not guarded with appropriate affect
- Life stress likely caused the brief psychosis
- He has taken time off work but plans to return soon and has the support of his wife
- He has continued his atypical antipsychotic monotherapy
- His prognosis is promising

Case outcome: follow-up at 1 month

- The patient is educated about the diagnosis being complicated due to his minor levels of several symptom clusters and his BPD
- He feels the current dose of olanzapine (Zyprexa) is effective and asks to keep it as it is
- He is not depressed or suicidal
- The patient is getting support from his wife and family

Case debrief

- The patient suffered a single brief psychotic episode that was severe in intensity
- He was a complete responder to atypical antipsychotic monotherapy
- He has continued on olanzapine (Zyprexa) for now
- He remains positive symptom free
- He returned to work shortly after discharge and had an appointment with a psychotherapist

Take-home points

- There are three essential elements of the history and physical in an individual with suspected BPD:
  - The presence of at least one positive psychotic symptom such as hallucinations, disorganized speech, delusions, or disorganized or catatonic behavior
  - Establishing that the symptoms have not been present for less than 1 day or more than 1 month
  - Investigating whether the disturbance in behavior is otherwise explainable by another mood disorder, medical condition, or substance/medication use
- There are a limited number of clinical trials evaluating the efficacy of specific treatment modalities in patients with BPD. Therefore, current recommendations for treatment of BPD relies on

pharmacological and psychotherapeutic interventions known to be effective in patients with other psychotic disorders
- Antipsychotics, especially second-generation ones, are the first-line treatment for BPD. Although BPD typically has complete resolution of symptoms within 1 month of symptom onset, it is suggested that treatment with antipsychotics is continued for 1–3 months after symptom remission
- Increased occurrence of BPD generally occurs in populations known to be under high stress such as natural disaster victims, those in military combat, those experiencing death, refugees, etc.
- In order to further clarify individual cases of BPD, it is necessary to recognize whether the triggering of psychotic symptoms was from a stressful event. Additionally, recognizing patient characteristics such as the presence of a personality disorder that can limit coping skills is important in identifying individuals at greater risk of developing disorders such as BPD. It is also necessary to recognize that the presenting symptoms of BPD can be very severe and, as a result, mimic the presentation of delirium
- Medication should be continued for approximately 6 months to prevent a relapse in addition to follow-up with outpatient psychiatry monthly. The patient should then be re-evaluated at 6 months to see if medication needs to be continued

- It is unclear how long the patient continued taking antipsychotic medication beyond our 1-month check-in as he was lost to follow-up
- For this patient, the coronavirus pandemic was a significant stressor. Extra stress factors during the COVID-19 pandemic that impact those at risk of BPD are social isolation, homelessness, unemployment, relationship stress from shelter-in-place orders, and domestic violence

Overview of brief psychosis
- Demographics
  - BPD is rare with an incidence of about 1.4 per 100,000 in the UK and up to 2% in a small county in the USA[10]
  - BPD is more common in women than men
  - BPD is often comorbid in those with personality or mood disorders (which are also more common in women)
  - Genetically, a family history of mental illness of schizophrenia or mood disorders with psychosis is also associated with an increased risk of psychosis
  - There is an increased frequency of BPD in high-stress environments such as in populations of immigrants, refugees, and victims of natural disasters

- Developing countries also have a ten times higher incidence of BPD than industrial countries according to the World Health Organization; although the etiology of this is unclear, it may result from a culturally bound expression of distress
- Risk factors for brief psychosis
  - Brief psychosis is most commonly triggered by severe stress factors or a preceding trauma such as violence, the death of a loved one, natural disasters, and sudden environmental changes (refugees/ immigrants)
  - Psychosis has an association with pandemics (influenza, severe acute respiratory syndrome (SARS), Middle East respiratory syndrome (MERS)), with "psychosis of influenza" being well documented
  - The stress associated with pandemic-related physical distancing measures has correlated with a rise in BPD due to rumination
  - Psychotic symptoms are positively correlated with virus symptom severity, amount of isolation with treatment, and steroid treatment. The human coronavirus strains HKU1 and NL63, two of the four most common coronaviruses, were also implicated as a risk factor for psychosis when compared with controls. This is difficult to parse due to patients with psychosis also being less willing to adhere to self-hygiene and appropriate hand washing or isolative behavior
  - Pandemic-related psychosis is correlated with higher suicide attempt rates
- Chance of recurrence of psychosis
  - Shorter duration of prodrome has a better outcome
  - The biggest predictor of relapse is non-adherence to medication, indicating the need to continue antipsychotic medication for 1–3 months after symptoms are in remission
  - There are some cases of remission without pharmaceutical therapy. In one study, 41% of patients refused medications, and 33% of these still achieved symptomatic remission without pharmacological treatment[11]
  - Patients that have residual psychotic symptoms for more than 1 month or relapse soon after stopping medication should be further evaluated
  - Patients with a diagnosis of cannabis abuse are more likely to experience relapse, as cannabis is an environmental risk factor that may induce further episodes of psychosis. Brief mindfulness-based practice in inpatients with psychosis may reduce relapse and readmission due to decreased stress

avoidance and changes in cognitive and behavioral response to perceived stressors

- Comorbid mental illness
  - The proportion of patients in Denmark diagnosed with a personality disorder after BPD at 1 year was as high as 29% with DSM-4 criteria[10]
  - There is no significant difference between groups in any of the five personality subscales[10]
- Additional information
  - There is no specific laboratory test to make a diagnosis of BPD, but considering the differential diagnosis of BPD, medical conditions should be ruled out by ordering an electrocardiogram (ECG), electrolytes, glucose levels, thyroid function, and urinalysis to rule out drugs or medications
- Additional questions:
  - Do people incorporate beliefs about the virus into their symptoms (delusions ruled by fear and distress of contamination)?
    - A common manifestation of BPD has been paranoid delusions about contamination or being in close contact with others who will be severely ill. Other delusions include somatic ideas of infection caused by any abnormal sensation being interpreted as having COVID-19, with subsequent "coronaphobic" behavior. Delusions may also be of persecution and punishment by spiritual beings
  - Is there an increased susceptibility of getting the virus from physical deterioration of psychosis?
    - Patients with psychosis are normally less willing to adhere to self-hygiene and appropriate hand washing or isolative behavior, especially those with disorganized thoughts, unless they have delusions of contamination

Tips and pearls

- Educational bullet points on differentiating BPD from late-onset schizophrenia (LOS):
  - The nomenclature for onset of schizophrenia in older adults is defined as LOS for patients age 40–60 years and very-late-onset schizophrenia-like psychosis (VLOSLP) for patients over 60 years
  - Inconsistencies regarding the age of diagnosis of schizophrenia (as skewed toward early adult onset) may be attributed to the diagnostic bias that causes of psychosis and symptoms of

schizophrenia in middle-aged patients are more likely due to organic factors rather than a primary psychiatric illness

- Individuals with a first diagnosis of schizophrenia after age 40 comprise about 23.4%, while individuals over 65 years comprise about 0.1–0.5%. Admission rates for patients over 60 years may have an annual incidence of psychosis increase by 11% per 5-year age increase. However, studies rarely included patients older than 40 so the data is scarce and likely skewed
- Gaps in discovering patients with LOS may be due to patient paranoia with reluctance to seek care for symptoms or because of healthcare issues that decrease access for older adults with mental illness
- Psychosocial stressors that can trigger symptoms of schizophrenia in older adults include financial difficulties, bereavement, physical disability, and retirement
- VLOSLP can be associated with sensory impairment and social isolation
- VLOSLP patients also have a higher prevalence of visual hallucinations but a lower prevalence of thought disorders or affective blunting
- Relatives of VLOSLP patients have a lower risk for developing schizophrenia compared with relatives of patients with early onset of disease
- There is no association of LOS with any progressive dementing disorder. Brain imaging has been found to be similar, no matter the age of onset (or does not show statistically significant differences between early-onset schizophrenia and LOS).
- Women are more likely to have later onset of symptoms than men
- LOS patients are more likely to be well organized but have persecutory delusions with greater conviction and poorer insight
- Some studies say that LOS patients have less-negative symptom severity, while others say there is no difference
- LOS has a lower daily antipsychotic dose requirement for control
- LOS has less impairment with abstract/ flexible thinking, processing speed, or verbal memory compared with early-onset patients
- Patients with high C-reactive protein levels may have a 6–11-fold increase in risk for developing LOS, with chronic inflammation as a potential risk factor
- There is not enough evidence to create a specific guideline for antipsychotics for LOS patients. Short-term benefit (6 months)

has been suggested with risperidone (Risperdal), olanzapine (Zyprexa), aripiprazole (Abilify), and paliperidone (Invega)
- There is no evidence for secondary antipsychotic medication benefit for long-term use due to safety and efficacy concerns
- In terms of psychosocial treatment, Functional Adaptation and Skills Training (FAST) was associated with functional improvement and decreased use of emergency medical or emergency psychiatric services in LOS patients

Posttest self-assessment question and answer

Which of the following are approved treatments for BPD?

A. Haloperidol (Haldol)
B. Risperidone (Risperdal)
C. Olanzapine (Zyprexa)
D. Psychotherapy
E. All of the above

Answer: E

Haloperidol can be used effectively to treat acute psychosis. In cases where it is difficult to differentiate BPD and delirium, it should be kept in mind that intravenous haloperidol is also effective for delirium. Unlike haloperidol, risperidone has serotonergic blocking effects that alleviate negative symptoms of psychosis (e.g. anhedonia, avolition, amotivation, and flat affect). It is well tolerated and has fewer extrapyramidal adverse effects than typical antipsychotics. Olanzapine efficacy is similar to that of risperidone; it has fewer dose-dependent adverse effects, but it is more likely to be associated with weight gain. Individual, family, and group psychotherapy may be considered to help cope with stressors and resolve conflict.

References

1. Bowtell M, Eaton S, Thien K, et al. Rates and predictors of relapse following discontinuation of antipsychotic medication after a first episode of psychosis. *Schizophr Res* 2018; 195:231–6. https://doi.org/10.1016/j.schres.2017.10.030
2. Bozikas V, Parlapani E. Resilience in patients with psychotic disorder. *Psychiatriki* 2016; 27:13–16.
3. Brown E, Gray R, Monaco SL, et al. The potential impact of COVID-19 on psychosis: a rapid review of contemporary epidemic and pandemic research. *Schizophr Res* 2020; 222:79–87.https://doi.org/10.1016/j.schres.2020.05.005
4. Caseiro O, Pérez-Iglesias R, Mata I, et al. Predicting relapse after a first episode of non-affective psychosis: a three-year follow-up

study. *J Psychiatr Res* 2012; 46:1099–105. https://doi.org/10.1016/j.jpsychires.2012.05.001

5. Howard R, Rabins PV, Seeman MV, Jeste DV. Late-onset schizophrenia and very-late-onset schizophrenia-like psychosis: an international consensus. The International Late-Onset Schizophrenia Group. *Am J Psychiatry* 2000; 157:172–8. https://doi.org/10.1176/appi.ajp.157.2.172

6. Huarcaya-Victoria J, Herrera D, Castillo, C. Psychosis in a patient with anxiety related to COVID-19: a case report. *Psychiatry Res* 2020; 289: 113052. https://doi.org/10.1016/j.psychres.2020.113052

7. Jacobsen P, Peters E, Robinson EJ, Chadwick P. Mindfulness-based crisis interventions (MBCI) for psychosis within acute inpatient psychiatry settings; a feasibility randomised controlled trial. *BMC Psychiatry* 2020; 20: 193. https://doi.org/10.1186/s12888-020-02608-x

8. Maglione JE, Thomas SE, Jeste DV. Late-onset schizophrenia: do recent studies support categorizing LOS as a subtype of schizophrenia? *Curr Opin Psychiatry* 2014; 27:173–8. https://doi.org/10.1097/YCO.0000000000000049

9. Martin EB Jr. Brief psychotic disorder triggered by fear of coronavirus? *Psychiatric Times*, 2020; 37, 8 May. Available from: https://www.psychiatrictimes.com/coronavirus/brief-psychotic-disorder-triggered-fear-coronavirus-small-case-series (accessed March 26, 2021).

10. Mojtabai R. Brief psychotic disorder. In: Melin JA, ed. *UpToDate*, 2018. Available from: https://www.uptodate.com/contents/brief-psychotic-disorder?search=brief%20psychotic%20disorder&source=search_result&selectedTitle=1~150&usage_type=default&display_rank=1#H863609256 (accessed March 26, 2021).

11. Rodriguez, T. Predictors of favorable outcomes in first-episode psychosis without medication. *Psychiatry Advisor*, 2017. Available from: https://www.psychiatryadvisor.com/home/topics/schizophrenia-and-psychoses/predictors-of-favorable-outcomes-in-first-episode-psychosis-without-medication/ (accessed April 3, 2021).

12. Stephen A, Lui F. Brief psychotic disorder. In: *StatPearls*. Treasure Island, FL: StatPearls Publishing, 2020. Available from: https://www.ncbi.nlm.nih.gov/books/NBK539912/(accessed March 26, 2021).

Case 12: Sunny with a chance of depression

The Question: Can stimulants be used in the treatment of major depressive disorder?

The Psychopharmacological Dilemma: How to treat recurrent major depression in patients who are resistant to various treatments and have specific comorbidities

Madeline Saavedra, Bo Ram Yoo, Douglas Grover, and Christopher G. Fichtner

Pretest self-assessment question (answer at the end of the case)

Which of the following is NOT a mechanism of action of phenelzine (Nardil)?

A. Amphetamine-like dopamine (DA)- and norepinephrine (NE)-releasing properties

B. Non-selective inhibition of both A and B forms of monoamine oxidase (MAO)

C. Irreversible inhibition of an enzyme that preferentially metabolizes NE and serotonin (5-HT)

D. Irreversible inhibition of an enzyme that preferentially metabolizes amines

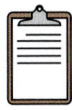

Patient evaluation on intake

- A 72-year-old male with the chief complaint of recurrent major depressive disorder (MDD)

Psychiatric history

- The patient has a 40-year history of MDD with a seasonal component (seasonal affective disorder, SAD) treated with phenelzine (Nardil) for 25–30 years. Doses were adjusted based on the season, with higher doses required during the fall and winter (as high as 45 mg twice per day), and lower doses required during the summer and spring (as low as 15 mg daily). He experienced periods of anxiety, elevated mood, and agitation when higher doses were taken going into the summer and spring
- His depression is characterized by features consistent with atypical depression, including fatigue, hypersomnia (sleeping about 12 hours or more per day), and lack of energy and motivation
- The onset of depressive symptoms coincided with a shift in his job, going from working outside as an agricultural appraiser to working primarily inside as a loan officer at the same bank, suggesting that there may be a seasonal component to his depression

- The patient has been hospitalized for severe depression and suicidal ideations on two occasions
- Phenelzine (a monoamine oxidase inhibitor, MAOI) was discontinued in preparation for cardiovascular surgery but restarted after several months of unsuccessful trials of duloxetine (Cymbalta) (the patient had hallucinations), aripiprazole (Abilify), and bupropion (Wellbutrin)
- He noted that in the 18 months after his surgery, his depression seemed "different" in that he felt it was less severe. His dose was decreased from 45 mg twice per day to 30 mg twice per day during his hospitalization for orthostatic hypotension
- The patient has also had a trial of fluoxetine (Prozac), paroxetine (Paxil), imipramine (Tofranil), desipramine (Norpramin), and lithium in the past. He was maintained on phenelzine due to his favorable response to the medication
- At various points, the patient took trazodone (Desyrel), alprazolam (Xanax), clonazepam (Klonopin), and risperidone (Risperdal) to help with sleep, although he typically did not need sleep aides due to his problem primarily being hypersomnia rather than insomnia
- The patient has not been treated with electroconvulsive therapy or had abnormal results on his thyroid function tests

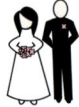

Social and personal history

- He is a former smoker and quit 28 years ago. He denies alcohol abuse or using any other recreational drugs
- He is happily married to his wife, who is a nurse
- The patient works as a loan officer at a bank

Medical history

- The patient has symptomatic idiopathic orthostatic hypotension, with a drop in blood pressure from 205/115 to 86/36 mmHg on standing. He has lost his balance a few times and had episodes of falls due to the drop in his blood pressure. However, he denies any full syncopal episodes
- He had paroxysmal atrial fibrillation, status post aortic valve replacement in 2012 with a pericardial tissue valve. Pulmonary vein isolation-ablation was performed at the time but was unsuccessful. He admitted he had syncopal episodes after his surgery
- He denied a history of stroke
- He admits fatigue, generalized weakness, and unsteadiness in the past, along with his labile blood pressure
- The patient underwent coronary angiography in the past, although the details are not quite clear

Family history

- His father passed away from kidney cancer
- There is no family history of sudden cardiac arrest
- There is no known psychiatric history

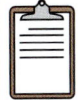

Patient evaluation on initial visit

- The patient presented with his wife who was well informed and helpful during the interview
- He was pleasant, cooperative, and relevant. He was alert and oriented to person, place, and time. He denied any psychotic symptoms and his thought process was normal
- He had normal affect, reported that he was in a good mood, and denied feeling "depressed", but noted that he was not in full remission. He denied any suicidal ideation
- He was diagnosed with recurrent MDD, severe without psychotic features, in partial remission. There was a possible past history of pharmacologically induced hypomania in response to a previous antidepressant, but the patient did not meet the diagnostic criteria for bipolar disorder

Question

Can individuals taking MAOIs use psychostimulants such as amphetamine derivatives?

- Yes
- No

Attending physician's mental notes: initial encounter

- Medications that increase NE should be used with caution with MAOIs
- Phenelzine (Nardil) is a non-selective inhibitor of both monoamine oxidase A and B. It does not have any amphetamine-like releasing properties of DA and NE. It preferentially metabolizes NE, 5-HT, and amines
- MAOIs can be very beneficial for many in the treatment of MDD. In this patient's case, however, he has had multiple side effects including symptomatic orthostatic hypotension, for which his current treatment with phenelzine cannot be ruled out as a potential contributing factor
- The patient has failed several trials of various medications including selective serotonin reuptake inhibitors (SSRIs), serotonin-norepinephrine reuptake inhibitors (SNRIs), and antipsychotics used for augmentation purposes

Question

The patient has a history of atypical depressive features including positive mood reactivity on occasion, hypersomnia but still feeling drowsy, and lack of energy, despite several trials of antidepressants and experiencing orthostatic hypotension with the current medication regimen. Which of the following would be your next step?

- Taper then stop phenelzine (Nardil) and attempt monotherapy with an SSRI
- Augment the current regimen with stimulants in addition to the phenelzine
- Augment the current regimen with mood stabilizers in addition to phenelzine
- Taper then stop phenelzine and attempt an SSRI and augment with stimulants

Attending physician's mental notes: initial encounter (continued)

- Many patients with atypical features can benefit from the addition of stimulants to their medication regimen. While this may be an acceptable strategy for some patients on MAOIs, in this patient's case, the side effects with the current medication regimen have already become worrisome

Case outcome

- Due to his depression having a seasonal component, the patient was advised to increase his amount of exposure to light (whether artificial or natural sunlight)
- The risk of a recurrent depressive episode while tapering the patient's phenelzine (Nardil), especially during the fall, was acknowledged and taken into account
- Because hypersomnia was a significant component of his depression, augmenting the patient's medication with a wakefulness-promoting medication such as modafinil (Provigil) or a stimulant was explored. The patient's ECG was normal
- Based on the above considerations, as well as the patient's past history of SSRI treatment failure, methylphenidate (Ritalin) was started initially at the low dose of 5 mg daily and increased to 10 mg three times per day, as phenelzine was concomitantly tapered and then discontinued; methylphenidate was switched to a once-a-day extended-release (ER) form (Concerta osmotic-controlled release oral delivery system (OROS)), which was then titrated against the patient's residual depressive symptoms. The methylphenidate ER

OROS was increased with continued improvement in mood and energy level, but at 72 mg every morning, the patient did not get to sleep as easily and on one occasion awoke early in the morning with intrusive anxious thoughts about being involuntarily psychiatrically hospitalized (an issue that had never been discussed or considered in the course of his treatment). Methylphenidate ER OROS was then decreased back to 54 mg every morning and risperidone (Risperdal) 0.25 mg at bedtime was added, with normalization of sleep and full remission of the patient's anxious ruminations. The patient reported feeling a little more vulnerable to dysphoric mood setbacks in the face of day-to-day situational stressors on the lower dose of methylphenidate ER OROS, and at that point escitalopram (Lexapro) was introduced at 5 mg and later increased to 10 mg every morning

- The patient has been stable and his depression in remission on this medication regimen without further adjustment for the past 7 years, even during the fall and winter

Current medications

- Methylphenidate (Concerta) ER OROS 54 mg every morning
- Escitalopram (Lexapro) 10 mg every morning
- Risperidone (Risperdal) 0.25 mg at bedtime
- Flecainide (Tambocor) 75 mg three times per day
- Fludrocortisone (Florinef) 0.1 mg three times per day
- Digoxin (Lanoxin) 0.125 mg daily
- Warfarin (Coumadin) 5 mg daily
- Aspirin 81 mg daily
- Midodrine (Amatine)
- Vitamin B complex
- Vitamin D_3

Case debrief

- A 72-year-old male presented to us with recurrent major depression with a seasonal component and atypical features
- The patient was put on a trial of various medications for his depressive symptoms, but none of them proved to be effective. Phenelzine (Nardil), an MOAI, was prescribed, which improved his symptoms. Due to the favorable effects of the medication, the patient was maintained on phenelzine, even though it is known to have several side effects including orthostatic hypotension, hypertensive crisis, and sympathomimetic effects
- The patient had a history of heart problems and noted significant orthostatic hypotension. He also admitted having falls and losing

his balance, likely due to his steep drop in blood pressure when he stands up

- His cardiologist recommended starting the patient on a different medication due to the contribution of phenelzine to the patient's orthostatic hypotension
- After much consideration, the patient was prescribed a stimulant along with an antidepressant, which he has been taking for 7 years
- The patient is currently doing well and is stable on his medications

Take-home points

- Many individuals with symptoms consistent with SAD benefit from a form of light therapy and increasing the amount of time outdoors in natural sunlight
- With the high prevalence of treatment-resistant depression, many first-line pharmacotherapies have been unsuccessful in improving patients' symptoms. Research suggests that augmenting antidepressants, such as with stimulants, may be an effective way to modality for treatment-resistant depression
- Methylphenidate (Concerta) and dextroamphetamine (Dexedrine), which inhibit the uptake of DA and NE, are used to treat attention-deficit/hyperactivity disorder (ADHD). However, several studies have explored their efficacy in treating depression, both as an adjunct to antidepressants and as monotherapy
- In a case series, patients with dysthymia and major depression showed a quick, sustained response to stimulant augmentation.[4] The response to these medications seems to vary, as another trial found that 30–34% of patients who received stimulants as monotherapy or augmentation reported mood improvement, while 36% reported no improvement.[4] When stimulants were offered to patients with bipolar depression, patients reported less depression and sedation
- Interestingly, patients with depression and traumatic brain injury showed a favorable response to methylphenidate as monotherapy. In one study, methylphenidate monotherapy reduced depression just as well as sertraline (Zoloft), improved cognition and fatigue, improved daytime sleepiness (while it did not with sertraline), and was better tolerated than sertraline[4]
- Stimulants are particularly effective in treating acute depression because they are quick acting and have generally been well tolerated. Stimulants should especially be considered for treatment of depression in those who are medically fragile or are recovering from a stroke

Tips and pearls

- MAOI myths debunked:
  - There is no absolute contraindication to using stimulants simultaneously; use with caution
  - To be used with caution with local or generalized anesthesia containing epinephrine, which could raise blood pressure
  - Sympathomimetic decongestants may also be used with caution
- Evidence for utilizing stimulants in the treatment of depression
  - Subjectively, a diagnosis of MDD is a culmination of various symptoms within a certain span of time. Each symptom is a piece of the puzzle that ultimately produces the complete picture
  - Each piece of the puzzle can theoretically be mapped to a certain area of the brain (Figure 12.1)

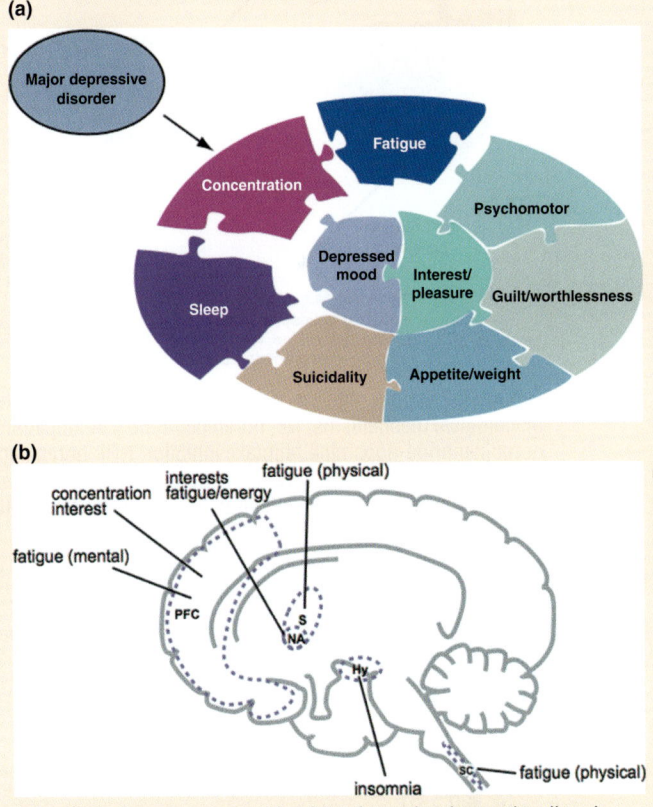

Figure 12.1. Symptom-based algorithm for major depressive disorder with hypothetical brain circuit mapping. (a) Symptom-based algorithm for antidepressants: deconstructing the most common residual diagnostic symptoms. (b) Match the most common residual symptoms to the hypothetically malfunctioning brain circuits. From Stahl (2013).

– Increases in NE and DA improve concentration and fatigue, which is affected by SNRIs, norepinephrine-dopamine reuptake inhibitors (NDRIs), and MAOI antidepressants but also by atypical antipsychotics, lithium, thyroid hormones, and stimulants – one of the reasons these are useful as augmenting agents in treatment-resistant depression (Figure 12.2)

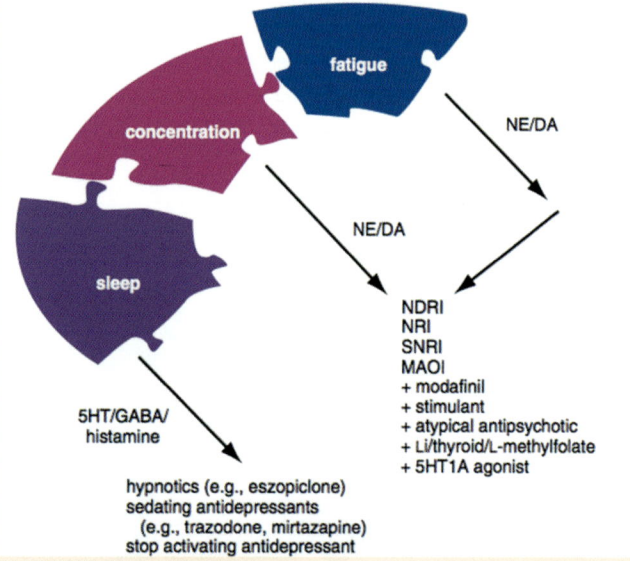

Target Regulatory Neurotransmitters With Selected Pharmacological Mechanisms

Figure 12.2. Target regulatory neurotransmitters with selected pharmacological mechanisms. NE: norepinephrine; DA: dopamine; NDRI: norepinephrine-dopamine reuptake inhibitor; NRI: norepinephrine-reuptake inhibitor; SNRI: serotonin-norepinephrine reuptake inhibitor; MAOI: monoamine oxidase inhibitor; Li: lithium; 5-HT: serotonin; GABA: γ-aminobutyric acid. From Stahl (2013).

Posttest self-assessment question and answer

Which of the following is NOT a mechanism of action of phenelzine (Nardil)?

A. Amphetamine-like DA- and NE-releasing properties
B. Non-selective inhibition of both A and B forms of MAO
C. Irreversible inhibition of an enzyme that preferentially metabolizes NE and 5-HT
D. Irreversible inhibition of an enzyme that preferentially metabolizes amines

Answer: A

While some MAOIs do have amphetamine properties such as tranylcypromine and selegiline, phenelzine does NOT have amphetamine properties. Phenelzine is non-selective and inhibits both MAO subtypes, A and B. The primary substrates of MAO subtype A are 5-HT and NE, the two monoamines most closely linked to depression. The primary substrates of MAO subtype B are trace amines including phenethylamine.

References

1. Grady M, Stahl SM. Practical guide for prescribing MAOI: debunking myths and removing barriers. *CNS Spectr* 2012; 17:2–10. https://doi.org/10.1017/S109285291200003X

2. Huffman JC, Stern TA. Using psychostimulants to treat depression in the medically ill. *Prim Care Companion J Clin Psychiatry* 2004; 6:44–6. https://doi.org/10.4088/pcc.v06n0109

3. Lee H, Kim S-W, Kim J-M, et al. Comparing effects of methylphenidate, sertraline and placebo on neuropsychiatric sequelae in patients with traumatic brain injury. *Hum Psychopharmacol* 2005; 20:97–104. https://doi.org/10.1002/hup.668

4. Pary R, Scarff J, Jijakli A, et al. A review of psychostimulants for adults with depression. *Fed Pract* 2015; 32:30S–37S.

5. Stahl SM. Antidepressants. In: *Stahl's Essential Psychopharmacology: Prescriber's Guide*, 4th edn. New York, NY: Cambridge University Press, 2013; pp. 335–58.

6. Stahl SM, Felker A. Monoamine oxidase inhibitors: a modern guide to an unrequited class of antidepressants. *CNS Spectr* 2008; 13:855–70. https://doi.org/10.1017/s1092852900016965

Case 13: A not-so-simple case of anxiety

The Question: What should you do when a patient with no history of mental illness presents with sudden psychiatric complaints, significant behavioral changes, and a variety of physical symptoms?

The Psychopharmacological Dilemma: How to appropriately evaluate patients presenting with a broad range of symptoms, including physical, psychiatric, and behavioral, in order to prevent misdiagnosis of a disease

Karla P. Furlong, Roberto Castaños, and Bo Ram Yoo

Pretest self-assessment questions (answers at the end of the case)

Which of the following is not a clinical manifestation that should raise suspicion for an autoimmune condition?

A. Headache
B. Psychosis
C. Seizures
D. Acute behavioral change
E. None of the above

Up to what percentage of autoimmune cases may present with psychiatric symptoms?

A. 5%
B. 10%
C. 50%
D. 70%
E. 95%

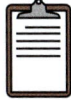

Patient evaluation on intake

- A 15-year-old female presents to the emergency room complaining of anxiety and panic attacks for over 1 month
- She admits to nervousness, intermittent sweating and hot flashes, fatigue, decreased appetite, vomiting, and unintended 20 lb weight loss during this time period

Psychiatric history

- The patient reports a history of anxiety and mild depression for 1 month. She has had no events of anxiety or depression prior to this
- She denies having any previous psychiatric hospitalizations, suicidal attempts, manic or psychotic episodes
- She admits to going to two therapy sessions to deal with anxiety without any benefit

- Specifically, she denies having any previous history of anxiety, anorexia, or bulimia
- No aversions to food are reported
- No body image issues are identified

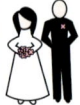

Social and personal history

- The patient is a high-school student, single, and with no children
- She reports having good grades in school throughout her life
- She denies having any history of behavioral issues
- She lives with her father, mother, and two brothers
- She admits to having a supportive family environment
- She admits to recent stress related to a bad grade in AP European History
- She denies any history of verbal, physical, or sexual abuse
- She denies any history of alcohol, tobacco, and/or drug use
- She denies being sexually active
- She denies any bullying at school
- Her family reports that she is very shy and has been nervous about going to school recently due to worsening grades

Medical history

- The patient has a history of asthma and allergic rhinitis

Family history

- The patient denies having any family history of mental illness
- She does, however, admit a family history significant for autoimmune diseases, including systemic lupus erythematosus (SLE), Grave's disease and juvenile rheumatoid arthritis in her brother
- There is a history of hypo- and hyperthyroidism in her uncle, aunt, and cousin

Current medications

- The patient denies being on any medications prior to her presentation

Patient evaluation on initial visit

- The patient reports that she started feeling severely anxious 1 month ago, resulting in decreased appetite. She had attributed her anxiety to stress from school, given her recent decline in academic performance

- Over the following month, she quickly deteriorated, and began experiencing hot flashes, sweating, severe fatigue, palpitations, and significant weight loss
- She eventually refused to go to school and became more withdrawn
- Her family noticed that she was staying in her room most of the day and was unusually tearful. She was not eating much, felt nauseated, and continued to rapidly lose weight
- Her mother became increasingly concerned as she witnessed her daughter's worsening physical and mental state. She could not find any explanation for the patient's sudden behavioral changes; they seemed quite out of character. She finally decided to bring the patient to the emergency room for a prompt psychiatric evaluation. She wanted her daughter to get help
- Upon arrival, the patient was admitted for workup, and the psychiatric consultation/liaison service was consulted

Attending physician's mental notes: initial evaluation

- The evaluation shows a young, thin, and tearful girl, with long brown hair in a hospital gown
- She is shy and appears embarrassed by all the attention from hospital staff
- She has some difficulty explaining her symptoms but admits to feeling most debilitated by her "nervousness" and sudden "panic attacks"
- After a detailed history was obtained, the consultation/liaison team recommended a thorough workup due to the patient's rapid decline, the absence of psychiatric history in both patient and family, and a positive family history for autoimmune disease
- The diagnosis given was "anxiety disorder due to another medical condition"
- Deep diaphragmatic breathing exercises were recommended by the psychiatry consult and liaison service

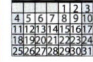

Case outcome

- Her laboratory results show leukocytosis, hematuria, proteinuria, microcytic anemia, elevated erythrocyte sedimentation rate and C-reactive protein, elevated blood urea nitrogen/creatinine, positive anti-nuclear antibodies, positive anti-myeloperoxidase antibodies, positive perinuclear anti-neutrophil cytoplasmic antibodies, and elevated factor VIII
- Days later, a kidney biopsy shows anti-neutrophil cytoplasmic antibody (ANCA)-associated crescentic glomerulonephritis

- Eventually, the workup confirms that the patient is suffering from microscopic polyangiitis
- In this patient, her autoimmune condition had initially manifested with symptoms of severe anxiety and perceived panic attacks
- She was treated with cyclophosphamide and mycophenolate

Tips and pearls

- ANCA-associated vasculitides comprises a group of diseases that occurs when neutrophils attack small and medium vessels throughout the body
- Clinical signs can vary widely, as they may affect several different organs, including the kidney, gastrointestinal tract, and lung
- Treatment of these diseases includes glucocorticoids, cyclophosphamide, and autoimmune drugs such as rituximab
- Once diagnosed, they are considered chronic diseases requiring long-term immunosuppressive therapy
- ANCA-associated vasculitides are rare, and pose diagnostic challenges, often resulting in a diagnostic delay of more than 6 months in one-third of patients
- A detailed history is necessary, as well as assessment of inflammatory markers, kidney function, and serological testing. A biopsy should be considered
- Differentiating autoimmune from psychiatric disorders can be challenging, especially as a large number of studies suggest that immune dysregulation plays a role in the pathogenesis of various psychiatric disorders. Additionally, inflammatory markers have been known to be elevated in the cerebrospinal fluid and blood of patients with psychosis. These have also been linked to an increased risk of psychotic disorders in children and adolescents
- Several autoantibodies have been identified to act on specific synaptic sites in the brain. Therefore, psychiatrists should remain vigilant for the possibility of mistaking an autoimmune disorder for a psychiatric disorder, as such cases can initially present to psychiatrists for evaluation
- One example is neuropsychiatric SLE (NPSLE), which often presents to psychiatrists first. Compared with patients diagnosed with SLE without neuropsychiatric symptoms, patients diagnosed with NPSLE have higher serum and cerebrospinal fluid levels of neuronal surface antibodies. Cases of NPSLE presenting as bipolar disorder have been reported previously, along with other common symptoms including headaches, seizures, mood disorders, psychosis, and movement disorders. The diagnosis of SLE is complicated in psychiatry by the fact that there is a

temporal component –SLE should present before neuropsychiatric symptoms. However, studies indicate that neuropsychiatric symptoms often present before the diagnosis of SLE. Furthermore, the lack of diagnostic tests for SLE as well as definitive clinical symptoms limits accurate diagnosis. Thus, an attempt to paint the full picture of the disease requires neuroimaging, immunoserological tests, and assessments from neurology, psychiatry, and rheumatology

- Clinical symptoms that should raise suspicion for autoimmune conditions include: atypical psychiatric presentations, acute/subacute behavioral or personality changes, a family history of autoimmunity, hypo- or hyperthyroidism, kidney disease, memory deficits, and autonomic instability

Case debrief

- A thin and tearful 15-year-old female was brought to the emergency room by her mother for psychiatric evaluation. The patient admitted to nervousness, intermittent hot flashes and sweating, unintended weight loss, and a decreased appetite for over 1 month
- Prior to the development of physical symptoms, the patient experienced mostly anxiety, which she attributed to stress from school
- Neither she nor her family had a prior psychiatric history
- The family history was significant for autoimmune diseases
- A thorough workup revealed microscopic polyangiitis, which had initially manifested as anxiety in this patient

Take-home points

- Failing to diagnose an autoimmune disease masked as a psychiatric disorder can have devastating consequences and in some cases be potentially fatal
- Journalist Susannah Cahalan aimed to raise awareness of her own experience with autoimmunity in her book, *Brain on Fire*.[1] In it, she describes her experience with anti-*N*-methyl-D-aspartate (NMDA) encephalitis and how it was misdiagnosed as bipolar disorder. Her disease initially presented with psychiatric symptoms and behavioral changes before it evolved into seizures and catatonia
- Forms of vasculitis, such as microscopic polyangiitis, are uncommon and thus may go unrecognized. Symptoms can be non-specific and result in delayed diagnosis or treatment. A high index of suspicion is essential for the prompt diagnosis and treatment of autoimmune diseases

- In summary, when a patient presents with a new onset of psychiatric symptoms associated with physical complaints, it is important to consider autoimmune causes

Posttest self-assessment questions and answers

Which of the following is not a clinical manifestation that should raise suspicion for an autoimmune condition?

A. Headache
B. Psychosis
C. Seizures
D. Acute behavioral change
E. None of the above

Answer: E

All of these are symptoms that should prompt additional workup of other possible diagnoses such as autoimmune disorders.

Up to what percentage of autoimmune cases may present with psychiatric symptoms?

A. 5%
B. 10%
C. 50%
D. 70%
E. 95%

Answer: E

It is estimated that up to 95% of patients with systemic lupus erythematosus can present with psychiatric symptoms.

References

1. Cahalan S. *Brain on Fire: My Month of Madness.* New York: Simon and Schuster, 2013.
2. Jeppesen R, Benros ME. Autoimmune diseases and psychotic disorders. *Front Psychiatry* 2019; 10:131. https://doi.org/10.3389/fpsyt.2019.00131
3. Kayser MS, Dalmau J. The emerging link between autoimmune disorders and neuropsychiatric disease. *J Neuropsychiatry Clin Neurosci* 2011; 23:90–7. https://doi.org/10.1176/jnp.23.1.jnp90
4. Psyche Scene Hub. Autoimmune diseases masquerading as psychiatric disorders – a paradigm shift. 2016. Available from: https://psychscenehub.com/psychinsights/autoimmune-diseases-masquerading-psychiatric-disorders-paradigm-shift-psychiatry/(accessed March 26, 2021).
5. Rege S, Hodgkinson SJ. Immune dysregulation and autoimmunity in bipolar disorder: synthesis of the evidence and its clinical

application.*Aust N Z J Psychiatry* 2013; 47:1136–51. https://doi
.org/10.1177/0004867413499077

6. Vaillant AAJ, Mohammed W, Vuma S, Anderson N. Autoimmunity in
   neurological and psychiatric disorders: participation of antibodies and
   cytokines in the immunopathogenesis of these diseases. *Immunome
   Res* 2015; 11:089. https://doi.org/10.4172/1745-7580.1000089

7. Vasculitis Foundation. Microscopic polangiitis. Available from:
   https://www.vasculitisfoundation.org/education/forms/microscopic-
   polyangiitis/ (accessed March 26, 2021).

Case 14: I'm a woman in a man's body

The Question: I'm not a specialist in this area. What can I do to help recognize and alleviate gender dysphoria?

The Psychopharmacological Dilemma: Finding an effective regimen for the treatment of gender dysphoria while juggling with comorbid depression and anxiety

Sarah Grace, Matt Jason V. Llamas, and Jami Woods

Prestest self-assessment question (answer at the end of the case)

Which of the following pharmacological regimens is NOT included in the treatment of gender dysphoria in transgender women?

A. Micronized progesterone
B. Estradiol
C. Testosterone
D. Spironolactone (Aldactone)

Patient evaluation on intake

- A 25-year-old transgender female with the chief complaints of recurrent depression and gender dysphoria

Psychiatric history

- The patient has a 15-year history of depressed mood, decreased interest, avolition, anhedonia, apathy, decreased self-worth, and passive suicidal ideations with one suicide attempt at age 17
- She has no history of manic episodes or psychosis. She denies any history of sexual abuse and reports no alcohol or drug use
- She realized she was a female on the inside when she was about 10 years old. She was assigned as male at birth and expressed as male for her entire life until 24 months ago
- She exhibited a preference for cross-dressing and, as a young child, "he" preferred make-believe play with the girls next door
- She has a very strong disgust for her lower body anatomy, causing her to suffer from a dysphoric mood and experience difficulty in social situations given her incongruence between her gender identity and her sexual anatomy

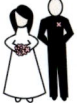

Social and personal history

- She is single
- She attended an evangelical school growing up
- She has had little contact with her family of origin after sharing her gender identity
- She has a strong preference for female friends over male friends

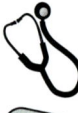

Medical history

- There is no history of medical illnesses

Current medications

- Bupropion extended-release (Aplenzin) 300 mg every morning
- Escitalopram (Lexapro) 10 mg daily

Attending physician's mental notes: initial evaluation

- The patient was awake, alert, friendly, and cooperative with good affective reactivity, good spontaneous movements, good expressive gestures, and good eye contact
- She denied any suicidal ideations, remained future-oriented, and displayed no evidence of any positive formal thought disorder, bizarre behavior, delusional thinking, internal preoccupation, flight of ideas, pressured speech, psychomotor agitation, or psychomotor retardation
- The best diagnosis for this patient may be recurrent major depressive disorder (MDD), moderate without psychotic features, and gender dysphoria

Further investigation

What steps can the healthcare provider take to help alleviate the patient's gender dysphoria?

- Assess for gender dysphoria using DSM-5 criteria
- Manage any coexisting mental health concerns. The presence of coexisting mental health issues does not necessarily preclude possible changes in gender role or access to feminizing/masculinizing hormones or surgery; rather, these concerns need to be optimally managed prior to concurrent treatments for gender dysphoria
- Provide information regarding options for gender identity and expression, and possible medical interventions
- While many interventions are outside the scope of practice for most psychiatrists, it is within every psychiatrist/psychiatric nurse practitioner's ability to provide these resources
- Assess for comorbid anxiety symptoms, substance abuse, eating disorders, and autistic spectrum disorders (as peer-reviewed data demonstrates that individuals with gender dysphoria are at higher risk for autism spectrum disorders)
- Assess the need for psychotherapy. Psychotherapy – although highly recommended – is not a requirement for hormone

confirmation therapy or gender confirmation surgery. The general goal of psychotherapy is to find ways to maximize a person's overall psychological well-being, quality of life, and self-fulfillment. Therapy may consist of: individual psychotherapy designed to identify core maladaptive assumptions, selective abstractions, errors in judgment, and overgeneralizations regarding their transition; couples psychotherapy designed to help the patient's significant other participate in the process; or family therapy. Psychotherapy is not intended to alter a person's gender identity; rather, it may help an individual to explore gender concerns and find ways to alleviate gender dysphoria if present[1]

- Educate and advocate on behalf of patients within their community and assist with making changes in identity documents
- Provide information and referral for peer support

What are the criteria for hormone therapy in patients with gender dysphoria?

- Persistent, well-documented gender dysphoria
- The capacity to make a fully informed decision and to consent for treatment
- Age of majority in the patient's given country (or younger, if World Professional Association for Transgender Health (WPATH) guidelines/standards of care are followed)
- If significant medical or mental health concerns are present, they must be reasonably well controlled
- Feminizing or masculinizing hormone therapy is a medically necessary intervention for many transgender individuals with gender dysphoria. Some people seek maximum feminization/ masculinization, while others experience gender dysphoria relief with a more androgynous/non-binary presentation resulting from more minimal hormonal manipulation of existing secondary sex characteristics. For the treating professional to initiate hormone therapy, a psychosocial assessment must have been completed and informed consent must have been obtained

Attending physician's mental notes: initial evaluation (continued)

- As mentioned, some form of feminizing hormone therapy in addition to antidepressants is likely necessary for this patient
- Transdermal estradiol does not appear to be associated with increased risk of blood clots or breast cancer in comparison with other forms of estrogen hormone therapy

- Testosterone blockers such as spironolactone (Aldactone), leuprorelin (Lupron), bicalutamide (Casodex), and finasteride (Proscar) diminish masculine characteristics such as body hair
- There is anecdotal evidence in the transgender female population that progesterone increases breast size and areolar maturation

Case outcome

- The patient was continued on bupropion extended-release (Aplenzin) 300 mg daily and escitalopram (Lexapro) 10 mg daily for MDD
- After screening laboratory tests, she was started on feminization hormone therapy
- She demonstrated almost immediate improvement, and after a period of about 8 months, she underwent vaginoplasty (removal of her penis and testicles in the formation of a neovagina and clitoris)
- After 1 year, her depression, which she had endured for approximately 15 years, was in remission

Tips and pearls

Pharmacological treatment of the transgender female

- Estrogen
    - Use of the birth control pill estrogen (ethinyl estradiol) appears to increase the risk of blood clots. Because of this, it is generally not recommended as a pharmacological treatment for the transgender female. Older conjugated estrogens also appear to have a very small but statistically significant increased risk of blood clots and breast cancer (Women's health initiative). However, as stated previously, transdermal estradiol does not appear to be associated with an increased risk of blood clots or breast cancer
    - WPATH guidelines recommend a 17β-estradiol level of 100–200 pg/ml. The estradiol tablets that are currently available are the bioidentical hormone and, if given sublingually, bypass the liver, giving a higher blood level with less activation of clotting mechanisms. Injectable estrogen appears to be relatively safe as it is also the bioidentical hormone
    - The decision was made in the patient's case to start her on transdermal estradiol 0.1 mg/24 hours, one patch weekly, and was raised to two patches weekly after a couple of months, which gave her a 17β-estradiol level of 153 pg/ml
- Testosterone blockers
    - A combination of estrogen and androgen-blocking medications is the most commonly studied regimen for feminization

These drugs block testosterone, thus diminishing masculine characteristics such as body hair. They also minimize the dosage of estrogen needed to suppress testosterone, thereby reducing the risks associated with high-dose exogenous estrogen administration[4]

- Examples of anti-androgens include spironolactone (Aldactone), gonadotropin-releasing hormone (GnRH) agonists such as leuprorelin (Lupron) and bicalutamide (Casodex), and 5α-reductase inhibitors such as finasteride (Proscar), which block the conversion of testosterone to its more active metabolite 5α-dihydrotestosterone. As such, they give a partial androgen reduction in activity but not as pronounced as the direct testosterone blockers. Spironolactone is a very old potassium-sparing diuretic, which, at normal doses, blocks aldosterone and is used as an antihypertensive and in congestive heart failure. However, at higher doses of about 200 or 300 mg daily, it seems to function as at least a partial antagonist at the testosterone receptor. Side effects include orthostasis, possible hyperkalemia, dizziness, and polyuria. Bicalutamide, in contrast, is a non-steroidal anti-androgen that is FDA approved for the treatment of prostate cancer in men. As it is specific for the testosterone receptor, there are very few unwanted side effects
- The patient chose bicalutamide 50 mg daily. Extraordinarily rare occurrences of elevated liver function enzymes have been associated with bicalutamide but the patient's liver function tests remained within normal limits

- Progesterone
  - The inclusion of progesterone is somewhat controversial because, as of 2020, there are no double-blind placebo-controlled randomized clinical trials that have evaluated the efficacy of micronized progesterone administration in the transgender female. There is, however, a wealth of data in the cisgender menopausal female that supports its usage and efficacy in treating depression, reducing cardiovascular risk, and improving sleep, and there is anecdotal evidence in the transgender female population that progesterone increases breast size and areolar maturation. It is important to use the bioidentical micronized progesterone over some of the progestins, such as medroxyprogesterone, as they appear to be associated with a very small increased risk of breast cancer and cardiovascular risk in cisgender women. Again, as is the case with estradiol, the bioidentical hormones appear to be associated with less risk

- The patient opted for micronized progesterone 200 mg PO at bedtime. She understands that a higher, more sustained blood level can be obtained with rectal administration

Pharmacological treatment of the transgender male

- Testosterone
  - Testosterone is available in the USA as the bioidentical hormone, which is preferred. While it can be given orally, this results in lower serum testosterone levels than non-oral preparations and has limited efficacy in suppressing menses.[3] Intramuscular (IM) testosterone may be given at a starting dosage of 20 mg IM per week with an average dose of about 50 mg IM per week. It is also available in creams and gels, although the IM preparation is much cheaper and gives 100% bioavailability
  - Concurrently, many transgender men choose to have oocyte freezing. The frozen gametes and embryo can later be used with a surrogate woman to carry to pregnancy

Case debrief

- It appears as though this patient had a partial response to bupropion extended-release (Aplenzin) 300 mg daily and escitalopram (Lexapro) 10 mg daily
- She was diagnosed with gender dysphoria by her treating health professional
- Because she has gender dysphoria, she was started on transdermal estradiol 0.1 mg/24 hours one patch weekly and increased to two patches weekly, in addition to bicalutamide (Casodex) 50 mg daily as a testosterone blocker. Additionally, she was administered micronized progesterone 200 mg at bedtime, which resulted in a significant improvement in her depressive symptomatology

Take-home points

- Gender dysphoria is frequently overlooked as a precipitating psychosocial stressor in patients with treatment-resistant depressive symptoms
- More than half of transgender individuals are forced to perform a false narrative at work
- Murders of transgender people in 2020 surpassed the *entire* murder rate of transgender individuals in 2019 in *just 7 months*, reflecting an emboldened stance against transgender individuals over the past 2 or 3 years

- 29% of transgender individuals said a doctor or other healthcare provider refused to see them because of their actual or perceived gender identity
- Approximately 40% of transgender individuals are rejected by their own families
- Depending on the age range, 40–73% of relationships end when a person transitions
- 13% of transgender women of color are currently homeless. They are 83 times more likely than the general population to be human immunodeficiency virus (HIV)-positive. They are denied visitation to see their children, and the average lifespan of a transgender woman of color is estimated to be 35–37 years
- Transgender individuals face horrific disparities in access to legal care, healthcare, education, and housing

Two-minute tutorial

Testosterone blockers

- Spironolactone (Aldactone)
  - A potassium-sparing diuretic that, at normal doses, blocks aldosterone and is used as an antihypertensive and in congestive heart failure
  - At higher doses of about 200 or 300 mg daily, it seems to function as at least a partial antagonist at the testosterone receptor
  - Side effects include orthostasis, hyperkalemia, dizziness, and polyuria
- Bicalutamide (Casodex)
  - A non-steroidal anti-androgen, that is FDA approved for the treatment of prostate cancer in men
  - It is specific for the testosterone receptor, with very few unwanted side effects
  - Rare occurrences of elevated liver function enzymes have been associated with its use
- Finasteride (Proscar)
  - A 5α-reductase inhibitor that blocks the conversion of testosterone to its more active metabolite 5α-dihydrotestosterone
  - It gives a partial androgen reduction in activity, but not as pronounced as the direct testosterone blockers

Physical effects of hormone replacement therapy

- Transgender male patients (female to male (FTM))

- Deepened voice
- Clitoral enlargement
- Growth of facial and body hair
- Cessation of menses
- Breast tissue atrophy
- Increased male libido
- Decreased percentage of body fat compared with muscle mass
- Transgender female patients (male to female (MTF))
  - Breast growth
  - Decreased male libido and erections
  - Testicular/penile atrophy
  - Increased percentage of body fat compared with muscle mass, with the body taking on a more gynoid appearance

Risk assessment and modification

- Absolute contraindications for feminizing hormone therapy (MTF)
  - Previous venous thromboembolism due to an underlying hypercoagulable state
  - History of estrogen receptor-positive breast cancer
  - End-stage chronic liver disease
- Absolute contraindications for masculinizing hormone therapy (FTM)
  - Pregnancy
  - Unstable coronary artery disease
  - Untreated polycythemia with a hematocrit of 55% or higher
- An increased risk of polycystic ovarian syndrome in transgender males has been noted, even in the absence of testosterone usage. Polycystic ovarian syndrome is associated with an increased risk of diabetes, cardiac disease, high blood pressure, and ovarian and endometrial cancers. Referral to an appropriate primary care physician for assessment of hypertension, weight, pulse, heart and lung examination, examination of the extremities for peripheral edema, localized swelling, a Pap smear for transgender males, and mammography for transgender female should be obtained

Posttest self-assessment question and answer

Which of the following pharmacological regimens is NOT included in the treatment of gender dysphoria in transgender women?

A. Micronized progesterone
B. Estradiol
C. Testosterone
D. Spironolactone (Aldactone)

Answer: C
Testosterone is the preferred treatment for transgender men, but testosterone blockers such as spironolactone reduce the effect of circulating testosterone, allowing a lower dose of feminizing estrogen for transgender women.

References

1. Bockting WO, Knudson G, Goldberg JM. Counseling and mental health care of transgender adults and loved ones. *Int J Transgend* 2006; 9:35–82. https://doi.org/10.1300/J485v09n03_03
2. Coleman E, Bockting W, Botzer M, et al. Standards of care for the health of transsexual, transgender, and gender-nonconforming people, version 7. *Int J Transgend* 2012; 13:165–232. https://doi.org/10.1080/15532739.2011.700873
3. Feldman J, Safer J. Hormone therapy in adults: suggested revisions to the sixth version of the *Standards of Care. Int J Transgend* 2009; 11:146–82. https://doi.org/10.1080/15532730903383757
4. Prior JC, Watson YM, Diewold P, Robinow O. Spironolactone in the presurgical therapy of male to female transsexuals: philosophy and experience of the Vancouver gender dysphoria clinic. *J Sex Info and Edu Cncl of Can* 1986; 1: 1–7.

Case 15: The spacey, fidgety son with overwhelming sadness

The Question: How to manage adolescent depression with comorbid attention-deficit/hyperactivity disorder (ADHD)?

The Psychopharmacological Dilemma: Being cognizant of possible drug interactions when selecting antidepressants in adolescents who also require treatment for ADHD

Niya Larios, Casey Lester, and Carl Feinstein

Pretest self-assessment (answer at the end of the case)

Which of the following are first-line, evidence-based pharmacological treatments for major depressive disorder (MDD) in adolescents?

A. Sertraline (Zoloft)
B. Escitalopram (Lexapro)
C. Citalopram (Celexa)
D. Fluvoxamine (Luvox)
E. Fluoxetine (Prozac)
F. Paroxetine (Paxil)

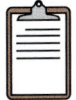

Patient evaluation on intake

- A 13-year-old male brought in by his mother with the chief complaints of depression, passive suicidal ideation, frequent depressed or irritable moods, decreased interest in previously pleasurable activities, social withdrawal, hypersomnia, fatigue, impaired concentration, and poor attention to activities of daily living for around 4 months

Psychiatric history

- The patient was diagnosed with attention-deficit/hyperactivity disorder (ADHD; combined presentation) in 5th grade, 3 years prior to presentation, and has been taking atomoxetine (Strattera) during that time
- He has been in therapy over the past 10 years
- There is no known history of suicide attempts or hospitalizations
- He is currently experiencing 4 months of continued ADHD symptoms, passive suicidal ideation, frequent depressed or irritable moods, decreased interest in previously pleasurable activities, social withdrawal, hypersomnia, fatigue, impaired concentration, and poor attention

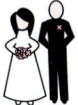

Social and personal history

- The patient is a child of a single mother
- He was in 8th grade at the time of evaluation

- Prior to this appointment, he earned grades of Cs, Ds, and Fs in his classes
- He has a 504 Plan, which is a civil rights law under the federal Rehabilitation Act of 1973 that requires that school districts construct a broad and informal free educational plan in accordance with a child's identified disability. He has never had an Individualized Education Plan (IEP) – a law under the Disabilities Education Act that requires a detailed and formalized educational plan for a student with disabilities that must be renewed yearly
- He is noted to have a history of being bullied, mainly verbal abuse by his peers
- His mother suspects he may have been sexually abused by an adult male around age 5. She noted that he occasionally made comments alluding to sexual trauma
- He has no known history of substance use
- He has no history of legal trouble
- Developmental history
  - His mother experienced domestic violence in the third trimester of pregnancy, placing the pregnancy in a higher risk category
  - There were no complications of labor and he was considered healthy at birth
  - His speech was initially delayed, improving around age 2–3, when he underwent ear canal therapy
  - Toilet training was delayed until age 4, and he experienced enuresis until age 12

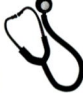

Medical history

- Vitamin D deficiency. He has been recommended by his primary care physician (PCP) to increase his sunlight exposure and vitamin D intake
- He has history of a hearing problem caused by scar tissue build-up around one ear, which led to early trouble with speech and hearing but improved after surgical repair around age 2–3
- He has a sulfa allergy
- He was noted to have unusually large ears
- He has no other known medical issues

Family history

- His biological father's family history is unknown
- Mother, maternal grandfather, and maternal aunt with depression
- Uncle and great uncle with bipolar disorder
- Great aunt and great uncle with schizophrenia

- Mother, grandmother, great aunt, and great uncle with anxiety
- Mother with ADHD

Current medications

- Atomoxetine (Strattera) 50 mg every morning

Question

To the best of your knowledge, is atomoxetine (Strattera) the first-line, evidence-based treatment for ADHD?

- Yes
- No

Attending physician's mental notes: initial evaluation

- A mental status examination was consistent with depression
- While terminal insomnia is classic for adult MDD, hypersomnia is common in adolescents with MDD
- The most likely diagnosis is MDD
- The patient has a family history of schizophrenia, and schizophrenia prodrome could explain his depressive and ADHD-like symptoms
- His family history of bipolar disorder should raise suspicion for bipolar depression
- This patient has experienced significant adverse childhood events (ACEs) such as possible sexual abuse, parental separation, and mental illness in the household. ACEs are linked to adverse mental health outcomes such as depression, anxiety, posttraumatic stress disorder (PTSD), and suicide
- PTSD should always be considered as an alternate explanation for depressive and ADHD-like symptoms in a patient with a history of trauma. However, there was no clear history of intrusion symptoms in this patient
- This patient's unusually large ears raise concern for fragile X syndrome, which is associated with hyperactivity, intellectual disability (ID), and deficits in social interaction. He could be referred for genetic testing
- Stimulants are the first-line treatment for ADHD and should be tried, unless there is a strong parental preference for a non-stimulant or if stimulants are contraindicated. Contraindications include a history of substance abuse, tics, and comorbid anxiety. Once the mood is stabilized, a trial of stimulants should be undertaken
- Fluoxetine (Prozac) is FDA approved for treatment of MDD in patients aged 8 and up
- Escitalopram (Lexapro) was FDA approved in 2009 for treatment of MDD in patients aged 12 and up

- Subsequent review articles pointed out that, at the time of FDA approval of escitalopram, only one randomized controlled trial had shown positive results, while another had shown negative results.[4,10] A previous trial of citalopram (Celexa; which is a racemic mix of *S*-citalopram and *R*-citalopram, while escitalopram is pure *S*-citalopram) had also been cited as indirect evidence of the efficacy of escitalopram

- Fluoxetine and escitalopram have never been directly compared in a high-quality randomized controlled trial

- A meta-analysis comparing the efficacy of different selective serotonin reuptake inhibitors (SSRIs) found no difference between escitalopram and fluoxetine, although the authors acknowledged statistical power was low due to the small number of studies available[22]

- The American Academy of Child and Adolescent Psychiatry (AACAP) continues to recommend fluoxetine as the first-line pharmacological treatment for adolescent MDD

- Fluoxetine is a potent inhibitor of cytochrome P450 2D6 (CYP2D6), while escitalopram is not

- Atomoxetine (Strattera) is a substrate of CYP2D6 and thus concurrent use with fluoxetine can lead to higher-than-expected blood levels of atomoxetine

- As fluoxetine was started in this case, the patient and his family were educated regarding the possibility that fluoxetine might lead to increased blood levels of atomoxetine, leading to worsened adverse effects. Escitalopram is also approved in adolescents for MDD and, unlike fluoxetine, does not inhibit CYP2D6

- In contrast to adolescents and children, adult psychopharmacological treatment of MDD is selected primarily on the side-effect profile, potential for toxicity, drug interactions, and properties such as weight gain and sedation. SSRIs lack some of the safety, adverse effects, and drug–drug interaction concerns of other classes of antidepressants, making them an ideal starting point for treatment

Further investigation

Is there anything else you would especially like to know about this patient?

- Has the patient undergone any psychosocial interventions for ADHD?

    - The patient has been treated with pharmacotherapy for ADHD and has a 504 Plan, but psychosocial interventions for ADHD, such as an IEP have yet to be employed

- Has the patient taken stimulants in the past and suffered adverse effects?
  - He has never taken stimulants; atomoxetine (Strattera) was the selected initial treatment agreed upon by the family and provider

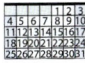

Case outcome: first interim follow-up at week 4

- He tolerated fluoxetine (Prozac) well
- His mood had improved and his mother observed that he was more socially interactive
- His inattention, poor task initiation, and poor organizational skills have persisted
- He continues to show vitamin D deficiency. He was advised to increase his sunlight exposure and vitamin D intake

Question

How would you manage the patient's residual ADHD symptoms despite previous success on atomoxetine (Strattera)?

- Discontinue atomoxetine and start a trial of a stimulant
- Increase the dosage of atomoxetine

Attending physician's mental notes: first interim follow-up at week 4

- While atomoxetine (Strattera) could be a good first-line treatment in some cases, this patient might benefit from a stimulant trial
- Methylphenidate (Concerta) and amphetamine, when tried sequentially, have an initial response rate of 85%. If the patient does not respond to one drug, the likelihood of a response to the other is high
- It is important to counsel parents regarding possible adverse effects of stimulants including insomnia, weight loss, anorexia, irritability, worsening of tics, nervousness, and dizziness

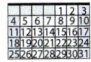

Case outcome: second and third interim follow-ups through weeks 10–14

- After the patient was tapered off atomoxetine (Strattera), his mother noticed that his hyperactivity seemed to worsen. He was suspended from school for disruptive classroom behavior
- Amphetamine/dextroamphetamine immediate-release 5 mg every morning (age-adjusted dosing) and amphetamine/ dextroamphetamine extended-release 5 mg daily were started
- The patient was adherent to this medication for 6 days, after which he discontinued due to feelings of anger and difficulty sleeping

- Atomoxetine was restarted and gradually increased to 40 mg in the morning and 25 mg in the afternoon

Question

Which of the following is the FDA maximum recommended daily dose of atomoxetine (Strattera) for children and adolescents who are normal metabolizers of CYP2D6 and who are not taking a CYP2D6 inhibitor?

- The lesser of 1.2 mg/kg/day or 60 mg
- The lesser of 0.75 mg/kg/day or 50 mg
- The lesser of 1.4 mg/kg/day or 100 mg

Attending physician's mental notes: second and third interim follow-ups through weeks 10–14

- Extended-release formulations of stimulants can present challenges concerning sleep, tics, appetite, and mood lability. Shorter-acting formulations present the challenge of continual dosing while the patient is taking classes, which would be disruptive to the learning environment
- If patients experience intolerable adverse effects of amphetamine/ dextroamphetamine, then the next most evidence-based step is a trial of methylphenidate (Concerta)
- As methylphenidate is not metabolized by CYP2D6, a trial of methylphenidate would have avoided potentially problematic drug– drug interactions with fluoxetine (Prozac)
- The needs of ADHD patients will vary depending on the developmental age. It is important to periodically review the patient's ADHD treatment plan and provide ongoing psychoeducational counseling. Strategies for managing ADHD also include behavioral training, use of daily report cards to motivate good behavior, establishing reward-based systems of positive reinforcement, and utilizing time outs

Case outcome: fourth through sixth interim follow-ups at weeks 20, 22, and 24

- After reaching the new dose of atomoxetine (Strattera), the patient started to report feeling sick, and his mother observed that he seemed unlike himself
- He had reduced back to the previous dose of 50 mg every morning due to intolerable side effects
- A 10 mg afternoon dose was added to address afternoon inattentiveness
- As fluoxetine (Prozac) had been effective for depression, it was continued

- He reported recently experiencing suicidal ideation with a plan, which had resolved by the time of evaluation
- Fluoxetine was increased to 20 mg daily
- He reported feeling less suicidal, and his mother noticed that he was spending more time outside
- His irritable moods continued, and he was noted to arrive late for his classes
- Fluoxetine was increased to 30 mg daily
- Two weeks later, he reported an improvement in his ability to get to school on time and socialize. His depressed mood persisted
- Fluoxetine was increased to 40 mg daily

Attending physician's mental notes: fourth through sixth interim follow-ups at weeks 20, 22, and 24

- Although the initial SSRI dosage for pediatric patients should be smaller than that for adults because of side effects, the suggested dosage between the groups is similar
- All SSRIs have a black box warning about possible increases in suicidal ideation in individuals under 24 years, but this patient's suicidal ideation has lessened overall. Also, although the risk of suicidal ideation is increased in this population, the risk of completed suicide has been found to be decreased
- For adults, if dose optimization fails to induce remission, an SSRI with adjunct treatment, such as bupropion (Wellbutrin) or buspirone (BuSpar), has been shown to increase remission rates in patients with MDD. Use of such adjunct treatments has not been sufficiently studied in adolescents

Question

Atomoxetine (Strattera) is metabolized by the CYP2D6 enzyme. Which SSRIs are known to have a strong inhibitory effect on this enzyme?

- Citalopram (Celexa)
- Sertraline (Zoloft)
- Fluoxetine (Prozac)
- Paroxetine (Paxil)

Case outcome: seventh, eighth, and ninth interim follow-ups at weeks 26, 29, and 34

- The patient complained of initial insomnia, poor appetite, racing thoughts, and increased disruptive classroom behavior
- Fluoxetine (Prozac) was stopped without taper due to its long half-life

- Escitalopram (Lexapro) was started due to its reduced tendency for CYP2D6 interactions compared with fluoxetine. It was titrated to 10 mg at bedtime
- Eight weeks after starting escitalopram, his mother reported that he seemed significantly better than when taking fluoxetine

Question

In your clinical experience, how important do you find a discussion on psychotropic medication non-adherence with adolescent patients and their families?

- It depends on the drug being administered
- I underscore the importance of medication adherence at every visit

Attending physician's mental notes: seventh, eighth, and ninth interim follow-ups at weeks 26, 29, and 34

- The patient's adverse effects were most likely due to atomoxetine (Strattera)
- As they occurred after an increase in fluoxetine (Prozac) dose and without a change in atomoxetine dose, one can infer that it is due to drug–drug interactions. Fluoxetine exerts a strong inhibitory effect on CYP2D6, the metabolic enzyme utilized by atomoxetine, resulting in higher serum concentrations of atomoxetine
- Consequently, the patient should stop taking fluoxetine and replace it with another SSRI. Escitalopram (Lexapro) may be a good choice here because it is FDA approved in a patient of this age and is associated with fewer drug–drug interactions than some of the other medications in its class

Case outcome: 10th through 14th interim follow-ups through weeks 48–82

- The patient reported that he was currently failing most of his classes
- The teachers had contacted his mother to inform her that he was not completing his schoolwork
- He had recently stopped taking escitalopram (Lexapro) as it was not available at his pharmacy
- Escitalopram was reinitiated and increased to 15 mg daily
- Atomoxetine (Strattera) was increased to 60 mg in the morning and 10 mg in the afternoon
- His depression appeared to enter remission

Attending physician's mental notes: 10th through 14th interim follow-ups through weeks 48–82

- It is important to have discussions with this patient's mother regarding the importance of regular dosing with escitalopram (Lexapro), which is necessary for the drug's effectiveness
- Escitalopram has a shorter half-life than fluoxetine (Prozac); the patient's mother should understand that SSRIs with shorter half-lives are associated with acute withdrawal symptoms
- Medication adherence is an important topic that requires the understanding and collaboration of the patient, provider, patient's family, therapists, and school administrators

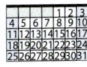

Case outcome: 15th through 37th follow-ups through weeks 86–186

- The patient presented to his PCP's office with scleral icterus and flattened affect, and his atomoxetine (Strattera) was reduced to 50 mg daily
- His symptoms improved; however, atomoxetine was tapered off due to concerns for hepatotoxicity. The patient subsequently began to struggle to complete schoolwork
- The results of a routine laboratory test showed elevated alkaline phosphatase. Over the next few months, the patient's alkaline phosphatase was followed (ranging from 293 to 443 IU/l, with a reported laboratory normal interval of 84–254 IU/l) as the patient was tapered off and later reinstated on atomoxetine due to its efficacy in managing the patient's ADHD symptoms. No elevations in transaminases were seen
- The patient's alkaline phosphatase level did not improve once atomoxetine was stopped. Next, escitalopram (Lexapro) was evaluated as the hepatotoxic causal medication and discontinued. His alkaline phosphatase levels began to trend down slowly (293 lowest assessed value), and the patient's depressive symptoms returned
- The patient's PCP suggested that the elevation in alkaline phosphatase might be related to a growth spurt, rather than to hepatotoxicity
- Escitalopram was reinstated, and the patient's depression entered remission and he remained stable upon transfer to an adult psychiatric clinic

Attending physician's mental notes: 15th through 37th follow-ups through weeks 86–186

- Elevated alkaline phosphatase is not always pathological in children and adolescents, especially in the absence of elevation of hepatic enzymes or bilirubin. Common benign causes include a growth spurt and transient hyperphosphatasemia of infancy and early childhood
- This patient has a history of vitamin D deficiency, and elevated alkaline phosphatase can be seen in rickets. Rechecking his vitamin D level would be useful in building a differential
- A full panel of hepatic function tests including aspartate transaminase/alanine transaminase (AST/ALT) and direct/indirect bilirubin would have been useful in understanding the significance of the patient's elevated alkaline phosphatase
- Serum γ-glutamyltransferase (GGT), which is specific to the liver, would have been useful in differentiating alkaline phosphatase from a bone source versus a hepatic source
- Aside from the elevated alkaline phosphatase, his episode of scleral icterus with lethargy is highly concerning for a more serious hepatic pathology
- Scant case reports indicate that atomoxetine (Strattera) may be a rare cause of hepatotoxicity
- Possible exposure to hepatotoxins such as alcohol or acetaminophen should be explored
- Some traditional herbal supplements such as pyrrolizidine alkaloids (e.g. *Echinacea purpurea*) can also be hepatotoxic and are often unreported by patients
- Risk factors for viral hepatitis, such as recent travel to endemic areas, should also be investigated. Acute hepatitis serological tests would be appropriate
- Wilson's disease is a cause of both psychiatric issues and hepatopathy. Taking a careful family history would be appropriate, and collecting serum ceruloplasmin would be reasonable

Question

Given the patient's elevated alkaline phosphatase and scleral icterus, should the patient continue on atomoxetine (Strattera)?

- Yes
- No

Case debrief

- The patient was diagnosed with MDD and comorbid ADHD and was initially treated with a combination of fluoxetine (Prozac) and atomoxetine (Strattera)
- The side effects of atomoxetine include irritability and disruptive behavior. These side effects were potentiated by the administration of fluoxetine, a CYP2D6 inhibitor
- With the discontinuation of fluoxetine and the start of escitalopram (Lexapro), the patient began to show signs of improvement
- The patient demonstrated signs of liver injury, scleral icterus, and lethargy, which are concerning for hepatotoxicity secondary to atomoxetine administration. Ongoing consultation with the child's PCP and ongoing monitoring of liver enzyme function laboratory results are very important. Alkaline phosphatase elevation may occur during periods of growth spurts and can otherwise be benign. It is important to continue to monitor the patient's laboratory results and symptoms until they return to normal levels

Take-home points

- Patients with ADHD often benefit from psychosocial interventions, such as an IEP. Psychiatrists play an important part in assessing patient needs and advocating for educational justice
- Stimulants are the first-line treatment for ADHD. When stimulants are poorly tolerated, a trial of atomoxetine (Strattera) is appropriate
- When treating juvenile ADHD patients for comorbid depression or anxiety, consider fluoxetine–CYP2D6 interactions
- Medication adherence can be challenging for patients for a variety of reasons. Discuss possible impediments to daily dosing and brainstorm possible solutions before they arise
- An increase in alkaline phosphatase in adolescents is not necessarily pathological and can be the result of normal growth
- The differential for icterus and lethargy is very broad, includes a variety of toxicological, infectious, toxic/metabolic, and developmental/congenital causes, and necessitates a careful patient history and thorough workup
- Any elevation in liver enzymes should be monitored, especially when prescribing a medication that may be hepatotoxic, such as atomoxetine. Discontinue if there is suspected liver disease mediated by medication use

Performance in practice: confessions of a psychopharmacologist

What could have been done better here?

- For extensive metabolizers, when atomoxetine (Strattera) is given with a strong CYP2D6 inhibitor such as paroxetine (Paxil) or fluoxetine (Prozac), the starting and target dosages of atomoxetine should be reduced by 50%
- After one failed stimulant trial, evidence-based practice guidelines support a trial of a different stimulant as the next step. In this case, a trial of methylphenidate (Concerta) prior to resuming atomoxetine would also have avoided problematic drug–drug interactions due to fluoxetine's strong inhibition of CYP2D6
- Discuss with the patient and his family the importance of medication adherence, identify any issues that may impede adherence, and discuss possible solutions to these issues
- Advocacy for implementation of an IEP or other psychosocial measures
- A thorough workup for causes of his potential hepatopathy

What are possible action items for improvement in practice?

- A review of drug interactions for first-line medications commonly prescribed in children
- Documentation of ACE scores can help inform patient care
- A complete workup for sources of liver pathology including infectious, toxic/metabolic, and developmental/congenital causes
- A workup for ID/intellectual developmental disorder (IDD) with tighter collaboration between parents, schools, and mental health professionals

Tips and pearls

- When selecting medication for children and adolescents, consider a medication regimen that is the least intrusive in or disruptive to their daily lives
- Consider the possibility that adolescent patients with apparent ADHD may have underlying ID. A patient who exhibits signs of developmental delay, difficulties with socialization, or behavioral issues should receive functional testing and be considered for genetic testing
- Drug-induced liver injury is only one of many possible explanations of abnormal liver enzymes or other hepatopathy in a patient taking a potentially hepatotoxic medication. Maintaining a broad differential is important

Two-minute tutorial: ADHD and ID

- Psychiatric disorders are at least threefold more prevalent in children and adolescents with ID/IDD than those of neurotypical development. ADHD is one of the most common psychiatric comorbidities in children and adolescents with ID/IDD. Fragile X syndrome is the most common inherited ID and is most frequently comorbid with ADHD. In general, ADHD, oppositional defiant disorder, and anxiety have the highest rates of comorbidities with intellectual deficiency and disability. Fragile X syndrome is a single-gene defect whose etiology lies in the expansion of a trinucleotide repeat in the *FMR1* gene located on the X chromosome. Consequently, male children comprise most of the severe cases

- Morphological traits associated with fragile X syndrome include a disproportionately large jaw, forehead, and ears. Other observable traits include a long and narrow face, macro-orchidism, pes planus, and unusual flexibility of the fingers. Cognitively, male patients with fragile X syndrome range from mild to moderate ID. Approximately one-third of female patients are intellectually disabled. Delayed speech by 2 years of age is commonly observed among individuals. Behavioral characteristics include social anxiety, impaired social cognition and communication, and hyperarousal

- Screening for ID is done in pediatric offices as a part of well-child examinations. Parents or caregivers are encouraged to complete screening tools such as the Ages and Stages Questionnaire (ASQ) and the Parents' Evaluation of Developmental Status (PEDS). Systematic screening does not continue into later childhood (there is a lack of screening tools), where behavioral and intellectual disorders may appear as a result of decreased ability to adapt to the increasing intellectual and social complexity of the child's environment. Children who are observed to struggle intellectually or behaviorally in a manner that is different from their peers should be referred for standardized intellectual functioning testing and assessment of adaptive functioning. Genetic testing for neurobiological etiology may also be warranted

- Most randomized controlled trials for the treatment of ADHD have been done in neurotypical children and adolescents. Of the few trials that have been conducted, the findings support the use of stimulants, in particular, methylphenidate (Concerta) in children and adolescents with and without ID/IDD. Large studies have also been conducted using stimulants in combination with atypical antipsychotics (e.g. risperidone (Risperdal)) in children with ID/IDD and disruptive behavior disorders that have shown improvements in irritability, aggression, and hyperactivity

Posttest self-assessment question and answer

Which of the following are first-line, evidence-based pharmacological treatments for MDD in adolescents?

A. Sertraline (Zoloft)
B. Escitalopram (Lexapro)
C. Citalopram (Celexa)
D. Fluvoxamine (Luvox)
E. Fluoxetine (Prozac)
F. Paroxetine (Paxil)

Answer: B and E

Fluoxetine is FDA approved for use in ages 8 and up. Escitalopram is approved for use in ages 12 and up. The AACAP recommends fluoxetine as the first-line treatment.

References

1. American Psychiatric Association. *Practice Guideline for the Treatment of Patients with Major Depressive Disorder*, 3rd edn. Arlington, VA: American Psychiatric Association, 2010. Available from https://www.guidelinecentral.com/summaries/practice-guideline-for-the-treatment-of-patients-with-major-depressive-disorder-third-edition/

2. Bangs ME, Jin L, Desaiah D, et al. Hepatic events associated with atomoxetine treatment for attention-deficit hyperactivity disorder. *Drug Saf* 2012: 31:345–54. https://doi.org/10.2165/00002018-200831040-00008

3. Birmaher B, Brent D, AACAP Work Group on Quality Issues. Practice parameter for the assessment and treatment of children and adolescents with depressive disorders. *J Am Acad Child Adolesc Psychiatry* 2007; 46:1503–26. https://doi.org/10.1097/chi.0b013e318145ae1c

4. Blankenstein MA. Reference intervals – ever met a normal person? *Ann Clin Biochem* 2015; 52:5–6. https://doi.org/10.1177/0004563214561563

5. Carandang C, Jabbal R, Macbride A, Elbe D. A review of escitalopram and citalopram in child and adolescent depression. *J Can Acad Child Adolesc Psychiatry* 2011; 20:315–24.

6. Dulcan MK, Benson RS. Summary of the practice parameters for the assessment and treatment of children, adolescents, and adults with ADHD. *J Am Acad Child Adolesc Psychiatry* 1997; 36:1311–17. https://doi.org/10.1097/00004583-199709000-00033

7. Dynamed. Abnormal liver function tests – approach to the patient. 2018. Available from: https://www.dynamed.com/topics/dmp~AN~T316452 (accessed March 26, 2021).

8. Eli Lilly and Company. *Medication Guide: Strattera*. Indianapolis, IN: Eli Lilly and Company, 2003. Available from: http://pi.lilly.com/us/strattera-ppi.pdf

9. Felitti VJ, Anda RF, Nordenberg D, et al. Relationship of childhood abuse and household dysfunction to many of the leading causes of death in adults. The Adverse Childhood Experiences (ACE) Study. *Am J Prev Med* 1998; 14:245–58. https://doi.org/10.1016/s0749-3797(98)00017-8

10. Fugh-Berman A. Herbal medicinals: selected clinical considerations, focusing on known or potential drug–herb interactions. *Arch Intern Medi* 1999; 159:1957–9. https://doi.org/10.1001/archinte.159.16.1957

11. Garland EJ, Kutcher S, Virani A, Elbe, D. Update on the use of SSRIs and SNRIs with children and adolescents in clinical practice. *J Can Acad Child Adolesc Psychiatry* 2016; 25:4–10.

12. Hagerman RJ, Berry-Kravis E, Hazlett HC, et al. Fragile X syndrome. *Nat Rev Dis Primers*, 2017; 3, 17065. https://doi.org/10.1038/nrdp.2017.65

13. Kratochvil CJ, Newcorn JH, Arnold LE, et al. Atomoxetine alone or combined with fluoxetine for treating ADHD with comorbid depressive or anxiety symptoms. *J Am Acad Child Adolesc Psychiatry*, 2005; 44: 915–24. https://doi.org/10.1097/01.chi.0000169012.81536.38

14. March JS. The Treatment for Adolescents with Depression Study (TADS). Washington, DC: American Academy for Child and Adolescent Psychiatry, 2006. Available from: https://www.aacap.org/aacap/families_and_youth/Resources/Psychiatric_Medication/The_Treatment_for_Adolescents_with_Depression_Study_TADS.aspx (accessed March 26, 2021).

15. March J, Silva S, Vitiello B. The Treatment for Adolescents with Depression Study (TADS): methods and message at 12 weeks. *J Am Acad Child Adolesc Psychiatry* 2006; 45:1393–403. https://doi.org/10.1097/01.chi.0000237709.35637.c0

16. Muhle RA, Reed HE, Vo LC, et al. (2017). Clinical diagnostic testing for individuals with developmental disorders. *J Am Acad of Child Adolesc Psychiatry* 56:910–13. https://doi.org/10.1016/j.jaac.2017.09.418

17. National Institute of Diabetes and Digestive and Kidney Diseases. Atomoxetine. In: *LiverTox: Clinical and Research Information on Drug-Induced Liver Injury*. Bethesda, MD: National Institute of Diabetes and Digestive and Kidney Diseases, 2012. Available from: https://www.ncbi.nlm.nih.gov/books/NBK548671/

18. Roberts EA, Schilsky ML. Diagnosis and treatment of Wilson disease: an update. *Hepatology* 2008; 47:2089–111. https://doi.org/10.1002/hep.22261

19. Rush AJ, Trivedi MH, Wisniewski SR, et al. Acute and longer-term outcomes in depressed outpatients requiring one or several treatment steps: a STAR*D report. *Am J Psychiatry* 2006; 163:1905–17. https://doi.org/10.1176/ajp.2006.163.11.1905

20. Siegel M, McGuire, K, Veenstra-VanderWeele J, et al. Practice parameter for the assessment and treatment of psychiatric disorders in children and adolescents with intellectual disability (intellectual developmental disorder). *J Am Acad Child Adolesc Psychiatry* 2019; 59:468–96. https://doi.org/10.1016/j.jaac.2019.11.018

21. Stahl SM. *Stahl's Essential Psychopharmacology: Prescriber's Guide*, 6th edn. Cambridge, UK: Cambridge University Press, 2017.

22. Varigonda, AL, Jakubovski, E, Taylor, MJ, et al. Systematic review and meta-analysis: early treatment responses of selective serotonin reuptake inhibitors in pediatric major depressive disorder. *J Am Acad of Child Adolesc Psychiatry* 2015; 54:557–64. https://doi.org/10.1016/j.jaac.2015.05.004

23. Whyte, MP. Physiological role of alkaline phosphatase explored in hypophosphatasia. *Ann N Y Acad Sci* 2010; 1192: 190–200. https://doi.org/10.1111/j.1749-6632.2010.05387.x

Case 16: The man who spent thousands online

The Question: Can antiemetics play a role in the treatment of psychiatric disease?

The Psychopharmacological Dilemma: How to diagnose and treat sedative-hypnotic use disorder in an elderly patient who is sensitive to medications

Saloni Singh and Carla Hammond

Pretest self-assessment question (answer at the end of the case)

Which of these psychotropic medications is used for the treatment of nausea/emesis?

A. Chlorpromazine (Thorazine)

B. Escitalopram (Lexapro)

C. Olanzapine (Zyprexa)

D. Clonazepam (Klonopin)

E. Prochlorperazine (Compazine)

F. Haloperidol (Haldol)

G. Hydroxyzine (Vistaril)

H. A and E

I. A, E, F, and G

J. D and G

K. A, C, E, F, and G

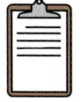

Patient evaluation on intake

• An 81-year-old man who has been dependent on lorazepam (Ativan) for 8 years and complains of severe withdrawal symptoms when he attempts to taper off

Psychiatric history

• The patient originally began taking lorazepam (Ativan) for the treatment of generalized anxiety disorder about 8 years ago, prescribed by his primary care physician (PCP), although he cannot personally recall the exact presentation of his anxiety at that time. Initially, the patient was taking 2 mg three times per day. He was successfully tapered down to 1 mg three times per day. Six months ago, he was tapered down further to 0.5 mg three times per day. At this stage of the taper, however, he has been taking more pills than prescribed and repeatedly running out before the refill date

- The patient complains of withdrawal symptoms if he misses a dose by even a few hours: nausea, irritability, restlessness, feelings of anxiety, headaches, and tremors. He has never experienced any seizures
- The patient's PCP decided he did not need to taper off completely and to "let him keep it because he's elderly"
- However, the patient's wife is struggling with the negative impact of the patient's sedative-hypnotic dependence. Because the patient has impaired mobility, he often pressures his wife to run to the pharmacy and get his medications filled early and often. If he misses his dose by even a few hours, he is intensely irritable, and his wife becomes the subject of his frustration
- The patient's wife complains that the lorazepam use has changed the patient's personality, as he no longer enjoys activities he used to. He no longer socializes with their friends, remaining hyper-focused on when and how he will obtain the lorazepam. This has been going on for about 2 years and has been worsening in the past 6–8 months
- The patient has a history of intermittent depressive episodes since he was 45 years old. He feels he is currently experiencing such an episode with symptoms of apathy, low appetite, hypersomnia, fatigue, and anhedonia with almost every activity. He derives joy/happiness only from his online sex chatting. The patient admits that he usually has comorbid anxiety with his depressive episodes. At this time, he admits symptoms of anxiety only when attempting to further taper from lorazepam
- The patient denies any suicidal ideation. He has never had this symptom in the past. He has no prior psychiatric hospitalizations or suicide attempts
- The patient also admits to a history of occasional visual/auditory hallucinations, usually at bedtime. He usually hallucinates that his wife is in the room and talking to him. He alludes to this in the morning only to discover that his wife was not in the room the night before. The patient denies any commanding hallucinations

Substance use history

- The patient has been on lorazepam (Ativan) for the past 8 years, requiring escalating doses up until the past year when he has attempted to taper off with his PCP. The patient meets 10/11 of the DSM criteria for substance use disorder (denies failure to fulfill major role obligations at work/school/home but wife's collateral suggests otherwise), qualifying as severe sedative-hypnotic use disorder

- The patient has no history of alcohol abuse. When the patient was still socializing, he would occasionally have one beer every 1–2 months in a social visit with friends
- The patient used to smoke half to one pack of cigarettes per day from age 18 to 21, but quit "cold turkey" with his wife at age 21
- The patient has previously tried cannabis (briefly) for nausea without a sufficient treatment response
- There is no history of other substance abuse. However, the patient has developed a sex addiction, as above

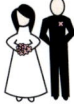

Social and personal history

- The patient has been married to his wife for 63 years. Together, they have three daughters, seven grandchildren, and 10 great-grandchildren
- The patient has had previous affairs and once nearly left his wife for another woman. However, the patient's wife does not feel that his current obsession with online sex chatting is in line with the patient's previous behaviors or his usual personality. She feels that this is a dramatic shift
- The patient worked in the construction industry for 25 years and then managed an amusement park for 25 years. He has been retired for over 10 years
- Over the past 6–8 months, according to the patient's wife, he has developed a new-onset computer/sex addiction. He has been purchasing internet chat time with women in Moscow and spent $1000 on this in the last month alone. He spends at least 8 hours a day on the computer flirting with these women or viewing pornography. When the couple's friends come to visit, the patient speaks with them only briefly before complaining of nausea and retiring to his room to spend time online. The patient has poor insight into this behavior and does not seem to realize that these women are only chatting with him because they are paid to do so. He feels that they are genuinely interested in him and he admits feeling excited to have them visit him in the USA. He has never exhibited this sort of behavior before
- The patient admits seeking out this sexual interaction with women because he and his wife no longer have intercourse. The patient's wife states that this behavior started when she moved to a different bedroom, as she could no longer share a bed with the patient who began thrashing about in his sleep

Medical history

- The patient has diagnoses of type 2 diabetes, atrial fibrillation, spinal stenosis, variable hypertension, benign prostatic hypertrophy, and spinocerebellar ataxia (SCA) type 3 (Joseph's disease)

Current medications

- The patient is currently prescribed lorazepam (Ativan) 0.5 mg PO three times per day, but has been taking two to three extra pills each day and routinely running out of medication days ahead of his refill date
- The patient is currently prescribed escitalopram (Lexapro) 10 mg PO daily but has never taken this medication for more than a few days due to lack of perceived efficacy (the patient noted no immediate effect on his anxiety)
- Metformin (Glucophage)
- Hydrochlorothiazide-valsartan (Diovan HCT)
- Tamsulosin (Flomax)
- Rivaroxaban (Xarelto)
- Pantoprazole (Protonix)
- Linaclotide (Linzess)
- Ferrous sulfate
- Vitamin D_3

Family history

- Sisters with severe recurrent major depressive disorder and suicidal ideation
- Father with alcohol use disorder

Question

Based on the patient's history, what symptoms and signs prompt you to consider a neurocognitive disorder?

Attending physician's mental notes: initial evaluation

- The patient's change in personality and hypersexual behavior (not consistent with baseline) could be secondary to the lorazepam (Ativan) abuse, as benzodiazepines (BDZs) may behaviorally (often sexually) disinhibit patients (known as a "paradoxical reaction"), especially those who are elderly
- The patient's change in personality could also be secondary to a neurocognitive disorder, such as frontotemporal dementia or Lewy body dementia. A diagnosis of Lewy body dementia could be supported specifically by the patient's nightly thrashing in his sleep

(which could indicate a rapid eye movement (REM) sleep behavior disorder), as well as auditory-visual hallucinations (although the exclusively hypnagogic nature makes this less likely). However, no increased tone or cogwheeling is observed on motor examination. Of note, a REM sleep behavior disorder is also seen in patients with SCA alone

- The patient's presentation could be a result of both above factors, as BDZs are more likely to disinhibit patients with underlying neurocognitive disorder
- Either way, the patient's pattern of lorazepam use is problematic and concerning, both for the patient and his wife
- The patient's relatively late onset of recurrent depression (age 45) may be secondary to his SCA symptoms (which also presented in middle age and resulted in progressive decline of function). This can arise either directly through neuropsychiatric changes or indirectly from adjustment to growing limitations on their instrumental activities of daily living (both seen in literature reviews of SCA)

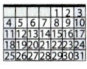

Case outcome: interim follow-up through 10 days

- The patient decided with the treatment team to taper the lorazepam (Ativan) down further to 0.5 mg every morning, 0.25 mg every day at 12 noon, and 0.25 mg every evening initially. He was provided with prescriptions that he could fill only every 7 days, to prevent significant time in withdrawal were he to overuse his medication (as he has done historically)
- The patient was also educated on the mechanism and proper dosing regimen of escitalopram (Lexapro) and encouraged to take it daily for 4–6 weeks to evaluate for any improvement of depression/ anxiety
- Prior to his scheduled follow-up, the patient calls the clinic a few days ahead of the interim refill date requesting that the refill be prescribed early as he has run out. He is educated on the importance of taking medication as prescribed and provided a refill on the originally discussed date
- The patient has been taking his escitalopram consistently for slightly over a week but has not yet noticed a difference in his depression or anxiety symptoms
- Given the patient's difficulty with the new regimen, he is switched to a lorazepam prescription, at the aforementioned doses, that he may fill only every 4 days. Thus, he would not need to endure multiple days of withdrawal symptoms

Performance in practice: confessions of a psychopharmacologist

What could have been done better here?

- In hindsight, it was not optimal to taper off the benzodiazepine while also initiating the selective serotonin reuptake inhibitor (SSRI), given the known possibility of increased anxiety during the first week of SSRI initiation. In fact, physicians often prescribe a short course of BDZ to manage this increased anxiety
- Given that patient's self-reported withdrawal symptoms include both anxiety and nausea, hydroxyzine (Vistaril) (indicated for both) might have been a wise choice to use as needed to minimize BDZ use/overuse

Attending physician's mental notes: interim follow-up through 10 days

- Given the patient's experience of withdrawal symptoms hours upon missing a dose, a long-acting BDZ such as chlordiazepoxide (Librium) or clonazepam (Klonopin) should be considered
- At this point, the patient is struggling with the lorazepam (Ativan) taper, physiologically and psychologically. However, given his success with tapering under his PCP as well as patient preference, we will continue the lorazepam taper with shorter-duration refills
- The most pressing concern is the risk of withdrawal seizures, but these are likely to occur a few days into withdrawal (not hours). The patient has no such history of seizures, despite being out of pills for days at a time before establishing with us. However, we must always look to mitigate the risk either through a long-acting BDZ or short-duration lorazepam refills to avoid lengthy withdrawals

Case outcome: interim follow-up at 3 weeks

- The patient has been taking the escitalopram (Lexapro) consistently for about 3 weeks, and has noticed an improvement in his baseline anxiety and depression symptoms
- With the shorter duration of 4-day refills, the patient has been doing better with his lorazepam (Ativan) use overall. However, he has still run out early twice since his last visit (for less than a day each time)
- The patient still complains of withdrawal symptoms within hours of missing a lorazepam dose – feeling nauseated, panicky, and frantic
- The patient admits to having tried just 2 mg of ondansetron (Zofran) (half of the prescribed dose), which effectively treated the nausea, but he felt "loopy" on this medication (although he denies clonus, hyperreflexia, or hyperthermia). However, his wife remarks that the

patient slept through the night after he took this medication (a rare occurrence)

- Given the patient's repeated struggle with overuse, his lorazepam dosing schedule is elicited in detail: he typically takes 0.5 mg when he awakens around 6 a.m., then 0.25 mg between 10 a.m. and 12 p.m. He does not typically take the third pill as scheduled in the evening, but instead when he awakens in the middle of the night at around 3 a.m.
- Surprisingly, the patient denies any withdrawal symptoms of nausea or anxiety in the evening or bedtime, despite routinely missing the evening lorazepam dose
- Due to an inability to progress with the planned lorazepam taper and ongoing withdrawal symptoms, the patient decides, with the team, to opt for a long-acting BDZ. Chlordiazepoxide (Librium) 5 mg three times per day is prescribed, with a plan to taper at the next visit
- The patient is encouraged to use ondansetron 1 mg as needed (a lower dose to prevent altered mental status), given its efficacy for his nausea

Further investigation

Is there anything else you would especially like to know about this patient?

- What about serotonin syndrome?
  - The patient had an adverse reaction to ondansetron (Zofran), complaining of altered mental status and feeling "loopy." As he is also taking escitalopram (Lexapro), there was initially a concern of serotonin syndrome due to combining these two medications for the first time. Although serotonin syndrome can present with agitation, this patient did not complain of any of the other symptoms
  - Serotonin syndrome is a clinical diagnosis based on the Hunter criteria. To fulfill the Hunter criteria, the patient must be taking a serotonergic agent and meet ONE of the following conditions:
    - Spontaneous clonus
    - Inducible clonus PLUS agitation or diaphoresis
    - Ocular clonus PLUS agitation or diaphoresis
    - Tremor PLUS hyperreflexia
    - Hypertonia PLUS temperature above 38·C PLUS ocular clonus or inducible clonus

Attending physician's mental notes: interim follow-up at 3 weeks

- At this point, we are suspicious of the patient's nausea truly being a symptom of BDZ withdrawal. Although nausea is a known symptom of BDZ withdrawal, the patient experiences this only when missing a morning/noon dose of lorazepam (Ativan), about 4–5 hours after his previous dose
- Meanwhile, patient denies nausea in the evenings or at bedtime, despite having gone without lorazepam for a minimum of 9 hours
- The patient has a long history of gastrointestinal issues, including acid reflux (resulting in Barrett's esophagus) and nausea. These symptoms date back to well before he began lorazepam 8 years ago. He has been to many gastrointestinal specialists without a clear diagnosis
- Further questioning of the patient reveals that he uses the lorazepam around 3 a.m. due to nausea, after having awakened from sleep. It is also clear that the patient had primary difficulty with nausea long before he was prescribed lorazepam 8 years ago. He posits that this may have been part of the original reason, along with anxiety, that he stayed on the lorazepam for so long
- After consulting with Internal Medicine, it is likely that the patient frontloads his lorazepam use at the beginning of the day due to nausea that is worse in the morning. This is likely secondary to acid reflux exacerbated after hours of lying prostrate during sleep. Nausea secondary to lorazepam withdrawal is becoming less likely

Case outcome: interim follow-up at 4 weeks

- The patient calls for telephone follow-up just 3 days after the visit due to difficulty with symptoms on chlordiazepoxide (Librium). He does not feel this medication helps at all with his "withdrawal" symptoms, specifically his nausea. This nausea remains an issue only in the morning hours after the patient has been lying down to sleep
- The patient is requesting another prescription of lorazepam (Ativan) instead. He is denied and informed that this is not indicated as his nausea is unlikely to be a symptom of withdrawal
- The patient is hesitant to continue ondansetron (Zofran), even at a lower dose, due to the adverse effect of altered mental status
- He is instead prescribed an alternate treatment for his primary nausea of metoclopramide 5 mg PO four times per day as needed and pyridoxine 10 mg PO every morning
- The patient is instructed to discontinue chlordiazepoxide, with no taper required

Further investigation

Is there anything else you would especially like to know about this patient?

- A review of the patient's medical records from gastrointestinal specialists would be helpful
- What medications has the patient already tried for nausea and what were the outcomes? He claims that he has tried every one but cannot recall the specifics. If that is true, why is it that he only found success with metoclopramide after over a decade? Is it because he was not titrated up slowly enough by the previous prescriber? Or was it due to a multifactorial, dynamic etiology of his nausea (a psychosomatic overlay that developed after long-term abuse of lorazepam (Ativan))?
- What do gastrointestinal specialists posit is the etiology of patient's nausea? Dysphagia is a known symptom of SCA, likely secondary to gastrointestinal tract dysmotility. Could the patient's nausea and acid reflux also be secondary to this? As the patient has type 2 diabetes, diabetic gastroparesis could also explain these symptoms
- What is the timeline of the patient's nausea presentation? How did it change after starting lorazepam?
- Some of the questions may seem extracurricular to a psychiatrist, but presently the patient's main deterrent to quitting lorazepam is his nausea. In order to achieve remission of his use disorder, a comprehensive history of pertinent symptoms is needed

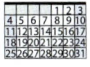

Case outcome: interim follow-up at 5 weeks

- The patient and his wife are delighted to share that he is "100% better" on his new regimen for nausea. He feels taking the pyridoxine daily has been helpful in reducing his nausea overall. He also takes the metoclopramide as needed two to four times per day, which resolves any breakthrough nausea
- The patient admits to being more active and doing more outside the house since he has been feeling better. His wife and friends feel that he is "a new man"
- The patient and wife also confide that he has discontinued the online sex chatting altogether, from about 1 week ago when he started the new regimen. He attributes this to "feeling better" and a return to intimacy with his wife. He even requests a prescription for sildenafil
- The patient feels liberated from his dependence on lorazepam (Ativan) and now feels "turned off" by it. He also feels liberated from being fixated on his nausea

Question

Why has the patient's sex chatting addiction suddenly remitted?

- Is this because he is no longer disinhibited by the BDZ? This presented about 4 days after discontinuing lorazepam (Ativan) and starting chlordiazepoxide (Librium)
- This "paradoxical reaction" of BDZ-induced disinhibition is more prevalent in elderly patients, especially those impacted by a neurocognitive disorder. This is why we must evaluate the patient for the latter
- The profound lack of insight into the nature of his sex chatting behavior (not understanding that he was paying these women thousands of dollars) invites a question of psychotic or near-psychotic thinking. As his remission started when he began the new regimen of metoclopramide, is there an anti-dopaminergic mechanism responsible for the resolution of this?
- The patient was referred to a geriatric psychiatrist for specialized evaluation of the above clinical questions
- Neuropsychological testing, a Montreal Cognitive Assessment (MoCA), and magnetic resonance imaging could be indicated, but the patient did not follow up with the geriatric psychiatrist

Case debrief

- This elderly patient was prescribed lorazepam (Ativan) for 8 years by a PCP to treat generalized anxiety symptoms without a sufficient trial of an SSRI. When he finally presented to addiction psychiatry, he saw remarkable improvement in his symptoms when treated with escitalopram (Lexapro) for a few weeks
- The patient had tried without success, with his PCP, to taper down and discontinue lorazepam. He struggled with self-reported "withdrawal" symptoms of primarily nausea, anxiety, tremors, and headaches. He denied any history of seizures
- It was discovered that in the past 6 months, the patient had become addicted to online sex chatting with very poor insight, paying women $1000 per month for their company. This could have been secondary to disinhibition from the BDZ and/or from a neurocognitive disorder
- After detailed history taking and frequent follow-ups, it became clear that the patient's nausea symptoms were not lorazepam withdrawal. They occurred exclusively in the morning (after only 4 or 5 hours from his last dose) and not in the evening or bedtime (despite 9 hours since his last dose). This assessment was confirmed when the patient found no benefit from the chlordiazepoxide (Librium)

for his nausea. The patient was prescribed ondansetron (Zofran) for nausea, to which he had an adverse reaction of altered mental status, even at a low dose. Metoclopramide was tried next, and it was effective. Once the patient's nausea was well controlled with this medication, he no longer felt the need to use the lorazepam. As soon as this occurred, the patient's online sex chatting addiction also remitted

- The etiology for the patient's nausea is unclear to even his gastrointestinal specialists. It could be attributed to gastrointestinal tract dysmotility secondary to his SCA type 3. It could also be secondary to diabetic gastroparesis, for which metoclopramide is FDA approved
- It is also possible that the patient's nausea had a psychosomatic component, so effectively treating his anxiety with escitalopram (he had had 4 weeks of therapy at that point) could have helped. However, the initiation of metoclopramide likely contributed more, as the remission occurred rather suddenly at that time
- The patient and wife felt liberated from his years-long struggle with lorazepam. They had a new-found love for each other and for life because the wife was no longer subjected to the patient's irritability and frustration when he missed his lorazepam. The patient became very active and engaged again. He and his wife lived happily ever after (as far as we heard)

Take-home points

- A holistic (and sometimes exhaustive) approach must be employed for patients with addiction (in this case yielding an intensive review of the dosing schedule by the patient, a review of systems yielding psychosomatic or primary non-psychiatric symptoms, a history of the caregiver burden, and the presence of thrashing in his sleep)
- Psychoeducation is an integral component of treating mental illness. The PCP prescribing the patient an SSRI should have explained what to expect when starting this medication (possible initial gastrointestinal upset, possible initial anxiety exacerbation, and weeks-long latency to achieve full effect). SSRIs have been proven the most effective for treatment of generalized anxiety, and trials of multiple agents in this class may be warranted. Instead, this elderly patient started a BDZ, which is not only less efficacious but is also more likely to result in abuse (especially with a family history of alcohol use disorder). A bit of teaching and patience could have averted 8 years of dependence
- Rapport building is crucial for patients struggling with addiction; otherwise, a minimized, deceptive, or incomplete history telling

could obscure the true presentation (the patient's actual use of lorazepam (Ativan) versus how it was prescribed, illuminating (un) likelihood of withdrawal)

- A patient's higher education level, more expansive vocabulary, or frequent engagement with physicians is a double-edged sword. It can often aid the psychoeducation process, as the patient's knowledge base can be built upon more easily. But, as they say, "a little knowledge is a dangerous thing." For example, this patient's self-report of "withdrawal" was initially taken at face value. However, after multiple visits and detailed history taking, several confounding variables and inconsistent chronicity illuminated that he was not actually suffering from physiological withdrawal (at least not intensely), and the nausea required independent/parallel treatment
- Patients may tolerate a medication for years before changes in their age or metabolism result in new-found adverse effects. This is especially true of benzodiazepines in the elderly
- Neurocognitive disorder must always be considered when an elderly patient presents as disinhibited compared with baseline. However, other causes (such as BDZ use) may also explain this, either partially or exclusively
- Non-psychiatric medications can often have psychotropic side effects, which could be adverse or beneficial. This is expected given the ubiquitous distribution of neurotransmitters in our body, especially in the gut. The beneficial side effects can be leveraged for treatment
- Patients with neurological disease often have comorbid psychiatric conditions, through direct mechanisms (e.g. depletion of dopamine in Parkinson's patients or, in this case, possibly the neuropsychiatric sequelae of SCA), and/or indirect mechanisms (poor (instrumental) activities of daily living affecting the patient's self-image, perceived independence, and life satisfaction). Patients who are sensitive to medications must be approached with an initial lower dosage, gentleness, and understanding. This will keep them engaged in early treatment of anxiety disorders

Posttest self-assessment question and answer

Which of these psychotropic medications is used for the treatment of nausea/emesis?

A. Chlorpromazine (Thorazine)

B. Escitalopram (Lexapro)

C. Olanzapine (Zyprexa)

D. Clonazepam (Klonopin)
E. Prochlorperazine (Compazine)
F. Haloperidol (Haldol)
G. Hydroxyzine (Vistaril)
H. A and E
I. A, E, F, and G
J. D and G
K. A, C, E, F, and G

Answer: K

Chlorpromazine, prochlorperazine, and hydroxyzine are each FDA approved for nausea/emesis. A review of off-label literature yields that olanzapine and haloperidol are used as antiemetics specifically in chemotherapy-induced and postoperative settings. Escitalopram and clonazepam are not useful in nausea/vomiting, unless it is psychogenic in nature (such as in anticipatory nausea due to psychological conditioning, or in psychosomatic presentations of depression/anxiety).

References

1. Bódizs R, Sverteczki M, Lázár AS, et al. Human parahippocampal activity: non-REM and REM elements in wake–sleep transition. *Brain Res Bull* 2005; 65:169–76. https://doi.org/10.1016/j.brainresbull.2005.01.002

2. Cassano GB, Petracca A, Cesana BM. A new scale for the evaluation of benzodiazepine withdrawal symptoms: Sessb: A pilot study. *Curr Ther Res* 1994; 55: 275–89. https://doi.org/10.1016/S0011-393X(05)80171-7

3. Chaparro C, Moreno D, Ramírez V, et al. Haloperidol as prophylactic treatment for postoperative nausea and vomiting: systematic literature review. *Colomb J Anesth* 2013; 41:34–43. https://doi.org/10.1016/j.rca.2012.07.010

4. Chi NF, Shiao GM, Ku HL, Soong B-W. Sleep disruption in spinocerebellar ataxia type 3: A genetic and polysomnographic study. *J Chin Med Assoc* 2013; 76:25–30. https://doi.org/10.1016/j.jcma.2012.09.006

5. Dunkley EJC, Isbister GK, Sibbritt D, et al. The Hunter Serotonin Toxicity Criteria: simple and accurate diagnostic decision rules for serotonin toxicity. *QJM* 2003; 96: 635–42. https://doi.org/10.1093/qjmed/hcg109

6. Galbiati A, Verga L, Giora E, et al. The risk of neurodegeneration in REM sleep behavior disorder: A systematic review and meta-analysis of longitudinal studies. *Sleep Med Rev* 2019; 43:37–46. https://doi.org/10.1016/j.smrv.2018.09.008

7. Hsu WY, Huang SS, Chiu NY. Escitalopram for psychogenic nausea and vomiting: a report of two cases. *J Formos Med Assoc* 2011; 110:62–6. https://doi.org/10.1016/S0929-6646(11)60010-7
8. Joffe RT, Levitt AJ, Sokolov ST. Augmentation strategies: focus on anxiolytics. *J Clin Psychiatry* 1996; 57:25–33.
9. Kamen C, Tejani MA, Chandwani K, et al. Anticipatory nausea and vomiting due to chemotherapy. *Eur J Pharmacol* 2014; 722:172–9. https://doi.org/10.1016/j.ejphar.2013.09.071
10. Lader M, Tylee A, Donoghue J. Withdrawing benzodiazepines in primary care. *CNS Drugs* 2009; 23:19–34. https://doi.org/10.2165/0023210-200923010-00002
11. Lai AX, Kaup AR, Yaffe K, et al. High occurrence of psychiatric disorders and suicidal behavior across dementia subtypes. *Am J Geriatr Psychiatry* 2018; 26:1191–201. https://doi.org/10.1016/j.jagp.2018.08.012
12. Lim KG, Morgenthaler TI, Katzka DA. Sleep and nocturnal gastroesophageal reflux: an update. *Chest* 2018; 154:963–71. https://doi.org/10.1016/j.chest.2018.05.030
13. Lo RY, Figueroa KP, Pulst SM, et al. Depression and clinical progression in spinocerebellar ataxias. *Parkinsonism Relat Disord* 2016; 22:87–92. https://doi.org/10.1016/j.parkreldis.2015.11.021
14. Mancuso CE, Tanzi MG, Gabay M. Paradoxical reactions to benzodiazepines: literature review and treatment options. *Pharmacotherapy* 2004; 24:1177–85. https://doi.org/10.1592/phco.24.13.1177.38089
15. McKenzie WS, Rosenberg M. Paradoxical reaction following administration of a benzodiazepine. *J Oral Maxillofac Surg* 2010; 68:3034–6. https://doi.org/10.1016/j.joms.2010.06.176
16. Naeim A, Reuben DB, Ganz PA, eds. *Management of Cancer in the Older Patient*. Philadelphia, PA: WB Saunders, 2012.
17. Reddy MSS, Achary U, Harbishettar V, et al. Paradoxical reaction to benzodiazepines in elderly – case series. *Asian J Psychiatry* 2018; 35:8–10. https://doi.org/10.1016/j.ajp.2018.04.037
18. Rüb U, Seidel K, Özerden I, et al. Consistent affection of the central somatosensory system in spinocerebellar ataxia type 2 and type 3 and its significance for clinical symptoms and rehabilitative therapy. *Brain Res Rev* 2007; 53:235–49. https://doi.org/10.1016/j.brainresrev.2006.08.003
19. Sani TP, Bond RL, Russell LL, et al. Sleep symptoms in frontotemporal dementia. *Alzheimer's & Dementia* 2017; 13: 726. https://doi.org/10.1016/j.jalz.2017.06.942
20. Spanemberg L, Nogueira EL, Belem da Silva CT, et al. High prevalence and prescription of benzodiazepines for elderly: data from psychiatric consultation to patients from an emergency

room of a general hospital. *Gen Hosp Psychiatry* 2011; 33:45–50.
https://doi.org/10.1016/j.genhosppsych.2010.12.004

21. Stahl SM. *Stahl's Essential Psychopharmacology: The Prescriber's Guide*, 6th edn. Cambridge, UK: Cambridge University Press, 2017.

22. Stanley M, Lautin A, Rotrosen J, et al. Metoclopramide: antipsychotic efficacy of a drug lacking potency in receptor models. *Psychopharmacology* 1980; 71:219–25. https://doi.org/10.1007/BF00433055

23. Tampi RR, Young JJ, Tampi D. Behavioral symptomatology and psychopharmacology of Lewy body dementia. *Handb Clin Neurol* 2019; 165:59–70. https://doi.org/10.1016/B978-0-444-64012-3.00005-8

24. Virtanen AI, Buckmaster PS, Galanopoulou AS, Moshé SL, eds. *Models of Seizures and Epilepsy*, 2nd edn. London, UK: Academic Press, 2017.

25. Yoodee J, Permsuwan U, Nimworapan M. Efficacy and safety of olanzapine for the prevention of chemotherapy-induced nausea and vomiting: a systematic review and meta-analysis. *Crit Rev Oncol Hematol* 2017; 112:113–25. https://doi.org/10.1016/j.critrevonc.2017.02.017

Case 17: The traumatized mother who can't stop bingeing

The Question: How do you treat refractory binge eating?

The Psychopharmacological Dilemma: Will the treatment of trauma and mood disorders help resolve this patient's binge eating, or is something more needed?

Kevin Simonson and Bo Ram Yoo

Pretest self-assessment question (answer at the end of the case)

Which medication is FDA approved for binge eating disorder (BED)?

A. Fluoxetine (Prozac)
B. Clomipramine (Anafranil)
C. Lisdexamfetamine (Vyvanse)

Patient evaluation on intake

- A 34-year-old woman with a traumatic history presents with worsening symptoms of posttraumatic stress disorder (PTSD), depression, anxiety, and binge eating who is struggling to manage her life and home school her five children

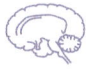

Psychiatric history

- The patient reports a history of PTSD, depression, and anxiety since the age of 6 following emotional, physical, and sexual abuse by her stepfather and mother
- At age 6, she "stopped eating and sleeping" and was psychiatrically hospitalized for 2 weeks. She states "I was held down and drugged for childhood bipolar disorder," which she reports caused further trauma. "I still can't drink orange juice because the psychiatric hospital gave me medications with orange juice"
- She denies a history of manic episodes, but admits to "complex PTSD"
- She has a history of burning her arms as a teenager and suicidal ideation by overdosing on medications
- The patient's mother "continues to insert herself into my life, and I feel disgust when around her"
- She has been binge eating for the last 3 years. She will occasionally binge until she vomits ("once per month"), but adamantly denies intentional purging behavior and a history of anorexia
- She gained over 100 lbs in a 12-month period
- She lost 40 lbs last year by calorie counting and then gained all of the weight back

- She has tried coping skills, relaxation techniques, time management, exercise, diet, mindfulness, and intermittent fasting, none of which have had lasting benefit. She was in Weight Watchers for 2 months, then had a binge cycle and quit

Social and personal history

- The patient's highest level of education was 11th grade
- She is married and a mother of five young children that she home schools while her husband is at work
- She denies all substance use

Medical history

- Obesity
- Denies history of seizure, heart palpitations, and panic attacks
- No allergies or surgical history

Family history

- Mother with bipolar disorder, borderline personality disorder, and a history of methamphetamine and cocaine abuse
- Father with schizophrenia, dissociative identity disorder, and a history of methamphetamine and cocaine abuse
- Maternal grandfather with bipolar disorder
- Maternal grandmother with fibromyalgia

Medication history

- Lithium
- Fluoxetine (Prozac)
- Diphenhydramine (Benadryl)
- Trazodone (Desyrel) ("Didn't help me sleep")
- She is unable to take sedatives or hypnotics due to "fear of losing control when I am too relaxed"

Current medications

- Sertraline (Zoloft) 100 mg daily for 2 years
- Bupropion (Wellbutrin) 75 mg daily started 1 year ago, increased to 150 mg daily 6 months ago
- Both medications were prescribed by a nurse practitioner

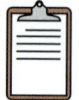

Patient evaluation on initial visit

- "I have no energy, sometimes I don't shower for 10 days, and the house is chaos"
- "It is very difficult to deal with the normal stressors of life"

- The patient sleeps only 3–4 hours per night, with difficulty initiating and maintaining sleep
- She has nightmares three or four times a week, especially when stressed
- She admits to 6 months of paranoid thoughts: "I know it's irrational, but I'm convinced that people are poisoning my food and watching me." "I only eat food that I prepare, and I have to shut the blinds when I am alone". She denies having had these paranoid symptoms before
- She binges on fast food, chocolate, and ice cream "eight or more times per week, to the point I'm sweating". "I'm emotionally overeating, it's the first thing I think about when I'm stressed." She has gained 30 pounds in the last 6 months
- "I have a lot of pain throughout my body. I think it's emotional and physical; my whole body weighs so much"
- Her depression is subjectively rated at 9/10
- She admits to sadness, irritable mood, anhedonia, excessive guilt, increased appetite, weight gain, decreased concentration, indecisiveness, fatigue, recurrent thoughts of death, intrusive negative thoughts, hopelessness, low self-esteem, tearfulness, decreased libido, excessive worry, restlessness, feeling on edge, fatigue, and muscle tension
- The patient has to drive a 120-mile round trip and find child care in order to attend psychiatry appointments

Attending physician's mental notes: initial evaluation

- This is a complicated case that can be difficult to tease apart diagnostically. While her presentation superficially suggests depression with psychotic features, her paranoid thoughts are thematically related to significant childhood trauma, and so may represent an exacerbation of chronic PTSD. The differential also includes a primary psychotic process, especially considering her family history, although this is less likely due to the late age of onset
- Bupropion (Wellbutrin) is a norepinephrine-dopamine reuptake inhibitor (NDRI), which may be causing/worsening her paranoid thoughts, anxiety, and insomnia
- Improving sleep quantity and quality is a top priority
- Her comorbid body pain may improve with replacement of sertraline (Zoloft), a selective serotonin reuptake inhibitor (SSRI), with a serotonin-norepinephrine reuptake inhibitor (SNRI)
- We will first address her sleep, paranoia, and mood symptoms, and then re-evaluate the status of her eating disorder

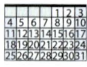

Case outcome: initial evaluation

- Discontinue (taper off) bupropion (Wellbutrin) due to insomnia, anxiety, and paranoid thoughts
- Start hydroxyzine (Vistaril) 25–50 mg every 8 hours as needed for anxiety and insomnia
- Stop sertraline (Zoloft) and start duloxetine (Cymbalta) 60 mg daily in a cross taper/titration to continue treating depression and anxiety but also to target body pain (possible fibromyalgia)

Case outcome: follow-up at week 4

- The patient's paranoid thoughts resolved soon after stopping bupropion (Wellbutrin). She was very relieved: "Thankfully, I'm not crazy"
- Her insomnia improved with hydroxyzine (Vistaril)
- Her mood improved, with her depression subjectively rated at 5/10
- Her body pain decreased after replacing sertraline (Zoloft) with duloxetine (Cymbalta)
- Her anxiety and stress continue
- Her bingeing continues unabated, with no change

Attending physician's mental notes: follow-up evaluation

- The patient responded surprisingly well to our medication changes
- In theory, it could have been helpful to make one change to this patient's medication regimen at a time, so that we would know exactly which changes were associated with which improvements (was it stopping bupropion (Wellbutrin), starting hydroxyzine (Vistaril), or switching sertraline (Zoloft) for duloxetine (Cymbalta) that had the greatest effect?). However, there are ethical limitations to this approach, and in this case, multiple changes were made at once due to the severity of her symptoms, the degree of her functional impairment, and the number of lives being affected (the patient's five children), as well as concern for the patient being lost to follow-up (due to the long commute and scheduling limitations)
- The patient's binge eating has not improved. She continues to feel stressed and anxious, and eats excessively to cope. We could start lisdexamfetamine (Vyvanse); however, there is concern that increasing norepinephrine and dopamine levels again will cause her paranoid thoughts, insomnia, and anxiety to return. We will watch and wait

Case outcome: follow-up at week 12

- Duloxetine (Cymbalta) increased to 90 mg daily
- Start buspirone (BuSpar) 15 mg twice per day for anxiety

- Her sleep is normalized with hydroxyzine (Vistaril)
- Her body pain decreased further with increased duloxetine
- Her anxiety improved
- Her bingeing continues unabated, with no change. The patient continues to gain weight
- She admits to improved mood, but has a continued lack of focus and concentration and has difficulty organizing and cleaning her home

Attending physician's mental notes: follow-up evaluation

- At this point, the patient's residual symptoms are unlikely to be affected by the current medication regimen
- Adding lisdexamfetamine (Vyvanse) now could address the binge eating as well as the lack of focus and organization
- We need to follow the patient closely and counsel her on the importance of stopping lisdexamfetamine and calling the clinic if her anxiety or insomnia worsens, her paranoia returns, or she has side effects such as a racing heart, seizures, or panic attacks

Case outcome: follow-up at week 20

- Start lisdexamfetamine (Vyvanse) 20 mg daily for BED
- "Lisdexamfetamine is incredibly helpful! My appetite has decreased and I'm no longer binge eating! Energy levels have improved, I can handle stress better, and I'm way less overwhelmed"
- She denies worsening anxiety and insomnia, paranoia, heart palpitations, panic, and seizures

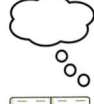

Attending physician's mental notes: follow-up evaluation

- We have arrived at a stable medication regimen

Case debrief

- A 34-year-old obese, married female with past history of PTSD, depression, and anxiety presented with worsening symptoms and binge eating
- She had been bingeing for 3 years, but denied any purging behavior or anorexia. Furthermore, she tried to lose weight, but gained all of it back due to her continuous binge eating cycle
- She had a significant history of mental illness in her family but had an unremarkable medical history
- On the initial visit, the patient was tearful and admitted to depressed mood, low energy, insomnia, nightmares, and paranoid thoughts. She would binge eat to the point of sweating and had low self-esteem, low motivation, and excessive guilt

- Addressing her sleep, paranoia, and mood were top priorities. Bupropion (Wellbutrin), which was thought to possibly be worsening her paranoid thoughts, anxiety, and insomnia, was tapered and discontinued. We also replaced her SSRI with an SNRI, duloxetine (Cymbalta) 60 mg, to treat her pain. Additionally, we started hydroxyzine (Vistaril) 25–50 mg to treat her anxiety and insomnia
- The patient responded well to the medication changes but continued bingeing in order to cope with her anxiety and stress. Her medications were adjusted on the next visit to duloxetine 90 mg and buspirone (BuSpar) 15 mg twice per day. The patient was kept on hydroxyzine for her sleep. These changes significantly improved her sleep and anxiety. Because the patient continued to gain weight and eat excessively, we carefully added lisdexamfetamine (Vyvanse) 20 mg to her medication regimen
- The patient reported that lisdexamfetamine was very helpful in decreasing her appetite and improving her energy levels. She was able to function better overall and denied side effects from the medication

Mechanism of action moment

- Lisdexamfetamine (Vyvanse), the first medication to be approved by the FDA to treat BED, is an inactive pro-drug of dextroamphetamine (*d*-amphetamine) (Dexedrine)
- While lisdexamfetamine is indicated for treating moderate-to-severe BED, it is not recommended for weight loss
- Lisdexamfetamine increases the half-life of *d*-amphetamine, which makes it possible to take it once per day. It is hydrophilic, does not cross the blood–brain barrier, and is absorbed quickly
- Upon absorption by the intestinal tract, lisdexamfetamine is hydrolyzed by red blood cell peptidases into its pharmacologically active form
- Data suggest that binge eating may involve dysfunction of the dopamine and norepinephrine pathways, which are involved in eating behavior and reward
- Dextroamphetamine increases the concentrations of neurotransmitters involved in regulating eating behaviors, appetite, and hunger by facilitating the release of dopamine, norepinephrine, and serotonin, and blocking the reuptake of norepinephrine and dopamine from the synaptic cleft. By doing so, it can help those struggling with BED, which is characterized by compulsive overeating

- The increase in dopamine and norepinephrine in certain regions of the prefrontal cortex may also improve depression, fatigue, and sleepiness, as well as wakefulness and concentration
- BED is considered an impulsive–compulsive disorder; it is thought to be associated with abnormalities in the cortical striatal circuitry where impulsivity eventually becomes compulsivity. Both impulsivity and compulsivity are components of various psychiatric disorders and may result from either excessive limbic emotional drive or lack of cortical inhibition
- While impulsivity and compulsivity originate from separate networks (impulsivity is regulated by a ventrally dependent learning system and compulsivity by a dorsally dependent habit system), these parallel circuits seem to overlap at certain points, which allows impulsive behavior to gradually shift to a compulsive behavior, and vice versa. This explains how behaviors that have their origins in the ventral loop, where impulses are driven by reward and motivation, can become compulsive behaviors as the brain adapts and engages in the dorsal loop
- Therefore, reversing this change seems to be critical in treating patients with impulsive–compulsive disorders such as BED, where the impulse of eating food to gain pleasure or nourishment becomes a mindless, habitual act. It may well be that lisdexamfetamine (Vyvanse), rather than suppressing appetite (as appetite is not what drives the disordered eating behavior seen in patients with BED), helps reverse this change by promoting striatal neuroplasticity

Two-minute tutorial

Can you become addicted to food?

- Although "food addiction" is not yet a formal DSM diagnosis, BED is. When maladaptive eating habits are performed despite apparent satiety and adverse health consequences, this defines a compulsion, with the formation of aberrant eating behaviors in a manner that parallels drug addiction
- Compulsive eating in obesity, BED, and bulimia can be mirrored by compulsive rejection of food, as in anorexia nervosa. BED is characterized by loss of control for eating, much as substance abuse has loss of control over seeking and taking a substance
- Briefly, BED is defined as having recurrent episodes of binge eating an amount of food larger than most people would eat in a similar amount of time under similar circumstances. What was once perhaps pleasurable eating to satisfy hunger and appetite has now

become compulsive eating that is out of control, and is associated with marked distress. About half of people with BED are obese

- BED is the most common eating disorder but is commonly undiagnosed. Many clinicians do not inquire about BED, even with obese patients. Most BED patients present to healthcare professionals for a comorbid psychiatric condition, rather than for binge eating. In fact, 80% of patients with BED meet the criteria for a mood disorder, anxiety disorder, other substance use disorder, or attention-deficit/hyperactivity disorder. One thing to remember for a clinician is to consider asking about binge eating in patients with any of these conditions, because treatment is available and the long-term complications of obesity are serious (discussed in Case 5 on drugs for psychosis)

- Lisdexamfetamine (Vyvanse) is the only currently approved treatment for BED. Several agents with limited efficacy and side effects used off label include topiramate (Topamax), several drugs used to treat depression, and naltrexone (ReVia). BED is another condition that belongs in the addictive disorders group and among the impulsive–compulsive disorders as it, too, is hypothesized to be linked to abnormalities in cortical striatal circuitry where impulsivity leads to compulsivity. The mechanism of *d*-amphetamine reversing binge eating symptoms may not be due to suppressing appetite, as appetite no longer really drives BED when it becomes compulsive. Instead, it is known that stimulants induce neuroplasticity, particularly in the striatum. Hypothetically, promotion of striatal neuroplasticity could help to reverse food-related behaviors that have their control migrate from ventral to dorsal when impulsive eating become compulsive. As for most impulsive–compulsive disorders, most studies adding various psychotherapies to drug treatment of BED report enhanced efficacy

Posttest self-assessment question and answer

Which medication is FDA approved for BED?

A. Fluoxetine (Prozac)
B. Clomipramine (Anafranil)
C. Lisdexamfetamine (Vyvanse)

Answer: C

Lisdexamfetamine is the only currently approved treatment for BED. Several agents with limited efficacy and side effects used off label include topiramate (Topamax), several drugs used to treat depression, and naltrexone (ReVia).

References

1. Chen Y, Baram TZ. Toward understanding how early-life stress reprograms cognitive and emotional brain networks. *Neuropsychopharmacology* 2016; 41:197–206. https://doi.org/10.1038/npp.2015.181

2. Guerdjikova AI, Mori N, Casuto LS, McElroy SL. Novel pharmacologic treatment in acute binge eating disorder – role of lisdexamfetamine. *Neuropsychiatr Dis Treat* 2016; 12:833–41. https://doi.org/10.2147/NDT.S80881

3. Hanson JL, Nacewicz BM, Suggerer MJ, et al. Behavioral problems after early life stress: contributions of the hippocampus and amygdala. *Biol Psychiatry* 2015; 77:314–23. https://doi.org/10.1016/j.biopsych.2014.04.020

4. Kundakovic M, Champagne FA. Early life experience, epigenetics and the developing brain. *Neuropsychopharmacology* 2015; 40:141–53. https://doi.org/10.1038/npp.2014.140

5. Marusak HA, Martin KR, Etkin A, et al. Childhood trauma exposure disrupts the automatic regulation of emotional processing. *Neuropsychopharmacology* 2015; 40:1250–8. https://doi.org/10.1038/npp.2014.311

6. McElroy SL, Hudson J, Ferreira-Cornwell MC, et al. Lisdexamfetamine dimesylate for adults with moderate to severe binge eating disorder: results of two pivotal phase 3 randomized controlled trials. *Neuropsychopharmacology* 2015; 41:1251–60. https://doi.org/10.1038/npp.2015.275

7. McEwen BS, Nasca C, Gray JD. Stress effects on neuronal structure: hippocampus, amygdala and prefrontal cortex. *Neuropsychopharmacology* 2016; 41: 3–23. https://doi.org/10.1038/npp.2015.171

8. McLaughlin KA, Sheridan MA, Gold AL, et al. Maltreatment exposure, brain structure and fear conditioning in children and adolescents. *Neuropsychopharmacology* 2016; 41:1956–65. https://doi.org/10.1038/npp.2015.365

9. Stahl SM. Impulsivity, compulsivity, addiction. In: *Stahl's Essential Psychopharmacology Online*, 4th edn, 2008. Available from: https://stahlonline.cambridge.org/essential_4th.jsf

10. Stahl SM. Lisdexamfetamine. In: *Stahl's Essential Psychopharmacology: Prescriber's Guide*, 6th edn. Cambridge, UK: Cambridge University Press, 2017; pp. 379–84.

11. Teicher MH, Anderson CM, Ohashi K, et al. Childhood maltreatment: altered network centrality of cingulate precuneus, temporal pole and insula. *Biol Psychiatry* 2014; 76:297–305. https://doi.org/10.1016/j.biopsych.2013.09.016

12. Tyrka AR, Burgers DE, Philip NS. The neurobiological correlates of childhood adversity and implications for treatment. *Acta Psychiatric Scand* 2013; 138:434–47. https://doi.org/10.1111/acps.12143

13. Ward K, Citrome L. Lisdexamfetamine: chemistry, pharmacodynamics, pharmacokinetics, and clinical efficacy, safety, and tolerability in the treatment of binge eating disorder. *Expert Opin Drug Metab Toxicol* 2018; 14:229–38. https://doi.org/10.1080/17425255.2018.1420163

14. Zhang JY, Liu TH, He Y, et al. Chronic stress remodels synapses in an amygdala circuit-specific manner. *Biol Psychiatry* 2019; 85:189–201. https://doi.org/10.1016/j.biopsych.2018.06.019.

Case 18: The man who couldn't stop hitting people

The Question: Is there a way to further optimize treatment of violent, psychotic agitation safely beyond the combination of clozapine (Clozaril) with a mood stabilizer in someone with significant cardiovascular history?

The Psychopharmacological Dilemma: How to reduce violent, psychotic behaviors in someone with an inadequate response to multiple empirical combinations of medications for treatment-resistant schizophrenia with behavioral agitation

Angharad Ames and Lawrence Faziola

Pretest self-assessment question (answer at the end of the case)

Which of the following are evidence-based treatments for psychotic aggression that is refractory to clozapine (Clozaril)?

A. Clozapine plus valproic acid (Depakote)
B. Clozapine plus a selective serotonin reuptake inhibitor
C. Valproic acid plus lithium
D. Clozapine plus lithium
E. A and D
F. All of the above

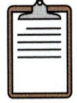

Patient evaluation on intake

- A 59-year-old male under mental health conservatorship presented to the hospital from a locked nursing facility after assaulting a peer in the context of worsening psychosis with delusions centered around themes of being raped by men
- The patient had been discharged just 6 weeks earlier after an 18-month psychiatric hospitalization for an identical presentation

Psychiatric history

- The patient's symptoms began at age 19 when he started hearing persecutory voices shortly after joining the Navy; he was honorably discharged 8 months later due to the severity of his symptoms
- His psychosis was characterized early on by auditory hallucinations of voices whispering degrading things about him and delusions of being raped by numerous non-specific males, that medications made him homosexual, that he was in a gang, and that he was sexually abused by male family members when he was an infant. Importantly, there was never any evidence to suggest past abuse or trauma. He often had manic symptoms, such as pressured speech, reduced need for sleep, significant irritability, grandiosity,

hypersexual behaviors, and labile affect, which could last for several weeks
- His mood was often depressed, as he ruminated on his inability to obtain affection from the opposite sex
- A review of past records revealed multiple hospitalizations beginning in his early 20s with a past diagnosis of schizoaffective disorder, bipolar subtype
- In his late 20s, he began demonstrating frequent and unpredictable aggressive behaviors, including physical assault against his father on two occasions; as he entered his 30s, his thought processes and behaviors became more disorganized, such that his parents could no longer take care of him due to fear for their personal safety
- At age 33, he was placed under mental health conservatorship for grave disability, as his behaviors became increasingly agitated and increasingly non-adherent to prescribed medications
- Numerous hospitalizations for severe psychotic agitation ensued, with placement in a variety of care facilities as his persecutory delusions became more severe and as he became more aggressive, with delusions that facility staff forced him to engage in sexual activities while he was asleep, strangling a peer who he believed raped him at a hospital, punching other residents, grabbing staff, and punching walls
- Neuropsychiatric testing was performed in 2013 in the setting of concerns for possible underlying cognitive impairment, suggesting developmental cognitive deficiency with non-specific attentional and executive dysfunction
- At baseline, there is an expression of strongly held persecutory beliefs that center around ego-dystonic sexual themes, such as being raped or molested by other male patients/residents and being sexually inadequate (e.g. feeling that his penis was shrinking and believing that female nurses talk about him having a small penis)

Medication history

- Numerous antipsychotics over the years
    - Fluphenazine (Prolixin)
    - Perphenazine (Trilafon)
    - Thiothixene (Navane)
    - Haloperidol (oral formulation and decanoate) (Haldol)
    - Olanzapine (Zyprexa) (caused weight gain and metabolic syndrome)
    - Risperidone (Risperdal)
    - Ziprasidone (Geodon)
    - Aripiprazole (Abilify)

- Clozapine (Clozaril) (initiated for the first time in 2013, later discontinued because it seemed he was still having aggression, then later restarted and discontinued in 2017 due to equivocal response and marginal effect on aggression)
- Quetiapine (Seroquel)
- Lurasidone (Latuda)
- Several mood stabilizers
  - Valproic acid (Depakote) 3000 mg per day at highest (at this level, his platelets dropped to 106×10^3 cells/ml, so the dose was decreased to 2500 mg per day)
  - Lithium
  - Topiramate (Topamax)
- Benzodiazepines
  - Clonazepam (Klonopin)
  - Temazepam (Restoril)
  - Alprazolam (Xanax)
  - Diazepam (Valium)
- Other
  - Gabapentin (Neurontin)
  - Trazodone (Desyrel) 300 mg every night; also later 100 mg four times per day for impulsivity (may have caused hyponatremia at high dose)
  - Propranolol (Inderal)
  - Diphenhydramine (Benadryl)
  - Sertraline (Zoloft)
  - Clonidine (Catapres)
  - Benztropine (Cogentin) 2 mg twice per day

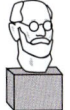

Psychotherapy history

- The overall severity of the patient's conceptual disorganization made most forms of psychotherapy impossible, although he sometimes had meaningful participation in inpatient recovery-oriented programming sessions. However, he often became too disruptive to remain for the full duration

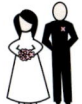

Social and personal history

- The patient was born in the South and moved to California as an infant; he was raised as an only child by his parents, who were married
- According to his parents' account, he developed normally and did not demonstrate any notable delays
- He experienced bullying from peers about having a large head

- He completed high school and 1 year of trade school, and then joined the military
- He was honorably discharged from the military after 8 months of serving in a non-combat role
- He lived with his parents until he was 34, at which age he attacked his father and broke his jaw; he was arrested for assault and battery of his father and served a 30-day jail sentence
- After becoming alienated from his father, he gradually lost contact with his mother, as his parents moved back to the South. He has generally become estranged from them over the last decade, with no other family connections
- He has never married and has no children
- He has never been gainfully employed
- His only source of income is Supplemental Security Income
- He has spent most of his adult life in care facilities for the mentally ill
- Although he experimented with cannabis and phencyclidine in his youth, and has periodically consumed alcohol, he did not have clear evidence of a substance use disorder

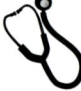

Medical history

- Coronary artery disease, status postmyocardial infarction 1 year ago
- Hypertension
- Hyperlipidemia
- Type 2 diabetes mellitus
- Normocytic normochromic anemia
- Gout
- Gastroesophageal reflux disease
- Head computed tomography (CT) scan and non-contrast magnetic resonance imaging (MRI) of the brain were grossly unremarkable; however, demonstrated enlarged sulci and ventricles

Current medications

- Non-psychotropic
  - Allopurinol (Zyloprim) for gout
  - Amlodipine (Norvasc) for hypertension
  - Aspirin for cerebrovascular disease
  - Atorvastatin (Lipitor) for hyperlipidemia
  - Benazepril (Lotensin) for hypertension
  - Budesonide-formoterol (Symbicort) inhaler for asthma
  - Cholecalciferol for prophylaxis
  - Fluticasone (Flonase) for asthma
  - Furosemide (Lasix) for hypertension

- Regular insulin for diabetes
- Isosorbide dinitrate (Isordil) for chest pain
- Magnesium oxide for prophylaxis
- Metoprolol (Lopressor) for hypertension
- Nitroglycerin for chest pain
- Pantoprazole (Protonix) for gastric reflux
- Psychotropic
  - Valproic acid (Depakote) extended-release 2500 mg at night for mood instability and irritability, with a serum level of 102 µg/ml (the patient weighs 278.6 lbs and his height is 72 inches)
  - Olanzapine (Zyprexa) 20 mg twice per day to manage psychotic symptoms
  - Lorazepam (Ativan) 1 mg twice per day for agitation
  - Hydroxyzine (Vistaril) 50 mg as needed for anxiety
  - Clonazepam (Klonopin) 1 mg as needed for agitation

Family history

- Mother, aunt, and three uncles had "mental breakdowns"
- Maternal great aunt died by suicide

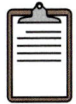

Patient evaluation on initial visit

- A 58-year-old conserved male with schizoaffective disorder, bipolar subtype, and several chronic medical conditions presents for stabilization of recurrent, violent, physical aggression that has made it impossible for him to sustain placement at a lower level of care for a meaningful period of time
- His symptoms were notable for auditory hallucinations of a persecutory nature, grandiose and paranoid delusions, disorganized speech, labile affect, disorganized thought processes, and unpredictable moods and behaviors
- Delusions abounded regarding being raped repeatedly in the night by other patients and people who had come onto the unit
- He required multiple emergency intramuscular medications due to violent behaviors, such as hitting other patients and attacking staff in the absence of provocation

Question

In your clinical experience, would you expect the patient to respond to any single medication regimen alone?

- Yes
- No

Attending physician's mental notes: initial evaluation

- The patient's initial laboratory results do not support a medical etiology of the patient's decompensation, or any acute medical issues
- Head CT and brain MRI reveal prominent cerebral volume loss and no acute process
- Decompensation may be due to medication non-compliance, which would make him more vulnerable to perceiving threats and reacting behaviorally
- Several psychotropic classes have been utilized in the past, both alone and in combination, none of which appeared effective in achieving durable and meaningful stability
- Either he has a consistent pattern of medication non-adherence outside of the hospital, which is less likely as he has been living in supervised mental health facilities, or, more likely, his illness is resistant to treatment
- Physical aggression is the reason for his repeated admissions, and if stabilized, he would be able to live outside of the hospital for a longer period of time
- The patient presents imminent risk of harm to others outside of the controlled hospital setting, which represents the least restrictive environment to maintain his safety, the safety of others, and to stabilize him on medications
- Strong consideration should be given to treatment with clozapine (Clozaril) for chronic aggression in schizophrenia spectrum illness with inadequate response to other antipsychotic agents, although this patient's absolute neutrophil count (ANC) on sequential testing has remained between 1000 and 1500/µl, which is too low for treatment initiation

Question

Despite taking several psychotropic medications at high doses, the patient does not appear to have robust efficacy, as evidenced by his inability to remain out of the hospital for a meaningful period of time, due to eventual and repetitive assaults on staff and/or peers in whichever facility he lives. Which of the following would be your next step?

- Get head imaging
- Get a serum valproic acid (Depakote) level
- Add a second antipsychotic
- Increase the clonazepam (Klonopin) dose
- Get a serum olanzapine (Zyprexa) level

Attending physician's mental notes: initial evaluation (continued)

- There is record of the patient responding well to the combination of olanzapine (Zyprexa) and valproic acid (Depakote) in the past
- It is prudent to limit polypharmacy as much as possible
- Valproic acid is at a marginally high level for the patient's weight, so it would be reasonable to decrease the dose to 1500 mg every night
- Although the patient seems to require benzodiazepines to control agitation, we should try to minimize long-acting formulations due to the patient's age, cardiovascular comorbidities, and fall risk
- The patient is switched from the long-acting clonazepam (Klonopin) to the shorter-acting lorazepam (Ativan) 1 mg twice per day for now
- For as-needed medication for acute anxiety, we will use hydroxyzine (Vistaril) instead of a benzodiazepine
- Due to the patient's diabetes and cardiovascular comorbidities, we should start a cross-titration from olanzapine to risperidone (Risperdal), with the hope that this might minimize his metabolic risk factors

Further investigation

Is there anything else you would especially like to know about this patient?

- What were the patient's clinical responses and side effects to prior trials of medications that might affect our pharmacological treatment choices?
  - Trazodone (Desyrel) 300 mg every night and 100 mg four times per day for impulsivity was suspected to have caused hyponatremia at the high dose
  - Haloperidol (Haldol) (oral formulation up to 20 mg twice per day and decanoate formulation 150 mg monthly) was discontinued after the patient was noted to have a worsening Parkinsonian gait
  - Olanzapine (Zyprexa) 20 mg PO twice per day plus 10 mg up to four times per day as needed for acute agitation caused weight gain and worsening metabolic syndrome markers

Case outcome: follow-up at week 12

- Over the prior weeks, olanzapine (Zyprexa) was cross-titrated to risperidone (Risperdal) 4 mg twice per day and the valproic acid (Depakote) dosage was reduced to 1500 mg every night, with a subsequent valproic acid serum level at 69 µg/ml. This level is above the minimum effective level, but the literature suggests that levels of 75–120 µg/ml are more effective in preventing manic episodes. Thus, the dose could be increased while bearing in mind that the patient experienced thrombocytopenia when his valproic acid serum level was approximately 100 μg/ml

- An improvement was noted in his psychotic symptoms, but the patient still experienced several paroxysmal behavioral outbursts, requiring emergency administration of injectable medications
- Olanzapine (Zyprexa) tablets as needed were not effective for acute agitation, but plasma blood levels at those doses were not determined; however, the combination of haloperidol (Haldol) with lorazepam (Ativan) and diphenhydramine (Benadryl) often showed efficacy
- With the consideration of pursuing dual antipsychotic therapy, low-dose haloperidol twice per day was initiated briefly but did not appear helpful
- Loxapine (Loxitane) was initiated and titrated to 75 mg twice per day but also appeared ineffective and was likewise stopped, and the patient was switched to chlorpromazine (Thorazine)
- In the last few days, the patient continued to demonstrate agitation fueled by persistent delusional beliefs, which endured despite staff verbal redirections and medication adherence, leading to physical injury to staff and a peer, which required that the patient be placed into physical restraints

Questions

Would you continue his antipsychotic regimen?

- Yes, continue both risperidone (Risperdal) and chlorpromazine (Thorazine)
- Continue risperidone, but discontinue chlorpromazine
- Continue chlorpromazine, but discontinue risperidone
- No, discontinue both risperidone and chlorpromazine
- Raise risperidone dose and monitor plasma drug levels to the point of tolerability or futility
- Try another trial of olanzapine (Zyprexa) with doses guided by plasma drug levels this time
- Try another trial of clozapine (Clozaril) with doses guided by plasma drug levels this time

Is there another antipsychotic medication you would try?

- Tables 18.1 and 18.2 provide the plasma levels of various antipsychotics and mood stabilizers
- Importantly, chronic exposure to maintenance lithium plasma concentrations greater than 1.0 mEq/l may increase the long-term risk of renal insufficiency

Table 18.1 Antipsychotic levels and expected plasma levels for given oral doses

Medication	Minimum response threshold (ng/ml)	Point of futility (ng/ml)
Aripiprazole Expected level = 12 × oral dose (mg/day)	150	500
Clozapine Male non-smoker: expected level = 1.08 × oral dose (mg/day) Female non-smoker: expected level = 1.32 × oral dose (mg/day)	350	1000
Fluphenazine Non-smoker: expected level = 0.08 × oral dose (mg/day)	0.8	4.0
Haloperidol Expected level = 0.78 × oral dose (mg/day)	5	30
Olanzapine Non-smoker: expected level = 2.0 × oral dose (mg/day)	40	200
Paliperidone Expected level = 4.7 × oral dose (mg/day)	28	112
Risperidone + 9-OH risperidone Expected level = 7.0 × oral dose (mg/day)	28	112
Perphenazine Expected level = 0.04 × oral dose (mg/day)	0.8	4.0

From Brunton et al. (2018).

Table 18.2 Plasma levels of effective mood stabilizers

Mood stabilizer	Plasma concentration	
	Acute mania	Maintenance
Lithium	1.0–1.4 mEq/l	0.8–1.2 mEq/l
Divalproex sodium, valproic acid	100–120 µg/l	80–120 µg/l
Carbamazepine	9–12 µg/ml	6–12 µg/l

From Brunton et al. (2018).

Attending physician's mental notes: follow-up at week 12

- Given the multitude of failed antipsychotic medication trials despite adequate doses and reasonable durations, it seemed sensible to either dose high to the point of futility by monitoring tolerability and plasma drug levels on any given antipsychotic *or* to attempt dual antipsychotic therapy in this patient, despite the inherent theoretical risk of increased adverse event burden, and with due consideration for this patient's cardiovascular risk factors, general physical deconditioning, and elevated fall risk
- Initiating chlorpromazine (Thorazine) combines an atypical antipsychotic (risperidone (Risperdal)) with a typical psychotic, with the hope that the relatively high level of antihistaminergic activity by chlorpromazine might improve the patient's severity of agitation

- Unfortunately, the patient remained steadfast in his belief of being persecuted by peers and staff, and consequently remained combative, even after the titration of chlorpromazine, with increasing frequency of emergency benzodiazepine and antihistamine administration to curtail his imminent risk of harm to others
- At this time, it would be reasonable to consider initiating clozapine (Clozaril) under the framework for benign ethnic neutropenia given the patient's ethnic ancestry (i.e. guidelines for dose scheduling and ANC monitoring in individuals who exhibit lower levels of white blood cells compared with normative values, but no increased risk of infection, and which reflect genetic variations exhibited more often in certain ethnic populations), and hematology consultation was sought
- Not only has the patient demonstrated clearly treatment-resistant schizoaffective disorder, for which clozapine is indicated, but there is also evidence suggesting clozapine is effective in treating treatment-resistant psychotic *aggression*, and even more so in combination with valproic acid (Depakote) or lithium
- Hematology did not believe that the patient met the parameters to be classified as having benign ethnic neutropenia
- However, with repeat testing, his ANC was found to have risen to 1790/µl, above the appropriate thresholds for the general population, and clozapine was initiated while tapering chlorpromazine to minimize the potential to induce an anticholinergic toxidrome, with a goal of achieving antipsychotic monotherapy on clozapine

Questions

How long does it take for clozapine (Clozaril) to become effective?
What would you expect the effect of clozapine in addition to valproic acid (Depakote) to have on this patient's behaviors?
Is the risk of enhanced sedation and increased risk of bone marrow suppression on each of the agents, valproic acid and clozapine, worth the potential benefit of this combination?

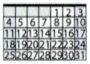

Case outcome: follow-up at week 24

- Over the last 12 weeks, clozapine (Clozaril) has been titrated to a therapeutic serum level of 768 ng/ml, achieved at a dose of 100 mg in the morning and 500 mg at night. Atropine drops were initiated as needed for sialorrhea
- Chlorpromazine (Thorazine) was discontinued simultaneously

- An electrocardiogram showed a normal sinus rhythm and a corrected QT interval of 464 ms
- Nursing staff took note of overnight gasping for air and found oxygen desaturations that prompted a recommendation for using a continuous positive airway pressure device during sleep
- A new goal of minimizing medications that might promote respiratory depression prompted a review of his as-needed medications for agitation, which were: hydroxyzine (Vistaril) as first line, olanzapine (Zyprexa) as second line, and lorazepam (Ativan) as third line, but olanzapine seemed to have minimal efficacy
- With the goal of having the patient take only one scheduled antipsychotic, risperidone (Risperdal) was tapered to discontinuation
- The patient seemed to improve, and appeared to have diminishing reactions to delusional beliefs, although his episodic aggression remained unpredictable and continued to occur, with the patient punching walls or peers
- Given that his clozapine serum level provided room for an increase, the clozapine dose was increased to target the positive symptoms of psychosis and episodic aggression; however, the patient felt extremely sedated and often dizzy at the higher dose and expressed feeling better at the lower dose. Thus, the dose was decreased back to 100 mg in the morning and 500 mg at night

Attending physician's mental notes: follow-up at week 24

- At this time, despite some marginal improvement, the patient remains prone to violent outbursts (hitting peers and staff, punching walls), seemingly due to the fixed belief that he is being raped by various male individuals on the unit, both seen and unseen
- He is tolerating clozapine (Clozaril) well, with a prophylactic bowel regimen effective in preventing constipation, his sialorrhea is tolerable with atropine drops, and his heart rate is regular, although, given that his positive symptoms are still not well controlled, he may benefit from further augmented therapy

Questions

What might you try as an augmentation strategy?
What concerns about further augmentation do you have?

Attending physician's mental notes: follow-up at week 24 (continued)

- Topiramate (Topamax) augmentation to an antipsychotic for psychosis was studied in two meta-analyses,[7,12] in which it demonstrated significant benefit

- Topiramate 50 mg twice per day was initiated with the goal of better controlling the continued aggressive outbursts and potentially reducing the overall severity of his psychotic beliefs, with close monitoring for paresthesia and worsened attention deficits
- Due to the lack of clear efficacy of olanzapine (Zyprexa) as needed and the superior response to chlorpromazine (Thorazine) historically, the as-needed medication regimen for agitation was altered to: hydroxyzine (Vistaril) 25 mg as first line, lorazepam (Ativan) 2 mg as second line, and chlorpromazine 50 mg as third line

Case outcome: follow-up at week 32

- Over the last few weeks, topiramate (Topamax) has been titrated to 100 mg twice per day, with minimal expected side effects of mild sleepiness and mental fogginess
- The patient had less irritability and fewer outbursts, which was appreciated by multiple staff, but the severity of his delusional beliefs persisted, and he remained fixated on certain male peers who he believed had raped him
- Fewer intramuscular administrations were being utilized, although multiple as-needed oral medications continued to be administered almost every day to maintain control of his agitation, with some days requiring three doses of hydroxyzine (Vistaril) as needed, often two doses of lorazepam (Ativan), and at least one dose of chlorpromazine (Thorazine)

Attending physician's mental notes: follow-up at week 32

- This patient continues to be exposed to dual antipsychotic agents, for which there are inherent dangers of higher all-cause mortality in older age groups and increased propensity for side effects
- Although chlorpromazine (Thorazine) is not a scheduled medication, the patient is requiring frequent enough administrations that he is receiving it on a nearly scheduled basis
- Chlorpromazine and clozapine (Clozaril) both significantly exert anticholinergic, anti-α-adrenergic, and anti-histaminergic effects, which, in combination with the weakly anticholinergic but frequently administered hydroxyzine (Vistaril), may lead to adverse effects of sedation, worsening tachycardia, dizziness, and cognitive deficits in older age groups
- These concerns prompt the need for aggressive prophylactic treatment of bowel motility to prevent the development of paralytic ileus

- These concerns are especially important in the setting of the patient's age, general weakness/elevated risk of falls, and cardiovascular comorbidities
- Ideally, the patient's behaviors would be stabilized on clozapine alone, but this seems unlikely because he continues to become fixated on certain peers, believing that they have raped him or are spreading lies about his sexuality, and he continues to issue threats
- The extant literature reveals evidence that potentially effective medication regimens for single agent-resistant psychotic aggression are clozapine in combination with valproic acid (Depakote) and clozapine in combination with lithium; however, there is no data on the efficacy of the combination of clozapine with valproic acid *and* lithium in treating psychotic aggression
- Trials such BALANCE (Bipolar Affective disorder: Lithium/ ANtiConvulsant Evaluation) have demonstrated the safety of combined lithium and valproic acid
- With continued aggression precluding discharge, it appears prudent to attempt additional augmentation with a so far unutilized mechanism of action, and thus lithium was initiated

Case outcome: follow-up at week 32 (continued)

- Start lithium augmentation for psychotic aggression at a low dose of 300 mg daily, given the patient's polypharmacy and age, monitoring for further alteration of mental status, diabetic ketoacidosis, and neuroleptic malignant syndrome, as the risk of these is higher when lithium is combined with clozapine (Clozaril)
- Recheck his lithium level, metabolic panel, thyroid studies, and urinalysis after 1 week
- The goal lithium level will be less than 1.0 mEq/l

Case outcome: follow-up at week 38

- The patient's initial lithium level was 0.15 mEq/l, and the dosage was increased to 600 mg daily, with subsequent lithium level of 0.65 mEq/l
- Achieving therapeutic serum levels, the patient's behavior was noticed to have improved in the following weeks, with fewer episodes of physical agitation and less-prominent delusions, and more linear thought processes
- Somnolence and sialorrhea became more prominent, with sleep reaching 10 hours per 24-hour period; atropine sublingual drops and oral trihexyphenidyl were required to reduce saliva overproduction

Attending physician's mental notes: follow-up at week 38

- In the month prior to the initiation of lithium, the patient's agitation required dosages of hydroxyzine (Vistaril) on 21 occasions, lorazepam (Ativan) on 19 occasions, and chlorpromazine (Thorazine) on six occasions, while in the month following a therapeutic serum lithium level, the patient required hydroxyzine on nine occasions, lorazepam on nine occasions, and chlorpromazine on two occasions, and in the month after that, the patient required hydroxyzine twice, lorazepam once, and chlorpromazine once
- Despite there being three female patients on the unit (an unusually high number on this particular unit), the patient has not demonstrated any fixation on them or any inappropriate behaviors toward them, which is in contrast to the tendency for the patient to expose himself to female patients several months prior to lithium augmentation
- The patient began doing so well that he was accepted into assisted living placement in lieu of state hospital placement

Case debrief

- A number of patients with severe schizophrenia exhibit violent episodes arising from their disconnection from reality-based thinking, which can be difficult to treat and is often the primary reason such patients require long-term care in locked psychiatric facilities
- Initial attempts to adjust the patient's medications, such as maximizing single antipsychotic therapy, mood stabilizer augmentation, and dual antipsychotic therapy, were all tried prior to re-initiation of clozapine (Clozaril), although clozapine initiation was initially precluded due to lower-than-acceptable neutrophil counts
- When clozapine failed to yield significant-enough improvements, augmentation with topiramate (Topamax) and as-needed medications were incorporated into the treatment plan
- The patient's age and medical comorbidities were a cause for concern when the patient's behavior continued to necessitate a second antipsychotic in addition to clozapine and his other medications
- When lithium was added to clozapine, valproic acid (Depakote), and topiramate, significant improvement in behaviors were notable
- Although the patient still occasionally has behavioral agitation, he requires far fewer as-needed rescue medications with significantly less frequency, which in turn reduces his overall risk of adverse medication outcomes

- The final psychotropic medication regimen on which the patient was discharged from the hospital to assisted living was:
  - Clozapine 100 mg PO every morning and 500 mg every evening
  - Valproic acid extended-release 1500 mg PO every night
  - Topiramate 100 mg PO twice per day
  - Lithium 600 mg PO daily
  - As-needed medications:
    ◦ First-line for agitation: hydroxyzine (Vistaril) 25 mg PO
    ◦ Second-line for agitation: lorazepam (Ativan) 2 mg PO
    ◦ Third-line for agitation: chlorpromazine (Thorazine) 50 mg PO

Take-home points

- Physical aggression due to severe psychosis may be difficult to treat and is often refractory to multiple psychotropic medications and pharmacological combinations
- Such physical aggression, often in the setting of severe schizophrenia, may be the primary reason a patient requires long-term hospitalization in a locked facility
- The use of two antipsychotics concurrently is associated with higher all-cause mortality in older age groups and an increased propensity for side effects, and thus ideally such a combination should be avoided or, at the very least, minimized
- Clozapine (Clozaril) in combination with lithium and valproic acid (Depakote) may be an effective alternative to dual antipsychotic use in treating these difficult cases
- There were multiple occasions in which it might have been helpful to obtain serum levels of antipsychotics, such as olanzapine (Zyprexa) and risperidone (Risperdal), before deciding that those medications were ineffective for the patient

Mechanism of action moment

- The mechanism of action of lithium is at this time not fully understood; however, there are several theories as to how it may exert its effects, including (Figure 18.1):
  - Stabilization of glutamate uptake
  - Normalization of low γ-aminobutyric acid (GABA) in cerebrospinal fluid
  - Antagonism at serotonin 5-HT$_{1A}$ and 5-HT$_{1B}$ autoreceptors, leading to increases serotonin in the synaptic cleft
  - Non-competitive inhibition of inositol monophosphate
  - Inhibition of glycogen synthase 3 (GSK3)

– Activates cAMP-response element binding protein (CREB), leading to increased expression of brain-derived neurotrophic factor (BDNF)

① In mice : Chronic lithium admin → ↑ and stabilization of glutamate uptake
② Normalization of low CSF levels of GABA
③ Enhances NE and 5HT function in the CNS:

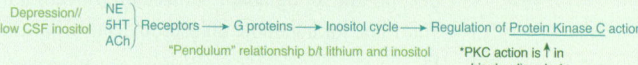

ANTAGONIST at 5HT$_{1A}$ and 5HT$_{1B}$ autoreceptors → ↑5HT availability in synaptic cleft
    MOOD SLEEP

④ Noncompetitive inhibitor of inositol monophosphatase → depletion of inositol W/in 5 d.

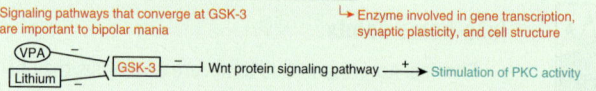

Depression// low CSF inositol
NE
5HT } Receptors → G proteins → Inositol cycle → Regulation of Protein Kinase C action
ACh
"Pendulum" relationship b/t lithium and inositol *PKC action is ↑ in bipolar disorder*

⑤ Lithium and VPA inhibit glycogen synthase 3 (GSK-3)

*Signaling pathways that converge at GSK-3 are important to bipolar mania → Enzyme involved in gene transcription, synaptic plasticity, and cell structure

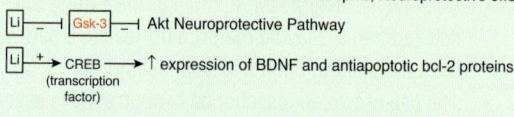

VPA –
Lithium – GSK-3 ─┤ Wnt protein signaling pathway ──+─→ Stimulation of PKC activity

⑥ Lithium treatment → Larger cortical and hippocampal volumes, independent of clinical treatment response
     ∴ Neurotrophic, Neuroprotective effect

Li –┤ Gsk-3 ─┤ Akt Neuroprotective Pathway

Li +→ CREB → ↑ expression of BDNF and antiapoptotic bcl-2 proteins
  (transcription factor)

Figure 18.1. The mechanism of action of lithium.

Posttest self-assessment question and answer

Which of the following are evidence-based treatments for psychotic aggression that is refractory to clozapine (Clozaril)?

A. Clozapine plus valproic acid (Depakote)
B. Clozapine plus a selective serotonin reuptake inhibitor
C. Valproic acid plus lithium
D. Clozapine plus lithium
E. A and D
F. All of the above
Answer: E

References

1. Brunton LL, Hilal-Dandan R, Knollmann BC. *Goodman & Gilman's: The Pharmacological Basis of Therapeutics*, 13th edn. New York, NY: McGraw-Hill Education LLC, 2018.
2. Buckley P, Miller A, Olsen J, et al. When symptoms persist: clozapine augmentation strategies. *Schizophr Bull* 2001; 27:615–28. https://doi.org/10.1093/oxfordjournals.schbul.a006901
3. Comai S, Tau M, Pavlovic Z, Gobbi G. The psychopharmacology of aggressive behavior: a translational approach: part 2: clinical

studies using atypical antipsychotics, anticonvulsants, and lithium. *J Clin Psychopharmacol* 2012; 32:237–60. https://doi.org/10.1097/JCP.0b013e31824929d6

4. Cummings M, Stahl SM. *Management of Complex Treatment-resistant Patients with Psychotic Disorders.* New York, NY: Cambridge University Press, 2021.

5. Ebenezer, I. *Neuropsychopharmacology and Therapeutics.* Chichester, UK/Hoboken, NJ: John Wiley & Sons,2015.

6. Geddes, JR, Goodwin, GM, Rendell, J, et al. Lithium plus valproate combination therapy versus monotherapy for relapse prevention in bipolar I disorder (BALANCE): a randomised open-label trial. *Lancet* 2010; 375: 385–95. https://doi.org/10.1016/S0140-6736(09)61828-6

7. Keck PE Jr, Bowden CL, Meinhold JM, et al. Relationship between serum valproate and lithium levels and efficacy and tolerability in bipolar maintenance therapy. *Int J Psychiatry Clin Pract* 2005; 9:271–7. https://doi.org/10.1080/13651500500305622

8. Meyer J, Stahl SM. *Clozapine Handbook.* New York, NY: Cambridge University Press, 2019.

9. Okuyama Y, Oya K, Matsunaga S, et al. Efficacy and tolerability of topiramate-augmentation therapy for schizophrenia: a systematic review and meta-analysis of randomized controlled trials. *Neuropsychiatr Dis Treat* 2016; 12:3221–36. https://doi.org/10.2147/NDT.S125367

10. Puzantian T, Balt S. *The Carlat Psychiatry Report: Medication Fact Book for Psychiatric Practice.* Newburyport, MA: Carlat Publishing,2014.

11. Schatzberg AF, Nemeroff CB, eds. *The American Psychiatric Association Publishing Textbook of Psychopharmacology*, 5th edn. Washington, DC: American Psychiatric Association Publishing, 2017.

12. Zheng, W, Xiang, YT, Yang, XH, et al. Clozapine augmentation with antiepileptic drugs for treatment-resistant schizophrenia: a meta-analysis of randomized controlled trials. *J Clin Psychiatry* 2017; 78:e498–505. https://doi.org/10.4088/JCP.16r10782

Case 19: Brexpiprazole: "an awakening"

The Question: Can the addition of brexpiprazole (Rexulti) to clozapine (Clozaril) reduce positive symptoms in a patient who has not fully responded to clozapine alone?

The Psychopharmacological Dilemma: Can "third-generation" antipsychotics, such as brexpiprazole, be utilized in combination with clozapine for treatment-resistant psychosis?

Troy Kurz, Lauren Kurz, and Samer Kamal

Pretest self-assessment question (answer at the end of the case)

Which of the following disorder(s) is brexpiprazole (Rexulti) FDA approved for?

A. Schizophrenia
B. Bipolar depression
C. Bipolar maintenance
D. Acute mania
E. Treatment-resistant depression (adjunct)

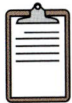

Patient evaluation on intake

- A 31-year-old woman with the chief complaint of diagnosed treatment-resistant schizophrenia disorder

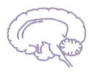

Psychiatric history

- The patient's first psychotic episode occurred at age 17 after her father died of cancer
- She was initially started on a second-generation antipsychotic, but her symptoms remained and different antipsychotics were thus trialed over many years
- Multiple psychotic episodes have occurred in the past, leading to multiple inpatient hospitalizations
- The family reports that the patient has been compliant with medications since moving in with them after initially living alone; they encourage the patient to take her medications daily
- The patient was trialed on long-acting injectables in the past when she lived by herself, including paliperidone (Invega) and haloperidol decanoate (Haldol Decanoate)
- Even with appropriate medication compliance, the patient continued to have positive symptoms while on both first- and second-generation antipsychotics, with frequent hospitalizations
- The patient eventually tried clozapine (Clozaril) a little over a year ago
- She admitted to manic-like symptoms in the past including episodes of grandiosity, high energy, and little sleep

- She reported multiple past psychiatric medication failures leading to the starting of clozapine roughly 13 months ago
- She denies past suicide attempts
- The patient's biological brother suffers from bipolar disorder, and she states that valproic acid (Depakote) was effective in treating him. Her biological father was diagnosed with schizophrenia

Medication history

- Several psychotropic medications have been tried over the last 10 years including antipsychotics and mood stabilizers
- Medication trials have included: quetiapine (Seroquel), asenapine (Saphris), lurasidone (Latuda), risperidone (Risperdal), haloperidol (Haldol), and valproic acid (Depakote)

Psychiatric history

- The patient has had numerous past psychiatric hospitalizations related to episodes of psychosis and suicidal ideation
- She denies a past history of trauma

Substance use history

- The patient previously used marijuana regularly from the age of 18 to 20
- She currently smokes one pack of cigarettes per day
- She denies illicit drug or alcohol use

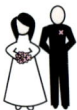

Social and personal history

- The patient's family is supportive and is actively involved with her care
- The patient is a second-generation Hispanic American
- The patient's biological father is deceased; he passed away when the patient was 16 years old
- The patient previously lived by herself in another city prior to moving back in with her parents last year
- The patient lives at home with her biological mother, eldest brother, and grandparents in an apartment
- The patient graduated high school and was previously enrolled in college with a stable job, prior to her first psychotic episode in 2010
- The patient is currently unemployed; she last worked as a hostess

Medical history

- The patient is obese with a body mass index (BMI) of 34 kg/m²
- Lipids: she has elevated cholesterol with low-density lipoprotein (LDL) 262 mg/dl and high-density lipoprotein (HDL) 42 mg/dl
- The patient appears overweight, but otherwise has a normal physical and neurological examination

- A white blood cell count is obtained monthly; her last result was normal (absolute neutrophil count 4.3)
- Vital signs: stable

Family history

- The patient's biological brother suffers from bipolar disorder, treated with valproic acid (Depakote)
- Her biological father was diagnosed with schizophrenia; he was never adequately treated with medications
- Her paternal uncle has depression
- There is no history of substance use in the family

Current medications

- Clozapine (Clozaril) 200 mg PO twice per day
- Oxcarbazepine (Trileptal) 600 mg PO twice per day
- Docusate (Colace) 250 mg PO daily for constipation

Patient evaluation on initial visit

- The patient is currently taking oxcarbazepine (Trileptal) 600 mg twice per day in combination with clozapine (Clozaril) 200 mg twice per day
- She has been taking clozapine for over a year, but continues to have ongoing positive symptoms such as auditory hallucinations
- She has been getting regular blood draws to evaluate for agranulocytosis
- The patient admits to current auditory hallucinations, which are command in nature, but not to hurting herself or others as evidenced by the patient's statement, "The FBI tells me to complete my job application for IBM"
- She displays multiple delusions during the intake appointment as evidenced by statements such as, "The FBI continues to contact me for a job" and "IBM has been sending me information through transmagnetic frequencies"
- She admits to depressive symptoms including depression, low energy, and poor sleep
- She denies suicidal ideation or self-harm thoughts
- She reports weight gain since starting clozapine and feels overly sedated some days

Further investigation

Is there anything else you would like to know about this patient?

- The patient denies issues with medication compliance due to family involvement in her care the last few years. However, she previously had issues with medication compliance when living by herself

- She takes clozapine (Clozaril) regularly with regular blood draws
- The family reports that they make sure she takes her medications regularly
- The patient has gained 20 lbs since starting clozapine

Attending physician's mental notes: initial evaluation

- The patient displays ongoing positive symptoms including delusions of persecution and auditory hallucinations
- She is responding to internal stimuli and mumbles to herself between questions
- She smokes one pack of cigarettes per day. Cigarette smoke can induce cytochrome 450 isoenzymes, especially CYP1A1, CYP1A2, and CYP2E1, and clozapine (Clozaril) is metabolized primarily by CYP1A2; thus, smoking could induce clozapine metabolism resulting in subtherapeutic plasma levels of clozapine
- She has several concerning symptoms for metabolic syndrome. Second-generation antipsychotics are notorious for their metabolic effects. Of these, clozapine has the highest risk for weight gain and the development of metabolic syndrome
- By blocking histamine H_1 receptors, clozapine causes excessive sedation and possibly weight gain

Question

Despite a high dose of clozapine (Clozaril), the patient continues to have positive symptoms. What would you do next?

- Order clozapine plasma drug levels
- Adjust her medications
- Refer the patient to therapy

Case outcome: initial evaluation

- The patient was started on metformin (Glucophage) 500 mg PO twice per day to help mitigate the metabolic side effects of clozapine (Clozaril)
- She was recommended to adjust her lifestyle management and exercise habits. The patient and family were educated on ways to help control weight gain, including nutrition and exercise
- Plasma levels of clozapine obtained and were subtherapeutic at 143 ng/ml
- The patient's clozapine level was low in the setting of smoking one pack of cigarettes per day

Question

Based on her plasma levels, what changes to the medications could you make?

- Increase the clozapine (Clozaril) dose, while monitoring the side effects and plasma drug levels
- Switch to another antipsychotic
- Add lithium, in addition to the clozapine
- Add another antipsychotic, in addition to the clozapine

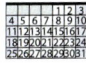

Case outcome: initial evaluation (continued)

- Due to subtherapeutic clozapine (Clozaril) levels, the clozapine dose was titrated to 300 mg PO twice per day over the next 4 weeks
- Her clozapine level is to be rechecked

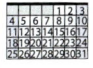

Case outcome: first interim follow-up visit at week 4

- The patient's plasma levels of clozapine (Clozaril) were rechecked and are now therapeutic at 255 ng/ml. However, the patient continues to display ongoing psychotic symptoms including grandiose delusions with flat affect, and moments of disorganized speech
- Since increasing the clozapine dose, the patient reports difficulty in completing tasks during the day and feels overly sedated. The family reports that she is sleeping over 10 hours per day
- The patient is responding to internal stimuli during evaluation and mumbles to herself between questions
- The patient and her family have been educated on smoking and its effect on the metabolism of clozapine, and if an extended (>1 week) period of smoking cessation occurs, the clozapine dose may need to be decreased to avoid supratherapeutic clozapine levels

Attending physician's mental notes: first interim follow-up visit at week 4

- The patient has failed multiple antipsychotic medications in the past and is currently on a therapeutic dose of clozapine (Clozaril), but continues to have ongoing psychotic symptoms
- One of clozapine's main side effects is excessive sedation. Dosing can be changed to nightly dosing to help mitigate daytime sedation

Question

Based on her rechecked plasma levels, what changes to the medications could you make?

- Increase the clozapine (Clozaril) dose, while monitoring the side effects and plasma drug levels

- Switch to another antipsychotic
- Add lithium, in addition to clozapine
- Add another antipsychotic, in addition to clozapine

Case outcome: first interim follow-up visit at week 4 (continued)

- Clozapine (Clozaril) was switched to 600 mg PO at bedtime to help mitigate daytime sedation
- Due to her ongoing psychotic symptoms, the addition of a partial dopamine D_2 receptor agonist medication to the patient's medication regimen was discussed with the family
- After discussing with the family and patient, brexpiprazole (Rexulti) was added to her medication regimen
- Brexpiprazole 1 mg PO daily was initiated, to be on a titration schedule where eventually the dose will be 4 mg PO daily. The schedule will occur over the next 2 weeks, with a follow-up appointment scheduled for 4 weeks

Case outcome: interim follow-up at week 8

- The patient is taking brexpiprazole (Rexulti) 4 mg PO in the morning and clozapine (Clozaril) 600 mg PO at bedtime
- She continues to take oxcarbazepine (Trileptal) 600 mg PO twice per day
- She subjectively states an improvement in psychosis
- She denies auditory hallucinations and is not responding to internal stimuli during the interview
- The patient does not make delusional references throughout encounter
- The family reports that the patient has been taking medications regularly and no side effects have been reported
- The patient reports more energy during the day and less sedation with nightly dosing of clozapine
- The family reports that initially the patient continued to display delusions and auditory hallucinations on brexpiprazole, but once titrated up to 4 mg PO daily, the positive symptoms resolved

Question

Which antipsychotic is a partial D_2 receptor agonist?

- Cariprazine (Vraylar)
- Iloperidone (Fanapt)
- Quetiapine (Seroquel)
- Lurasidone (Latuda)

Attending physician's mental notes: interim follow-up at week 8

- Some consider the partial D_2 receptor agonists as third-generation antipsychotics because their mechanisms of action do not directly antagonize D_2 receptors like first- and second-generation antipsychotics
- Brexpiprazole (Rexulti) has the benefit of being a partial D_2 receptor agonist and a potent serotonin 5-HT_{2A} receptor antagonist, 5-HT_{1A} receptor partial agonist and α_1- and α_2-adrenergic receptor antagonist
- Partial D_2 receptor agonists, such as brexpiprazole and aripiprazole (Abilify), are considered to have fewer side effects than first- and second-generation antipsychotics. Overall, partial D_2 receptor agonists have more favorable tolerability profiles compared with other antipsychotics, which leads some providers to use partial D_2 receptor agonists in combination with other antipsychotic medications to help mitigate the potential for negative side effects. The patient in this case could eventually show much improved metabolic side effects due to the addition of brexpiprazole
- Brexpiprazole is structurally similar to aripiprazole, but it has more affinity for 5-HT_{2A} receptors and more affinity for the D_2 receptors (Figure 19.1). Figure 19.2 shows how brexpiprazole is more potent

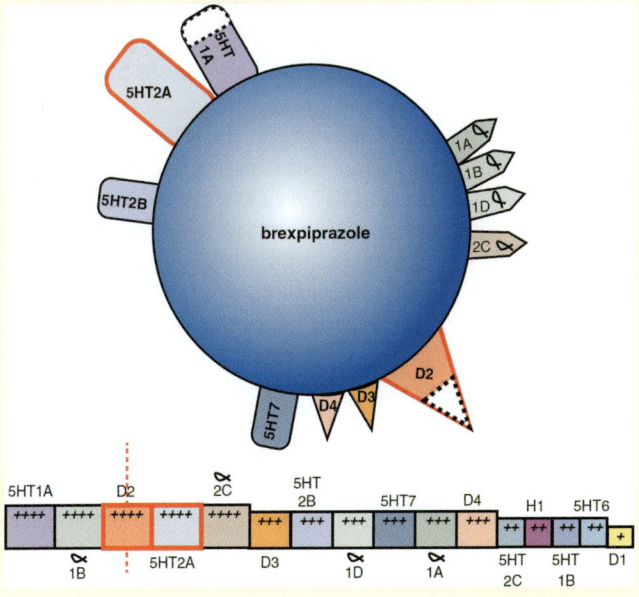

Figure 19.1. Brexpiprazole. The relative binding affinities of the different receptors are shown below. The dashed outline indicates that brexpiprazole is a partial agonist at these receptors.

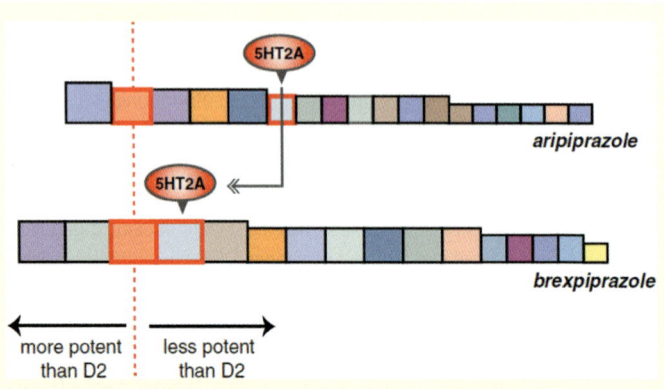

Figure 19.2. Comparison of serotonin 5-HT$_{2A}$ receptor binding by brexpiprazole and aripiprazole.

at the D$_2$ receptors compared with aripiprazole. The improved positive symptom improvements made possible by brexpiprazole, via binding to the D$_2$ receptors, were seen with this case

Case debrief

- The patient stated that she had an "awakening" (i.e. a very robust therapeutic effect on psychotic symptoms) with the addition of brexpiprazole (Rexulti) to the previous clozapine (Clozaril) treatment. She referred to this awakening as a positive experience where she felt fewer symptoms than she had prior to starting the medication
- As the patient was a smoker, it was important to educate her about how smoking cigarettes or using tobacco can affect the metabolism of clozapine and lead to subtherapeutic clozapine levels. It was critical to encourage the patient to refrain from smoking because if the clozapine was ineffective, her providers could only increase it to a certain therapeutic dosage (if the patient remains a smoker and with no symptom improvements). In addition, increases in antipsychotic medication can likely cause more or worsened metabolic side effects that could further worsen the patient's overall health
- Two of the main side effects of clozapine are metabolic syndrome and excessive sedation; the symptoms are most likely due to clozapine blocking the H$_1$ receptors (also known as the clozapine blockade)
- The patient's BMI should be monitored monthly for the first 3 months after starting clozapine, with quarterly BMI checks thereafter

- Brexpiprazole has a high affinity for D_2 receptors through partial agonism and is also a potent $5\text{-}HT_{2A}$ receptor antagonist, $5\text{-}HT_{1A}$ receptor partial agonist, and both α_1- and α_2-adrenergic receptor antagonist
- Clozapine most likely improved the patient's psychotic symptoms via glutamate signaling activity in the frontal lobe, based on multiple researched theories about how effective clozapine is in treating positive symptoms of schizophrenia, as well as how it has been proven not to have a strong affinity toward D_2 receptors

Take-home points

- In conclusion, brexpiprazole (Rexulti) most likely improved the patient's positive symptoms through D_2 receptor partial agonism, as the therapeutic effects of clozapine (Clozaril) are not thought to be mediated via D_2 receptor antagonism but by other mechanisms. More case studies and research on the combination of clozapine and brexpiprazole medications could be beneficial in proving the medication is truly working via the receptors and areas of the brain proposed in this case study
- The reason for the effectiveness of clozapine on psychosis for patients who do not respond to other antipsychotics first is not very well understood but is presumed to involve a mechanism other than D_2 receptor antagonism. Possible glutamate transmission is suggested to be involved[4]
- Patients who develop metabolic syndrome while taking antipsychotic medications could benefit from starting metformin (Glucophage). Metformin can be started at 500 mg PO daily and then titrated up. Consideration of better lifestyle management and exercise should also be recommended for all patients
- Patients suffering from excessive sedation while taking clozapine could have the medication switched to a night-time dose in lieu of a daytime dose
- Although similar in structure, brexpiprazole is a more potent $5\text{-}HT_{2A}$ receptor antagonist than aripiprazole (Abilify). Brexpiprazole is also a more potent D_2 receptor partial agonist than aripiprazole
- Clozapine has low D_2 receptor blocking ability (only ~30% of D_2 receptors are blocked), and thus the addition of brexpiprazole (with its partial D_2 receptor agonism) had little effect on clozapine's mechanism of action. However, when brexpiprazole is combined with other antipsychotics that work primarily through D_2 receptor antagonism, brexpiprazole will mostly outcompete the other medications at the D_2 receptor sites

- Due to their potent affinity for D_2 receptors, aripiprazole and brexpiprazole will both outcompete other antipsychotics at the D_2 receptor sites and should best be avoided in combination with other antipsychotics, aside from clozapine
- The pathophysiology of schizophrenia is more complicated than simply needing to decrease brain dopamine levels; glutamate systems most likely also play a vital role in symptom pathology, in addition to systems controlling serotonin levels

Tips and pearls

- Partial agonist medications such as cariprazine (Vraylar), aripiprazole (Abilify) and brexpiprazole (Rexulti) are valid options to combine with clozapine (Clozaril) because clozapine is most likely effective via the use of alternative mechanisms, rather than the D_2 receptor blockade
- Some clozapine side effects, such as excessive sedation and metabolic side effects, can be mitigated by the aforementioned agents
- Clozapine has multiple side effects needing regular monitoring such as patient sedation, metabolic effects (checking weight, height, BMI, and hemoglobin A1c (HbA1c) levels) and checking for agranulocytosis (monitoring white blood cell counts)
- Brexpiprazole is one of the more viable medication options due to its potency at both the D_2 and $5\text{-}HT_{2A}$ receptors in comparison with the other partial agonists
- Combining brexpiprazole with other antipsychotics, other than clozapine, may be of little utility due to brexpiprazole's high potency for D_2 receptors such that brexpiprazole will essentially replace the other antipsychotics at the D_2 receptor (rendering the additional medications useless, and adding increased costs to patients and/or insurance companies)
- Smoking induces cytochrome P450 isoenzymes. Clozapine is primarily metabolized by CYP1A2, and clozapine levels can thus be affected by continuous smoking (decreasing clozapine levels quicker and causing reduced effectiveness). Smoking cessation should thus be discussed with all patients; if patients have an extended period of smoking cessation (>1 week), clozapine levels can increase up to 50%, and thus the clozapine dose needs to be appropriately adjusted and blood levels monitored

Performance in practice: confessions of a psychopharmacologist

- Oxcarbazepine (Trileptal) has been shown to have minimal effectiveness in stabilizing mood, especially in comparison with other mood stabilizers. The patient in this case had been trialed on a few mood stabilizers in the past. Therefore, a more robust mood stabilizer, such as lithium, could have provided remission for the patient and could have been considered
- Valproic acid (Depakote) could also have been retried for the patient. The patient's brother had been treated effectively with valproic acid (although this was for his bipolar disorder and not schizophrenia). Familial medication effectiveness could render a medication useful for another family member as they have similar genetic make-up. The patient had also been treated previously with valproic acid, but it is unclear which dosage she tried, or for how long, therefore it is unknown if therapeutic levels had in fact been reached, nor whether it was tolerated. Valproic acid can be difficult to tolerate in combination with clozapine (Clozaril) both in terms of sedation and from the effects on bone marrow
- Psychotherapy could also have been recommended, but with the patient's acute psychotic state, stabilization on medications was considered to be of utmost importance and the first priority
- The patient appeared to be developing metabolic syndrome as evidenced by her elevated BMI and lipids. Fasting glucose levels and HbA1c should have been checked. It is recommended that blood pressure, fasting plasma glucose, and fasting lipids should be checked within 3 months of starting clozapine
- One of the main side effects of clozapine is constipation, which can lead to toxic megacolon if untreated. Every patient should be started on docusate (Colace) daily and screened regularly for constipation. This patient had already been started on docusate, which was beneficial
- Metformin (Glucophage) initiation at a dose of 500 mg PO daily could have been considered to help mitigate the metabolic side effects of clozapine and other second-generation antipsychotics
- Lastly, the patient smoked daily, and therefore educating the patient on smoking cessation, the reasoning for the need due to the medication regimen, and as the different treatment options available could have been explored

Posttest self-assessment question and answer

Which of following disorder(s) is brexpiprazole (Rexulti) FDA approved for?

A. Schizophrenia
B. Bipolar depression
C. Bipolar maintenance
D. Acute mania
E. Treatment-resistant depression (adjunct)

Answer: A and E

References

1. Meyer J, Stahl SM. *Clozapine Handbook.* New York, NY: Cambridge University Press, 2019.
2. Stahl M. Mechanism of action of brexpiprazole: comparison with aripiprazole. *CNS Spectr* 2016; 21:1–6. https://doi.org/10.1017/S1092852915000954
3. Stahl SM. *Stahl's Essential Psychopharmacology: Prescriber's Guide*, 6th edn. Cambridge, UK: Cambridge University Press, 2017.
4. Uno Y, Coyle JT. Glutamate hypothesis in schizophrenia. *Psychiatry Clin Neurosci* 2019; 73:204–15. https://doi.org/10.1111/pcn.12823

Case 20: Treatment-resistant depression and opioid dependence

The Question: How can we pharmacologically address refractory major depressive disorder in a patient on buprenorphine-naloxone (Suboxone) maintenance for opioid dependency?

The Psychopharmacological Dilemma: Does ketamine interact with buprenorphine-naloxone?

Kevin Simonson and Alexander H. Truong

Pretest self-assessment question (answer at the end of the case)

What is the primary mechanism of action of ketamine?

A. NMDA (*N*-methyl-ᴅ-aspartate) agonism
B. AMPA (α-amino-3-hydroxy-5-methyl-4-isoxazolepropionic acid) antagonism
C. NMDA antagonism
D. Opioid antagonism

Patient evaluation on intake

- A 24-year-old male with a history of benzodiazepine use disorder, opioid use disorder, treatment-resistant depression, and anxiety who is currently on buprenorphine-naloxone (Suboxone)

Psychiatric history

- The patient was diagnosed with major depressive disorder (MDD) and anxiety at age 15. His MDD has been recurrent with numerous failed antidepressant trials, including fluoxetine (Prozac), bupropion (Wellbutrin), vortioxetine (Trintellix), aripiprazole (Abilify), paroxetine (Paxil), venlafaxine (Effexor), and duloxetine (Cymbalta)
- There is no history of self-harm or suicidal ideation
- He took lorazepam (Ativan) sparingly from age 16 to 20: "Ten 1 mg tablets would last 6 months"
- At age 18, the patient began suffering from terrible daily cluster/migraine headaches that occasionally caused him to "pass out". He did not experience relief from triptans, nortriptyline, gabapentin (Neurontin), or oxygen therapy
- At age 19, the patient also began suffering from right-sided facial pain, diagnosed as trigeminal neuralgia. Carbamazepine (Equetro) relieved the headaches and facial pain but caused intolerable side effects ("The sluggishness felt like a walking coma"). Magnetic resonance imaging showed an inflamed optic nerve but no brain lesions. Multiple sclerosis has been ruled out for now. Prednisone was helpful but was not a sustainable treatment long term

- The summer before university started at age 20, his anxiety worsened and his "lorazepam use went out of control". He began taking lorazepam 1 mg up to three times per day
- The "pressure to get good grades" and the difficulty of math and physics courses continued to exacerbate his anxiety, insomnia, and headaches/facial pain
- He started on hydrocodone/acetaminophen 6 months into university, with limited relief. His tolerance increased over the next 2 years and doctors ended up prescribing hydrocodone/acetaminophen 10 mg/325 mg up to six times per day. The patient was also obtaining hydrocodone/acetaminophen from the street, and took up to ten doses of 10 mg/325 mg per day
- During the same period of hydrocodone/acetaminophen use, he was also taking diazepam (Valium) 10 mg at bedtime. He eventually tapered the lorazepam and settled on clonazepam (Klonopin) 1 mg three times per day, which he took for 3 years
- At age 23, he completed outpatient detox, came off the hydrocodone/acetaminophen and benzodiazepines, and started on buprenorphine-naloxone (Suboxone) 8 mg twice per day. According to the patient, benzodiazepines were "psychologically more challenging quitting than opiates"

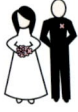

Social and personal history

- The patient is single, with no children
- He is currently in vocational school. He finished high school in a virtual program. He attended university to study electrical engineering, but due to difficulties with procrastination, inattentiveness, and feeling overwhelmed, he dropped out after 1.5 years. He attempted junior college and working at the same time, but ultimately quit these as well
- He denies alcohol, tobacco, or drug use other than hydrocodone/acetaminophen and benzodiazepines
- There are no legal issues

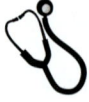

Medical history

- Cluster/migraine headaches
- Trigeminal neuralgia
- Inflamed optic nerve

Family history

- Both parents suffer from depression and take antidepressants
- Past medications:
  - Diazepam (Valium)

- Alprazolam (Xanax)
- Lorazepam (Ativan)
- Hydrocodone-acetaminophen
- Fluoxetine (Prozac)
- Venlafaxine XR (Effexor)
- Paroxetine (Paxil)
- Bupropion extended-release (XL) (Aplenzin)
- Vortioxetine (Trintellix)
- Aripiprazole (Abilify)
- Duloxetine (Cymbalta)

Current medications

- Buprenorphine-naloxone (Suboxone) 4 mg/1 mg three times per day
- Sertraline (Zoloft) 100 mg PO daily

Patient evaluation on initial visit

- The patient is currently on sertraline (Zoloft) but reports the lack of a noticeable effect and complains of sexual dysfunction
- He continues to complain of insomnia, low concentration, depressed mood, and anhedonia
- No trials of brexpiprazole (Rexulti) or Vilazodone (Viibryd) have been done
- Given the numerous failed antidepressants, he may be a candidate for esketamine (Spravato)

Attending physician's mental notes: initial evaluation

- Start the patient on a trial of brexpiprazole (Rexulti), and consider vilazodone (Viibryd)
- Apply for esketamine (Spravato) authorization
- Conduct pharmacogenomic testing

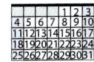

Case outcome: first interim follow-up at week 3

- The patient reported intolerable akathisia on brexpiprazole (Rexulti), and stopped taking it
- His pharmacogenomic results revealed normal folate metabolism but he was homozygous for poor metabolism through cytochrome P450 2D6 (CYP2D6)
- His affect is still restricted
- Start vilazodone (Viibryd), and taper sertraline (Zoloft)
- The patient was educated on serotonin syndrome

Case outcome: interim follow-up at week 6

- The patient continues to feel depressed, with prominent anhedonia and moods ranging from sad to numb to irritable. He denied suicidal ideation
- There was an initial improvement after starting vilazodone (Viibryd) at the 10 mg dose, but he currently feels about the same as he cross-titrates through current dosing of vilazodone 20 mg plus sertraline (Zoloft) 100 mg
- He is currently taking buprenorphine-naloxone (Suboxone) 4 mg/1 mg three times per day. Following a discussion with the prescribing physician, his nightly buprenorphine-naloxone will be reduced on the days he is receiving esketamine (Spravato)
- He reports having had some headaches in connection with taking vilazodone, but these usually remit on their own
- He started esketamine 56 mg twice per week. He reports no nausea, vomiting, or sedation. He reported some dissociation and visual changes (reported seeing two images of his mother who accompanied him to the session), and reported "feeling weird, but hard to describe"

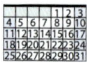

Case outcome: interim follow-up at week 9

- The patient reports continuing to feel better since starting esketamine (Spravato) (dose increased to 84 mg), particularly in terms of decreased anxiety and improved sleep, with possibly some improvement in mood. He reports feeling "great" today
- He states that he had a slight headache in the afternoon after the last esketamine session but no other side effects in the interim
- The plan was to continue on sertraline (Zoloft) 100 mg and vilazodone (Viibryd) 20 mg at bedtime; however, the patient self-discontinued vilazodone because he felt it was making him feel "foggy-headed"
- He continues to take only an evening dose of buprenorphine-naloxone (Suboxone) on the days he receives esketamine

Questions

How might you titrate buprenorphine-naloxone (Suboxone) down?
What common side effects of esketamine (Spravato) should a prescriber look out for?
What potential side effects of vilazodone (Viibryd) could explain the subjective feeling of being "foggy-headed" in this patient?

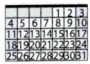

Case outcome: interim follow-up at week 12

- The patient reports continuing to feel better since increasing his dose of esketamine (Spravato), reporting decreased anxiety and decreased negative thoughts, as well as improvement of his depressive mood overall
- No side effects are reported following the last treatment session
- He is currently taking sertraline (Zoloft) 100 mg at bedtime but has not been continuing with vilazodone (Viibryd)
- His buprenorphine-naloxone dose has been reduced to 4 mg/1 mg twice per day with a plan for continued titration to be completed in the following weeks
- His mother reveals that the patient had an evaluation as a child for attention-deficit/hyperactivity disorder (ADHD) and limited treatment experience (he was tried briefly on amphetamine/dextroamphetamine but did not tolerate it well). The patient reports chronic difficulties with time management, self-organization, and task initiation and completion
- The plan is to continue esketamine 84 mg twice per week and sertraline 100 mg PO daily, start psychotherapy, and submit a neuropsychology referral

Case outcome: interim follow-up at week 15

- The patient reported continuing to do better in the interim since the last visit
- He has been sleeping better, his mood is improved overall, and he is not depressed. His anxiety has been gradually but markedly improving – he noted that when he recently went to the pharmacy, a situation that normally provokes somatic manifestations of anxiety (e.g. increased sweating), he did not feel particularly anxious
- He reports some benefit from the psychotherapy sessions
- The plan is to continue sertraline. Following FDA guidelines, esketamine (Spravato) dosing was decreased from 84 mg twice per week to once per week with continued positive effect

Case outcome: interim follow-up at week 19

- The patient acknowledges a significant improvement in anxiety following esketamine (Spravato) treatments
- However, he reports a mild increase in anxiety now that he is receiving esketamine weekly rather than twice per week
- He notes reduced "negative intrusive thoughts" and "feeling stiff around other people", which lasts for several days after esketamine treatment
- His sleep is good, with improvement from baseline

- He denies recurrence of depression
- There has been a dramatic reduction in his facial pain, despite titrating off buprenorphine-naloxone (Suboxone)
- The patient has begun exploring romantic relationships with peers but remains cautious, as he reports a history of "being taken advantage of" in previous relationships where his partner would "take and not give back"
- He is doing well in vocational school

Case outcome: interim follow-up at week 24

- The patient reports doing well over the past week, with his depression continuing to decrease
- His anxiety resurfaced as the week progressed prior to his next esketamine (Spravato) treatment, but today he notes that anxiety has not been a problem in the past week; however, he does note that left knee pain and right facial pain recurred at a low level
- He is eating and sleeping well
- He has been diagnosed with ADHD and is now taking dextroamphetamine (Dexedrine) capsules 10 mg twice per day (every morning and daily at noon)
- His is maintained on sertraline (Zoloft) 100 mg PO daily, buprenorphine-naloxone (Suboxone) 4 mg/1 mg three times per day, and esketamine 84 mg weekly

Case outcome: interim follow-up at week 28

- The patient's depression and anxiety continue to improve
- He is sleeping 7–8 hours nightly and typically eating two to three meals per day
- He reports that his medications are helpful and would like to continue on the current doses
- He continues to do well in vocational school and is beginning to seek friendship with peers in his classes

Case debrief

- Two-thirds of patients have treatment-resistant depression, which is defined as a lack of response to two trials of antidepressants given adequate dosing and treatment duration
- Treatment resistance in this patient was likely multifactorial from school stressors, difficulty with social relationships, homozygous lack of receptor at CYP2D6 leading to poor metabolization and side effects, and opioid dependence
- The patient showed improvement of his depression and anxiety with triple therapy consisting of esketamine (Spravato) 84 mg weekly,

sertraline (Zoloft) 100 mg PO daily, and buspirone (BuSpar) 5 mg PO daily

- His opioid dependence improved, as indicated by decreasing buprenorphine-naloxone (Suboxone) dosing
- With initial improvements in depression and anxiety, the patient was then able to participate meaningfully in psychotherapy

Mechanism of action moment

- Ketamine is a non-competitive open-channel inhibitor of the NMDA receptor; specifically, it binds to the phencyclidine site of the NMDA receptor, leading to downstream glutamate release and consequent stimulation of other glutamate receptors, including AMPA receptors
- Ketamine may also produce analgesia and modulate central sensitization, hyperalgesia, and opioid tolerance
- Recent studies have suggested that opioid receptor antagonism prior to administration of intravenous ketamine attenuates its acute antidepressant effects, as demonstrated by significantly lower reductions in Hamilton Depression Rating Scale (HAM-D) scores in participants receiving ketamine plus naltrexone (ReVia) versus ketamine plus placebo[15]
- It is theoretically possible that opioid agonists could potentiate NMDA antagonists, as the μ-opioid receptor (MOR) and the NMDA receptor are antagonistic to each other when they dimerize. Thus, buprenorphine-naloxone (Suboxone) may have enhanced the therapeutic action of ketamine in this case

Two-minute tutorial: ketamine and the opioid system

- Williams' group concluded that ketamine's antidepressant effects require opioid system activation, either as "a weak mu opioid receptor agonist or by releasing endogenous opioids".[15] Following the response by Sanacora[9] and Wang and Kaplin,[14] Schatzberg's group clarified their narrative to include the possibility of "an indirect interaction at the cellular level, perhaps mediated by cross-talk between [NMDA] and opioid receptors" and the need for "a normally functioning endogenous opioid system to express an antidepressant response to ketamine".[4] It is worth noting that the idea of cellular cross-regulation between naltrexone (ReVia) and ketamine, elucidated by Wang and Kaplin,[14] does not require the release of endogenous opioids. Naltrexone is not a true neutral antagonist but also has intrinsic inverse agonist activity at the MOR,[8,11] thus naltrexone antagonism/inverse agonism of the MOR could interfere with constitutive signal transduction needed for the downstream antidepressant effect of ketamine. This hypothesis is corroborated by recent research, which concluded that ketamine is not acting as an opioid to produce antidepressive effects but that tonic action of the MOR alters the biophysical properties of the NMDA receptor to gate antagonism of ketamine[6]

- Additionally, Williams et al. acknowledged that naltrexone does not have substantial selectivity for the MOR over the κ-opioid receptor (KOR), and that their data could not distinguish between the two in mediating ketamine's antidepressant effects.[15] Recent research suggests that activation of KORs may indeed contribute to the protracted clinical antidepressant effects of ketamine[5]

- There is new evidence for the rapid release of vascular endothelial growth factor (VEGF) in response to ketamine, a novel mechanism not demonstrated by classical antidepressants.[2] While the mammalian target of rapamycin (mTOR) protein seems to play a critical transduction role, research also suggests that production and release of brain-derived neurotrophic factor (BDNF) and inhibition of glycogen synthase kinase 3 (GSK3; shared in common with lithium) may also be required for ketamine's unique antidepressant effects.[10] While much is still unknown about ketamine's complex mechanism, what does appear certain is that "the mechanisms of ketamine's rapid and more persistent antidepressant effects are undoubtedly multifactorial", thus precluding simplistic explanations.[7]

Take-home points

- In treatment-refractory depression with concomitant opioid dependence, esketamine (Spravato) should be a consideration for safe and efficacious treatment of both depressive symptoms and opioid dependence
- Furthermore, esketamine provides quick but sustained effects that may be maintained with once or twice per week dosing
- The perception of pain and opioid dependence may improve with adequate treatment of depressive symptoms
- Ultimately, high-dose antidepressant monotherapies, combinations, and augmentations were utilized leading to a sustained response

Posttest self-assessment question and answer

What is the primary mechanism of action of ketamine?

A. NMDA agonism
B. AMPA antagonism
C. NMDA antagonism
D. Opioid antagonism
Answer: C

Ketamine is primarily an uncompetitive antagonist of the NMDA ionotropic glutamate receptor, although its complex mechanism of action does secondarily interact with several other receptor systems.

References

1. Berman RM, Cappiello A, Anand A, et al. Antidepressant effects of ketamine in depressed patients. *Biol Psychiatry* 2000; 47:351–4. https://doi.org/10.1016/s0006-3223(99)00230-9
2. Deyama S, Bang E, Wohleb ES, et al. Role of neuronal VEGF signaling in the prefrontal cortex in the rapid antidepressant effects of ketamine. *Am J Psychiatry* 2019; 176:388–40. https://doi.org/10.1176/appi.ajp.2018.17121368
3. Duman R, Li N, Liu R, et al. Signaling pathways underlying the rapid antidepressant actions of ketamine. *Neuropharmacology* 2012; 62:35–41. https://doi.org/10.1016/j.neuropharm.2011.08.044
4. Heifets BD, Williams NR, Blasey C, et al. Interpreting ketamine's opioid receptor dependent effect: response to Sanacora. *Am J Psychiatry* 2019; 176:249–50. https://doi.org/10.1176/appi.ajp.2018.18091061r
5. Jacobson ML, Simmons SC, Wulf HA, et al. Protracted effects of ketamine require immediate kappa opioid receptor activation and long-lasting desensitization. *FASEB J* 2020; 34: 1. https://doi.org/10.1096/fasebj.2020.34.s1.04214
6. Klein ME, Chandra J, Sheriff S, Malinow R. Opioid system is necessary but not sufficient for antidepressive actions of ketamine in rodents. *Proc Natl Acad Sci U S A* 2020; 117:2656–62. https://doi.org/10.1073/pnas.1916570117
7. Mathew SJ, Rivas-Grajales AM. Does the opioid system block or enhance the antidepressant effects of ketamine? *Chronic Stress (Thousand Oaks)* 2019; 3: 2470547019852073. https://doi.org/10.1177/2470547019852073
8. Raehal KM, Lowery JJ, Bhamidipati CM, et al. In vivo characterization of 6β-naltrexol, an opioid ligand with less inverse agonist activity compared with naltrexone and naloxone in opioid-dependent mice. *J Pharmacol Exp Ther* 2005; 313:1150–62. https://doi.org/10.1124/jpet.104.082966
9. Sanacora G. Caution against overinterpreting opiate receptor stimulation as mediating antidepressant effects of ketamine. *Am J Psychiatry* 2019; 176:249. https://doi.org/10.1176/appi.ajp.2018.18091061

10. Scheuing L, Chiu C-T, Liao H-M, Chuang D-M. Antidepressant mechanism of ketamine: perspective from preclinical studies. *Front Neurosci* 2015; 9:249. https://doi.org/10.3389/fnins.2015.00249

11. Shader, R. Antagonists, inverse agonists, and protagonists. *J Clin Psychopharmacol* 2003; 23:321–2. https://doi.org/10.1097/01.jcp.0000087502.38434.6c

12. Stahl SM. *Stahl's Essential Psychopharmacology*, 4th edn. New York, NY: Cambridge University Press, 2013.

13. Stahl SM. *Stahl's Essential Psychopharmacology: The Prescriber's Guide*, 6th edn. Cambridge, UK: Cambridge University Press, 2017.

14. Wang M, Kaplin A. Explaining naltrexone's interference with ketamine's antidepressant effect. *Am J Psychiatry* 2019; 176:410–11. https://doi.org/10.1176/appi.ajp.2019.19010044

15. Williams NR, Heifets BD, Blasey C, et al. Attenuation of antidepressant effects of ketamine by opioid receptor antagonism. *Am J Psychiatry* 2018; 175:1205–15.https://doi.org/10.1176/appi.ajp.2018.18020138

Case 21: A stiff patient

The Question: What are the main clinical considerations when discontinuing clozapine (Clozaril) due to side effects?

The Psychopharmacological Dilemma: How to improve quality of life and minimize medication side effects in a patient with medication-resistant psychotic symptoms

Angharad Ames, Joshua Valverde, and Gerald Maguire

Pretest self-assessment question (answer at the end of the case)

Which of the following may cause abnormal movement disorders?

A. Aripiprazole (Abilify)
B. Haloperidol (Haldol)
C. Clozapine (Clozaril)
D. Valproic acid (Depakote)
E. A and B
F. All of the above

Patient evaluation on intake

- A 55-year-old male with reported Asperger's disorder and schizoaffective disorder presents to the emergency department with the chief complaints of "100 seizures," "chewing movements in his face," and bowel continence. He was diagnosed with schizoaffective disorder many years earlier by an outside psychiatrist
- He has been living mostly independently until 3 months ago, at which time his ability to function began to decline. Over the last 3 months, he began having bradykinesia, hypokinesia, muscle rigidity, intermittent tremors, and progressive postural instability, and has had two falls
- He had been taking a medication regimen consisting of clozapine (Clozaril) (for 30 years), duloxetine (Cymbalta), and clonazepam (Klonopin)
- Two weeks ago, his father (a retired physician) discontinued the patient's clozapine due to concern it was contributing to instability/falls, dizziness, and potential autonomic instability. Four days later, after learning about this change, the patient's outpatient psychiatrist began tapering duloxetine (to try minimizing polypharmacy) and started lurasidone (Latuda), as the patient had failed trials of nearly every other antipsychotic
- Around this time, the patient began experiencing loss of bowel continence and excessive sweating. He quickly became non-verbal and unable to walk

- His parents took him to an outside hospital, where he presented with altered mentation, inability to swallow, move, or speak, and an elevated plasma creatine kinase (over 2000 U/l). He was treated for possible rhabdomyolysis in the setting of probable neuroleptic malignant syndrome (NMS) and sepsis. Lurasidone and clonazepam were placed on hold. With the help of physical therapy, he regained his ability to walk minimally. He was transferred home briefly but soon began experiencing intermittent episodes of shaking in his extremities that his parents worried were seizures. He was readmitted to the outside hospital and transferred to a local hospital for further psychiatric evaluation and management

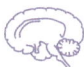

Psychiatric history

- The patient has a long history of Asperger's disorder, panic attacks, and obsessive–compulsive disorder (OCD) that were diagnosed decades ago by a former psychiatrist. His OCD symptoms were related to germ contamination and he tended to hoard magazines
- At age 17, he was diagnosed with schizophrenia, which was characterized by bizarre obsessive thoughts, auditory hallucinations of whispering voices, paranoia, and disorganized behavior. At his most recent baseline, he had tangential perseverative thoughts and blunted affect
- He has undergone exhaustive psychotropic medication trials. Until 3 weeks ago, he had been taking clozapine (Clozaril) 100 mg three times per day for 30 years. For the first 15 years on clozapine, he tolerated it well and showed improvement in his symptoms, but in the last 15 years, he has become slower and less independent. In the last 5 years, however, he demonstrated progressive worsening of panic attacks, obsessive thoughts, and difficulty with activities of daily living. He began experiencing motor side effects, including abnormal movements in the major muscle groups and fleeting tardive dyskinesia-like movements in his tongue. His constipation worsened. Many attempts were made to switch him from clozapine to a different atypical antipsychotic, as there was concern that clozapine was causing his movement abnormalities while controlling his symptoms ineffectively, but discontinuation of clozapine always resulted in near-immediate worsening of panic attacks and a decline in overall mobility
- Three months ago, the patient started having falls (with no witnessed loss of consciousness), progressive gait difficulty, bradykinesia, and muscle rigidity

- Clozapine was discontinued 12 days ago by his father, with the knowledge of the outpatient psychiatrist, because of concern that clozapine may be a major driver of the patient's gait instability, poor motor functioning, and potential autonomic instability
- The patient had two prior psychiatric admissions 30 years ago
- There is no history of suicide attempts.

Medication history

- Fluoxetine (Prozac)
- Escitalopram (Lexapro)
- Paroxetine (Paxil)
- Venlafaxine (Effexor)
- Duloxetine (Cymbalta)
- Bupropion (Wellbutrin)
- Buspirone (BuSpar)
- Imipramine (Tofranil)
- Amitriptyline (Elavil)
- Amoxapine (Asendin)
- Diphenhydramine (Benadryl)
- Hydroxyzine (Atarax, Vistaril)
- Trazodone (Desyrel)
- Haloperidol (Haldol)
- Risperidone (Risperdal)
- Quetiapine (Seroquel)
- Fluphenazine (Prolixin)
- Chlorpromazine (Thorazine)
- Trifluoperazine (Stelazine)
- Thiothixene (Navane)
- Thioridazine (Mellaril)
- Lurasidone (Latuda) for 3 days
- Clozapine (Clozaril)
- Benztropine (Cogentin) for extrapyramidal symptoms (EPS)
- Valproic acid (Depakote)
- Phenytoin (Dilantin)
- Gabapentin (Neurontin)
- Alprazolam (Xanax)
- Prazepam (Centrac)
- Clonazepam (Klonopin)

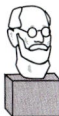

Psychotherapy history

- The patient has had supportive psychotherapy

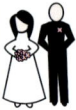

PATIENT FILE

Social and personal history

- The patient's highest level of education was at college. He obtained a General Educational Development (GED) qualification and then completed 10 college semesters, taking a couple of classes at a time
- Prior to last 3 months, he was living fairly independently on his own in an apartment 1 mile away from his parents' house. He has never driven a car. More recently, he has been living with them
- He has never been married and has no children
- He is not employed
- He denies use of alcohol, recreational drugs, or tobacco products

Medical history

- Obesity
- Hypothyroidism, on levothyroxine (Synthroid)
- Chronic constipation
- Recent loss of appetite and unintentional weight loss
- No history of seizures or head trauma

Family history

- No psychiatric history or medical history

Patient evaluation on initial visit

- On examination, the patient's vital signs were: blood pressure 125/82 mmHg, heart rate 72 bpm, temperature 98.7°F, respiration 26 breaths/min, and oxygen saturation 97%
- On laboratory tests, his white blood cell count was elevated to 15.2 × 10^3/µl and urinalysis was suggestive of urinary tract infection; otherwise laboratory tests were normal. A urine drug screen was negative
- A head computed tomography (CT) scan showed no evidence of acute intracranial hemorrhage, mass, or acute infarction. A 22 min electroencephalogram (EEG) was unremarkable
- In the emergency department, he was started on ceftriaxone empirically for a suspected urinary tract infection
- His neurological examination was notable for spontaneous eye tracking of movements, tardive dyskinetic movements of the tongue, hand tremor bilaterally, the presence of muscle rigidity, and ataxic gait. He was able to stand with support, but otherwise was off balance and falling to the side. He was alert and oriented to person and place

Current medications

- The patient has had no medications for the last 2 weeks. Prior to this, the patient had been taking clozapine (Clozaril) for nearly 30 years, clonazepam (Klonopin) 1 mg three times per day, and duloxetine (Cymbalta) 60 mg daily
- After clozapine was discontinued 2 weeks ago, the patient took lurasidone (Latuda) for 3 days but stopped when admitted to the first hospital

Question

In your clinical experience, what are some of the side effects you might expect to see in someone who has been taking clozapine (Clozaril) for many years?

- EPS
- Myocarditis
- Tardive dyskinesia
- Neutropenia
- Tachycardia
- Orthostatic hypotension

Attending physician's mental notes: initial evaluation

- The patient is encephalopathic, drowsy, and lethargic, and has leukocytosis. He is unable to answer questions or follow commands. The patient may have delirium, possibly due to an infectious etiology. If this were the case, it would be expected that his mentation would improve as the infection resolves
- An EEG does not suggest epileptiform activity, but the report of "100 seizures" at home, in the setting of recent abrupt discontinuation of clonazepam (Klonopin) at the outside hospital after chronic use (>12 weeks), is concerning for benzodiazepine withdrawal seizures
- The patient demonstrates behavioral withdrawal, moderate immobility/stupor, and mutism. Due to these observations, and within the wider setting of the patient's recent and sudden discontinuation of clozapine (Clozaril) and clonazepam, it is worth considering catatonia
- It is important that we rule out NMS. This was likely the explanation for his presentation to the outside hospital several days ago, as NMS can occur after sudden discontinuation of clozapine. There is data to suggest that NMS may be a form of severe catatonia
- Tremors, hypokinesia, and muscle rigidity can also be adverse effects of clozapine; however, if these were indeed caused by clozapine, they would be expected to have worsened prior to the

discontinuation of clozapine as opposed to after. Additionally, while clozapine can cause seizures at high doses, the patient's report of "100 seizures" occurred after clozapine was discontinued. Thus, it is unlikely that these symptoms are due to the use of clozapine

- Given the patient's reported progressive postural instability, bradykinesia, muscle rigidity, and intermittent tremors, and with his progressive decline in independent functioning, the differential diagnosis also includes Parkinson's disease and drug-induced Parkinsonism; however, the relative rapidity of symptom onset argues against the former, and the lack of a current antipsychotic argues against the latter

Question

Given the considerations above, what would be the most reasonable next step in evaluating the patient?

- Start intravenous dantrolene (Dantrium)
- Restart clozapine (Clozaril)
- Initiate bromocriptine (Parlodel)
- Perform a lorazepam (Ativan) challenge

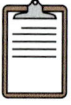

Patient evaluation on initial visit (continued)

- The patient receives lorazepam (Ativan) 1 mg intravenously. On re-evaluation 45 minutes later, the patient is verbal but slow, no longer withdrawn or immobile, and is oriented to self, time, and place, but not situation
- On mental status examination, his affect is blunted and he has impoverished speech, a paucity of ideas, and limited insight

Attending physician's mental notes: initial evaluation (continued)

- The patient seems to have responded well to lorazepam (Ativan) 1 mg, which supports the initial suspicion of catatonia
- If the patient had true NMS, we would not expect him to improve with simple antibiotics and benzodiazepines
- It is reasonable to continue the standing doses; however, his parents have requested that this be discontinued because they recalled the patient having a Parkinsonian-like reaction to lorazepam as a teenager
- This may be an example of catatonia due to clozapine (Clozaril) withdrawal/sudden discontinuation. Because there is no longer concern for NMS or severe Parkinsonism, it is reasonable to start an atypical antipsychotic at this time. Due to the historically medication-resistant severity of the patient's symptoms, we will initiate olanzapine (Zyprexa) 5 mg at night with the plan to titrate to a high dose as tolerated

Further investigation

Is there anything else you would especially like to know about this patient?

- What about details concerning his response to past medication treatments?
  - Valproic acid (Depakote) caused Parkinsonian symptoms a few years ago
  - Alprazolam (Xanax) caused Parkinsonian symptoms when he was a child
- Has he ever shown signs of catatonia in the past?

Case outcome: first interim follow-up evaluation on hospitalization day 3

- The patient's leukocytosis is downtrending
- His vitals are within normal limits and are stable
- The patient has been more interactive and verbal since starting olanzapine (Zyprexa)
- He remains with blunted affect and fairly impoverished speech and thought content. Tardive dyskinetic movements of his tongue also remain apparent
- He continues to have poor appetite and trouble staying asleep/ having frequent night-time awakenings
- He has demonstrated some mild verbal and behavioral agitation toward his mother. He wants to go home and does not like being in the hospital. According to his parents, he appears to have nearly returned to his baseline level of mental status and functioning
- Given the available information, it seems likely that the patient's original presentation to the outside hospital represented a mixed picture of catatonia and NMS in the setting of sudden discontinuation of first clozapine (Clozaril), and then lurasidone (Latuda) and clonazepam (Klonopin). Although he seemingly recovered at the outside hospital, he quickly decompensated and presented to our hospital with catatonia, likely still explained by the aforementioned abrupt discontinuation of medications

Questions

Would you continue the patient's olanzapine (Zyprexa)?

- Yes, continue olanzapine at the same dose
- Yes, and increase the dose
- No, discontinue olanzapine
- Yes, continue olanzapine and add a second antipsychotic

Would you consider adding any other medications at this time?

- No, we should focus on maximizing the dose of olanzapine first
- Yes, we should start mirtazapine (Remeron)
- Yes, we should valbenazine (Ingrezza)
- Yes, we should restart clonazepam (Klonopin)

Attending physician's mental notes: first interim follow-up evaluation on hospitalization day 3

- Given the necessity of clozapine (Clozaril) for controlling the patient's symptoms for so long, it may be challenging to find an alternative medication that will have similar efficacy. Due to concerns surrounding orthostatic hypotension, dizziness, and overall gait instability over the last few months, it is not appropriate to restart clozapine and it would be ideal to stay away from antipsychotics with a significant amount of α_1-adrenergic receptor blockade
- Although it is rare for clozapine to cause NMS, it does block some dopamine D_2 receptors in the striatum and can cause motor side effects, such as the rigidity the patient was experiencing. Thus, it is important to choose an atypical antipsychotic with a relatively low incidence of EPS side effects
- There is evidence that high-dose olanzapine (Zyprexa), even beyond the FDA-approved maximum of 20 mg daily, may be efficacious in treating medication-resistant psychosis and agitation
- It is appropriate to continue titrating olanzapine as tolerated to treat the patient's long-standing paranoia and behavioral agitation. An increase in the dose at this time may also help his appetite and sleep interruption. We will increase olanzapine to 15 mg daily (from 10 mg daily). If the patient continues to have trouble with sleeping despite increasing olanzapine, we can initiate something like mirtazapine (Remeron), melatonin, or suvorexant (Belsomra)
- We should hold off on making any other medication adjustments at this time and instead focus on one change at a time, so as to avoid confusion over which outcomes are due to which changes

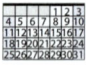

Case outcome: second interim follow-up visit at week 3 (outpatient clinic)

- The patient was discharged from the hospital 2 weeks ago. His discharge medications were olanzapine (Zyprexa) 15 mg daily and levothyroxine (Synthroid) 88 μg daily
- He presents as less paranoid and is ambulating better. His parents attend his appointment and agree. He still has some involuntary jerky movements of his tongue and a mild intention tremor in his hands bilaterally. He continues to have trouble sleeping at night and

wakes up several times. He also has episodes of agitation and his thoughts are often loosely associated
- The patient is tolerating olanzapine well, and he and his parents are amenable to continuing to increase the dose to target his paranoid thoughts. They are also amenable to initiating valbenazine (Ingrezza) for tardive dyskinesia

Question

Would you expect the patient to continue to respond well to olanzapine (Zyprexa) alone?

- Yes, especially if higher doses are used
- Yes, if he starts receiving regular cognitive remediation psychotherapy
- No, he will likely need augmentation with a mood stabilizer, such as valproic acid (Depakote) or lithium
- No, olanzapine will not be enough to treat his OCD and panic disorder, and he will require a benzodiazepine and selective serotonin reuptake inhibitor (SSRI)

Attending physician's mental notes: second interim follow-up visit at week 3 (outpatient clinic):

- If the patient continues to tolerate olanzapine (Zyprexa), we may plan to continue titrating, as there is documented utility in using higher doses with treatment-resistant patients, associated with increased efficacy without many more side effects
- Occasionally, for some patients who do not respond to other antipsychotics, a use of doses over 30 mg daily, and perhaps even over 90 mg daily in the short term, may be justified by an experienced clinician as long as it is tolerated and plasma drug levels remain below the point of futility (200 ng/ml)[4]
- We will increase olanzapine to 20 mg daily and provide 2.5 mg daily as needed for acute agitation

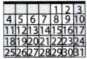

Case outcome: third interim follow-up visit at week 7 (outpatient clinic)

- Over the last month, the patient's father called the office and expressed concern that the patient was demonstrating catatonic and agitated behavior. A short-term prescription of lorazepam (Ativan) was provided. While the catatonic symptoms resolved, he seemed to be more agitated. He hit his mother twice in the past month. Olanzapine was increased to 25 mg daily
- His father began giving the patient extra 5 mg doses of olanzapine as needed to treat this agitation. He was taking up to 35 mg daily

- Fortunately, his appetite was improved and he was eating more normally. The severity of his tardive dyskinesia also notably diminished

Attending physician's mental notes: third interim follow-up visit at week 7 (outpatient clinic)

- Lorazepam (Ativan) may have precipitated the patient's worsening behavioral agitation by virtue of making him more disinhibited. It is reasonable to switch him back to clonazepam (Klonopin) for a longer-acting formulation, especially if we intend to continue using this as a longer-term treatment for panic disorder and as an augmentation agent to olanzapine (Zyprexa) for psychosis/behavioral agitation and recurrent catatonia
- The patient is still tolerating olanzapine and does not report side effects. It is worth increasing the dose to 50 mg daily with 2.5 mg available as needed
- The patient will discontinue lorazepam and start clonazepam 1 mg three times per day
- Given the patient's historic medication resistance, we will pursue genomic testing

Case outcome: fourth interim follow-up visit at week 12 (outpatient clinic)

- The patient's mood, paranoia, and severity of obsessive thoughts were all improved. He was noted to be interacting more with his family. The patient has had fewer episodes of agitation over last few weeks
- Most of his concerns were related to feeling like he had lost a lot of autonomy and was not able to live as an independent adult
- On examination, he had mild bilateral lower-extremity edema, likely caused by olanzapine (Zyprexa), as mild pedal edema has been a reported as a side effect
- Genomic studies revealed that the patient shows rapid metabolism by cytochrome P450 1A2 (CYP1A2). This explains why the patient has needed higher doses of olanzapine in order to experience improved effects

Question

What would you do now?

- Increase olanzapine (Zyprexa) further to 70 mg daily in divided doses
- Keep olanzapine at the current dose

- Obtain a serum olanzapine level
- Start an SSRI or serotonin-norepinephrine reuptake inhibitor (SNRI)
- Increase the frequency of psychotherapy sessions

Case debrief

- Many patients with autism spectrum disorders comorbid with OCD and psychotic symptoms demonstrate resistance to medication treatment, with variable resistances over time
- Some medications that were tolerated for extended periods of time can cause delayed onset of adverse effects that further complicate the clinical picture
- In order to alleviate the adverse autonomic side effects that were observed to be caused by clozapine (Clozaril), this medication was discontinued quickly; however, the sudden discontinuation itself precipitated other medical concerns, notably NMS and catatonia. These phenomena were likely exacerbated by the simultaneous discontinuation of a benzodiazepine. Although the intent was to remove the medication responsible for the patient's gait instability and risk of falls, the sudden removal carried with it its own risks
- Once the patient's NMS and catatonia were treated, high-dose olanzapine (Zyprexa) was used as a substitute for clozapine in treating his paranoia and intermittently assaultive agitation
- Genetic testing revealed that the patient was a rapid metabolizer by CYP1A2, the enzyme that metabolizes olanzapine, and thus he required much higher doses than he would have required otherwise, and his symptoms improved as the dose was increased to 70 mg daily
- At the end of this case, the patient's symptoms were stable and he was taking a regimen of olanzapine 70 mg daily, clonazepam (Klonopin) 1 mg three times per day, and melatonin 3 mg at bedtime

Questions

If the patient's obsessive thoughts and anxiety worsen, how would you change your treatment plan?

If the patient's paranoia and psychotic agitation worsen, would you make any further changes to your treatment?

Take-home points

- Although we focus a lot on early detection and minimization of the adverse effects associated with starting clozapine (Clozaril) and treating a patient with it over the course of months and years, it is just as important to consider the adverse effects of rapid discontinuation of clozapine, especially in a patient who has been taking it for a long time

- If rapid discontinuation of clozapine occurs, watch for rebound NMS, seizures, and catatonia
- High-dose olanzapine (Zyprexa) may be an effective treatment for medication-resistant psychotic symptoms and behavioral disruption in patients with autism spectrum disorder
- A long-acting benzodiazepine may be an effective augmenting agent in this type of patient

Performance in practice: confessions of a psychopharmacologist

- When discontinuing clozapine (Clozaril) or switching to a different antipsychotic, slow off-titration is preferred in order to avoid cholinergic rebound, rebound psychosis, and the risk of excited catatonia[5]
- It is understood, as in some cases related to agranulocytosis, that it may be necessary to abruptly stop the compound, but consideration of the emergence of the symptoms described above should be considered
- If abrupt discontinuation of clozapine is necessary, the patient should be covered with anticholinergic medications to prevent delirium and other symptoms associated with severe cholinergic rebound

Tips and pearls

- When patients seem to require much higher doses of medication than a typical individual would in order to demonstrate a meaningful response, this is the time to consider genetic testing
- For high doses of olanzapine (Zyprexa) in treatment-resistant patients, monitor therapeutic drug levels and target generally higher than the usual range of 50–75 mg/ml (generally >125 mg/ml), but keep below the toxic range associated with corrected QT interval prolongation (700–800 mg/ml). The risk of motor side effects also increases with higher doses

Posttest self-assessment question and answer

Which of the following may cause abnormal movement disorders?

A. Aripiprazole (Abilify)

B. Haloperidol (Haldol)

C. Clozapine (Clozaril)

D. Valproic acid (Depakote)

E. A and B

F. All of the above

Answer: E

Aripiprazole may cause akathisia and EPS, while haloperidol can cause EPS and tardive dyskinesia. Clozapine has a lower relative risk of EPS and tardive dyskinesia, but risk is still present. Valproic acid can cause Parkinsonian movements.

References

1. Ahmed, S, Chengappa, KN, Naidu, VR, et al. Clozapine withdrawal-emergent dystonias and dyskinesias: a case series. *J Clin Psychiatry* 1998; 59:472–7. https://doi.org/10.4088/jcp.v59n0906

2. Bobolakis, I. Neuroleptic malignant syndrome after antipsychotic drug administration during benzodiazepine withdrawal. *J Clin Psychopharmacol* 2000; 20:281–3. https://doi.org/10.1097/00004714-200004000-00033

3. Brown M, Freeman S. Clonazepam withdrawal-induced catatonia. *Psychosomatics* 2009; 50:289–92. https://doi.org/10.1176/appi.psy.50.3.289

4. Cummings M, Stahl S., *Management of Complex Treatment-resistant Psychotic Disorders*. New York, NY: Cambridge University Press, 2020.

5. Galova A, Berney P, Desmeules J, et al. A case report of cholinergic rebound syndrome following abrupt low-dose clozapine discontinuation in a patient with type I bipolar affective disorder. *BMC Psychiatry* 2019; 19:73. https://doi.org/10.1186/s12888-019-2055-1

6. Lee, JW, Robertson, S. Clozapine withdrawal catatonia and neuroleptic malignant syndrome: a case report. *Ann Clin Psychiatry* 1997; 9:165–9. https://doi.org/10.1023/a:1026230024656

7. Meyer J, Stahl SM. *Clozapine Handbook*. New York, NY: Cambridge University Press, 2019.

8. Nayak, V, Chogtu, B, Devaramane, V, Bhandary, PV. Pedal edema with olanzepine. *Indian J Pharmacol* 2009; 41:49–50. https://doi.org/10.4103/0253-7613.48883

9. Rosebush, PI, Mazurek, MF. Catatonia after benzodiazepine withdrawal. *J Clin Psychopharmacol* 1996; 16:315–19. https://doi.org/10.1097/00004714-199608000-00007

10. Stahl, SM. *Essential Psychopharmacology: The Prescriber's Guide*. New York, NY: Cambridge University Press, 2005.

11. Stonecipher, A, Galang, R, Black, J. Psychotropic discontinuation symptoms: a case of withdrawal neuroleptic malignant syndrome. *Gen Hosp Psychiatry* 2006; 28:541–3. https://doi.org/10.1016/j.genhosppsych.2006.07.007

12. Wadekar, M, Syed, S. Clozapine-withdrawal catatonia. *Psychosomatics* 2010; 51:355. https://doi.org/10.1176/appi.psy.51.4.355

13. Yeh, AWC, Lee, JW, Cheng, TC, et al. Clozapine withdrawal catatonia associated with cholinergic and serotonergic rebound hyperactivity: a case report. *Clin Neuropharmacol* 2004: 27:216–18. https://doi.org/10.1097/01.wnf.0000145506.99636.1b

Case 22: An adolescent awakening

The Question: How to manage an adolescent with treatment-resistant psychosis, underlying attention-deficit/hyperactivity disorder (ADHD) symptoms, daytime sedation, insomnia, and a propensity for weight gain?

The Psychopharmacological Dilemma: Finding an effective regimen for treatment-resistant psychosis in an adolescent while managing underlying ADHD symptoms, daytime sedation, insomnia, and weight gain

Monish Parmar and Richard J. Lee

Pretest self-assessment question (answer at the end of the case)

Which of the following is not an FDA-approved treatment for adolescent psychosis?

A. Aripiprazole (Abilify)
B. Chlorpromazine (Thorazine)
C. Olanzapine (Zyprexa)
D. Quetiapine (Seroquel)
E. Haloperidol (Haldol)
F. Perphenazine (Trilafon)
G. Lurasidone (Latuda)
H. Risperidone (Risperdal)
I. Paliperidone (Invega)
J. Clozapine (Clozaril)

Patient evaluation on initial visit

- A 13-year-old girl who has been experiencing dizziness for the last 1 year
- She has also been experiencing headaches in different regions of her head and visualizing colors
- She has felt rib pain, wrist pain with pressure, and muscle cramps, all without injury
- Additionally, she reports having hair loss
- She reports no social activity for the last 4 months by choice
- She chooses not to be around her friends because "they may say something I don't like"
- She believes her diagnosis is "depression and anxiety"
- She feels she is too fat and has been refusing certain foods
- She has been wanting to wear clothing to cover her whole body, even when it is hot outside

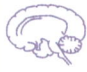

Psychiatric history

- None

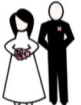

Social and personal history

- She is a second-generation Hispanic American
- Her biological mother and father are divorced
- She lives at home with her biological mother and oldest sister
- Her other older sister is out of the house at university
- She has a history of getting straight As in school; she is currently in the 8th grade
- She enjoys reading, playing the violin, studying, soccer, and playing with her dog
- Her biological father is from Mexico; her biological mom is Hispanic and was born in America

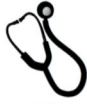

Medical history

- Irregular menstrual periods

Family history

- Mother with anxiety; not on any medication

Current medications

- None

Questions

Based on the current history, would you consider a primary psychotic disorder in the differential?

- Yes, she is keeping away from her friends (believes they may say things she does not like) and is wearing lots of clothing, despite it being hot outside
- No, it is too early to consider a primary psychotic disorder in someone so young

Would you consider initiating psychotropic medication?

- Yes, the benefit of initiating a selective serotonin reuptake inhibitor (SSRI) to treat her "anxiety or depression" outweighs the risks
- No, there is not enough history to initiate a psychotropic medication and more workup needs to be performed first

Attending physician's mental notes: initial evaluation

- The patient is likely experiencing an exacerbation of her underlying psychotic disorder or an anxiety disorder of some variety, and/or depression in addition to her psychotic disorder

- Basic laboratory and thyroid function tests all came back negative
- An SSRI does not seem warranted at this point; the patient was counseled on stress-reduction strategies, mindfulness, daily physical activity, and healthy eating

Case outcome: admission to psychiatric hospital at 5.5 months after initial presentation

- The patient, now 14 years old, is brought to the psychiatric emergency room by her biological sister
- Her sister tells the psychiatrist that the patient "has been acting bizarre at home for the last 5 days"
- The sister reports that the patient "does not sleep at home, talks to herself, and laughs randomly"
- The patient was aggressive toward her mother this morning
- In the triage of the psychiatric emergency room, she is pacing, responding to internal stimuli, and appears paranoid
- When asked to come inside the psychiatric emergency room, the patient runs out of the triage and requires emergency intramuscular (IM) olanzapine (Zyprexa) 5 mg to treat her agitation and paranoia
- She is subsequently placed on an involuntary hold and admitted to the inpatient psychiatric hospital
- During the inpatient evaluation, the patient reports that she has not been sleeping well for 2 weeks but cannot recall any further details
- She reports having thoughts of stabbing herself with a knife because her teacher and classmates are sexually harassing her and want to rape her

Further investigation

Is there anything else you would like to know about this patient?

- What about collateral information from her mother?
  - Her mother reports that the patient is making statements like "the tree is talking to me"
  - Her mother states that she wanted to keep the patient from going to school because of the accusations she was making about her teacher and classmates – this is what prompted the patient to become aggressive with her mother
- Did she ever have any viral or flu-like illness prior to the onset of her changes in behavior?
  - Her mother cannot rule out any infectious process prior to the onset of the patient's bizarre symptoms about 5.5 months ago

- Remember, however, that she did experience the rib pain, wrist pain with pressure, and muscle cramps 5 months ago
- Her mother reports that the patient may have had weakness on one side of her body, but she cannot remember

Attending physician's mental notes: first hospitalization

- Mental status examination reveals a teenager who is thought-blocking, disheveled, internally preoccupied, and paranoid
- The working diagnosis at this point is schizophrenia because of the characteristic prodromal phase and subsequent psychotic decompensation
- Bipolar disorder and schizoaffective disorder also need to be ruled out because of her 2-week period of not sleeping well (her urine drug screens have been normal and there is no suspicion for drug abuse)
- Lowest on the differential is posttraumatic stress disorder – her belief about being raped appears to be a persecutory delusion
- It is unusual for florid psychosis to present in a 14-year-old; therefore, it is important to rule out potential underlying medical etiologies
- A video electroencephalogram (EEG) should be obtained to rule out underlying epilepsy leading to her presentation
- Anti-*N*-methyl-D-aspartate (NMDA) receptor encephalitis should also be ruled out by testing for antibodies in the patient's cerebrospinal fluid via a lumbar puncture. This is worth considering because of her young age, possible previous one-sided weakness on her body, and a possibility of a viral etiology prior to the prodrome
- Hashimoto's encephalopathy should also be ruled out by testing for thyroid-stimulating hormone (TSH), T4, thyroglobulin antibody, and thyroid peroxidase antibodies (also known as steroid-responsive encephalopathy associated with autoimmune thyroiditis, or SREAT). This is worth considering because it is easy to screen for, easily treatable, and could present like a first-break psychosis
- Brain magnetic resonance imaging (MRI) should be obtained to rule out any structural process that could be leading to her presentation

Question

Would you start any psychotropic treatment at this point?

- Despite many potential underlying medical issues that could be leading to her presentation, a primary psychotic disorder appears to be highest on the differential because of the classic prodromal phase followed by further deterioration
- As a result, the patient is started on risperidone (Risperdal) 1 mg PO daily and is titrated up to 1 mg PO twice per day for her psychosis

PATIENT FILE

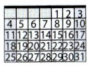

Case outcome: first psychiatric hospitalization

- The patient presents as less disorganized and less paranoid after being treated with risperidone (Risperdal) for 5 days during the hospitalization
- She no longer believes that her classmates or teachers are raping her
- She continues to present as odd, is slow to respond to questions, and is not interacting as well as she had been prior to her prodrome
- All her general medical workup came back negative

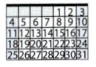

Case outcome: second hospitalization at 7 months after last hospitalization

- The patient is hospitalized again because she is refusing to take her risperidone (Risperdal) and deteriorates further
- She now believes that her parents and siblings are raping her physically and mentally
- After her last hospitalization, the patient had initiated psychotherapy
- The therapist notes that the patient smiles inappropriately during the session and responds to internal stimuli, despite being adherent to risperidone
- The patient believes that her neighbors are speaking to her while she is in her bedroom, despite her neighbors being too far away to do so
- The patient also believes that students at school are spying on her locker
- The patient stops her basic hygiene, including showering, brushing her hair, or changing her clothes
- She was previously a straight-A student, but her grades have now completely deteriorated
- Upon evaluation, she is disheveled and refusing/unable to speak
- Her mother reports that the patient refuses to take any medications by mouth
- Her mother states that she took the patient to another psychiatric hospital, but the psychiatrist there stated that he could not provide any treatment if the patient refuses to accept medication by mouth

Question

What else can be done for this patient?

- A long-acting injectable (LAI) can be considered for this patient as she has tolerated risperidone (Risperdal) by mouth previously
- The two LAIs worth considering at this point are (best options because of her good response to risperidone when adherent):

Oral equivalence (approximate)	
Oral paliperidone	1-month Sustenna
3 mg	39–78 mg
6 mg	117 mg
9 mg	156 mg
12 mg	234 mg

Figure 22.1. Oral equivalence for Invega Sustenna.

- Paliperidone (Invega Sustenna)
  - Dosing range of 39–234 mg monthly (Figure 22.1)
  - Advantages are that it does not require oral coverage, and is a monthly injection; once stable for 4 months on Invega Sustenna, the patient can switch to Invega Trinza (paliperidone) injection once every 3 months
  - The disadvantage is that a booster is required (second injection) approximately 8 days after the first injection
- Risperidone (Risperdal Consta)
  - Dosing range of 12.5–50 mg IM every 2 weeks
  - An advantage is that this is risperidone in an injectable form (unlike Invega Sustenna, which is the active metabolite of risperidone and therefore has many different pharmacokinetic and pharmacodynamic properties)
  - A disadvantage is that the time to reach maximum concentration in the blood (T_{max}) is long (21 days) and therefore there needs to be a 3–4 week oral overlap
  - Dosing tip: 2 mg of oral risperidone is equivalent to approximately 25 mg of Risperdal Consta every 2 weeks

Case outcome: second hospitalization at 7 months after last hospitalization (continued)

- The patient was treated with paliperidone (Invega) LAI 234 mg and administered the booster dose of 156 mg IM 5 days later
- Her persecutory delusions improved and she no longer believed her family was raping her
- She began to complete her activities of daily living without prompting
- However, she continues to present as odd and appears to be internally preoccupied
- The patient continues to have the following negative symptoms: blunting of affect, poverty of speech and thought, apathy, anhedonia, reduced social drive, loss of motivation, lack of social interest, and inattention to social or cognitive input

- Nonetheless, she is in a much better place psychiatrically than she has been for the last several months
- Her mother is pleased with the treatment outcome

Attending physician's mental notes: second hospitalization

- Although the patient's positive symptoms have decreased (paranoia, hallucinations, and persecutory delusions), her negative symptoms mostly persist

Two-minute tutorial

- Positive symptoms are believed to be the result of too much dopamine activity in the mesolimbic pathway
- Negative symptoms are thought to be related to hypofunctioning in the mesocortical pathway
- The negative symptoms and cognitive deficits in schizophrenia are often a result of a lack of dopamine stimulation in the prefrontal cortex, which are primarily dopamine D_1 receptors and some D_3 receptors
- The mesocortical pathway is believed to be involved in the physiology of:
  - Cognition and executive function via the dorsolateral prefrontal cortex
  - Emotions and affect via the ventromedial prefrontal cortex
- Negative symptoms predict a poor functional outcome for patients with schizophrenia (alarming in this patient because she is only 14 years old)
- Negative symptoms are believed to be treated with serotonin $5-HT_{2A}$ receptor antagonism, present in most second-generation antipsychotics (including paliperidone (Invega), as in this patient)
- $5-HT_{2A}$ receptor agonism is thought to cause the inhibition of dopamine release
- $5-HT_{2A}$ receptor antagonism is believed to promote dopamine release in the following regions of the brain: nigrostriatal areas (reducing extrapyramidal symptoms), the prefrontal cortex (reducing negative symptoms), and the ventromedial prefrontal cortex (having an antidepressant effect)

Case outcome: third hospitalization at 8 months after last hospitalization

- The patient has been deteriorating despite her paliperidone (Invega) LAI increasing from 234 mg IM monthly to every 3 weeks
- She is also taking risperidone (Risperdal) 2 mg PO daily to augment the LAI

- She is experiencing voices that are telling her to hurt herself and others
- Prior to this hospitalization, she had acted on the voices and attempted to hurt her niece with a knife because "she was playing with my puppy"
- The patient is experiencing visual hallucinations of duplicating people in front of her – if there is one person in the room, she will see five of them
- She is no longer physically going to school
- She is granted home hospitalization due to worsening psychosis at school
- Her grades have deteriorated and her ability to learn new information is poor
- Her mother has stopped working to take care of the patient at home full-time
- The patient has been started on bupropion extended-release (Aplenzin) 150 mg every morning, by the outpatient psychiatrist, for low energy (started after her psychotic symptoms started worsening)
- The thought of the bupropion worsening the psychosis was considered; however, bupropion was continued because the patient's psychosis had already worsened before bupropion's initiation
- The patient is noted to have significant oro-buccal-lingual acute dystonia during the hospitalization, which was suggestive of extrapyramidal symptoms (EPS) and drug-induced Parkinsonism rather than tardive dyskinesia
- She is also experiencing dropping of the jaw, mild protrusion of the tongue, muscle stiffness, and slowness in her movements (all likely EPS)

Question

How should one proceed at this point?

- The patient appears to be deteriorating despite treatment with paliperidone (Invega) LAI at an appropriate dose and for a reasonable period (at least 6 weeks)
- She also did not do well with risperidone (Risperdal), although she only went up to a total daily dose of 2 mg because of refusal of her medication by mouth
- At this point, she is willing to take pills by mouth, which increases the treatment options considerably

- A switch can be considered to the antipsychotic cariprazine (Vraylar), which can boost energy and motivation and has some evidence of efficacy in the negative symptoms of schizophrenia
- Benztropine (Cogentin) 1 mg PO twice per day is added to her regimen to treat her EPS/drug-induced Parkinsonism
- Clozapine (Clozaril) is initiated, despite a lack of two failed trials of other antipsychotics, because of its low propensity for EPS, its ability to treat negative symptoms, and its potential for a better response than other neuroleptic agents
- Her worsening psychosis despite high doses of paliperidone augmented with risperidone, muscle stiffness, and negative symptoms make this decision rational
- She does not meet the strict criteria for treatment-resistant schizophrenia (failing at least two adequate trials of other antipsychotics for a minimum duration and dose): she has only failed paliperidone LAI and did not have a long enough adherence period with risperidone
- Nevertheless, clozapine is started at 25 mg every night and increased to 50 mg every night after 48 hours

Tips and pearls

- Clozapine (Clozaril) is the gold-standard treatment for refractory schizophrenia
- It is not used as a first-line treatment due to side effects and monitoring burden
- However, some studies have shown that clozapine is associated with the lowest risk of mortality among antipsychotics, causing some study authors to question whether its use should continue to be restricted to resistant cases
- It may improve tardive dyskinesia
- It causes little or no prolactin elevation, motor side effects, or tardive dyskinesia
- It causes more weight gain than many other antipsychotics
- To treat constipation and reduce the risk of paralytic ileus and bowel obstruction, taper off other anticholinergic agents and start all patients routinely on docusate (Colace)
- Patients can have much better responses to clozapine than any other agent, but not always
- Clinical improvements often continue slowly over a number of years

- Clozapine requires a baseline absolute neutrophil count, and weekly blood draws for the first 6 months of treatment, followed by biweekly for the next 6 months and monthly thereafter
- This strict monitoring is necessary because the medication can cause agranulocytosis, especially early on during treatment

Case outcome: interim follow-up visit 1 month after discharge from the third psychiatric hospitalization (outpatient clinic)

- The patient is having intermittent derogatory auditory hallucinations and has visions of scary things (both of which are less intense and less often than previously)
- She continues to have muscle stiffness
- She continues to have negative symptoms
- The patient has constipation

Question

Would you attempt to pursue antipsychotic monotherapy for the patient?

- Yes
- No

Attending physician's mental notes: interim follow-up visit 1 month after discharge from the third psychiatric hospitalization (outpatient clinic)

- At this point, the psychiatrist decides to stop the paliperidone (Invega) LAI and further treat the patient with clozapine (Clozaril) monotherapy (it has been approximately 1 month since the last administration – there had been an overlap of a few weeks of both antipsychotics)
- In its place, risperidone (Risperdal) 2 mg PO twice per day is started to help with tapering off paliperidone's strong D_2 receptor blockade
- The goal will be to have her on clozapine monotherapy with a gradual taper of risperidone (she has had EPS, low motivation, lots of negative symptoms, and an overall poor response to D_2 receptor blockers so far)
- Clozapine is increased from 50 mg every night to 100 mg every night to address her psychosis
- It is best to treat with clozapine once daily, preferably at night, if possible, because of its propensity for sedation secondary to inverse agonism/antagonism at the histamine H_1 receptor

- Some patients may require twice per day dosing initially because of clozapine's strong α-adrenergic receptor antagonism, which can lead to significant orthostasis (the patient is not experiencing these issues and therefore is given a once-nightly dosing)
- The patient has been having constipation, likely secondary to clozapine and/or benztropine (Cogentin)
- As a result, docusate (Colace) 250 mg up to twice per day is initiated
- Benztropine is tapered from 1 mg PO twice per day to 1 mg daily (less EPS potential because of a reduction in dose of D_2 receptor blockade via the switch to a lower equivalent dose of risperidone)
- Clozapine provides strong anticholinergic activity and therefore should also help with any EPS secondary to risperidone (100 mg of clozapine has approximately the same anticholinergic activity as 2 mg of benztropine)
- Bupropion extended-release (Aplenzin) 150 mg is continued for the patient but it is unclear what, if anything, is being accomplished by it
- Bupropion does have the potential to raise energy levels, motivation, and concentration by increasing catecholamine transmission – it could be counteracting sedation from clozapine and paliperidone LAI via this action
- However, bupropion can also worsen psychosis

Case outcome: interim follow-up visits over the next 7 weeks

- At next visit, at 5 weeks postdischarge, the patient remains at her baseline from the last visit (having intermittent auditory and visual hallucinations)
- Her mother is giving her risperidone (Risperdal) 4 mg in the morning instead of 2 mg twice per day
- Her clozapine (Clozaril) is increased from 100 mg PO at bedtime to 150 mg PO at bedtime
- At the next two visits, at 6 and 7 weeks postdischarge, the patient remains at her baseline, continuing to have intermittent hallucinations
- Clozapine is further increased from 150 mg PO at bedtime to 200 mg PO at bedtime at 6 weeks postdischarge
- At 9 weeks postdischarge, the patient's insight has improved dramatically
- She begins talking about how behind she is in school, something she has not done previously, indicating that her insight is improving
- For the first time in about 2 years, she does not appear to be responding to internal stimuli and is fully present in her interaction with her mother and the psychiatrist

- She does have intermittent auditory and visual hallucinations at 9 weeks postdischarge
- Risperidone is tapered from 4 mg every morning to 2 mg every morning
- At 10 weeks postdischarge, her mother stops giving the patient risperidone 2 mg
- Her mother has noticed significant improvement with clozapine and does not feel that risperidone is necessary, which is why she abruptly stops it
- At 11 weeks postdischarge, the patient appears to be doing much better
- She is now having more productive thinking
- She is quick to respond to questions and her affect is appropriately reactive
- Her motivation in life has increased – she is exercising with her mother, playing her instruments again, and reading books
- She continues to have baseline hallucinations
- Interestingly, she is better able to talk about the hallucinations now – she describes the daytime auditory hallucination as a voice that is derogatory
- At night, she experiences a vision that is scary and tells her to hurt herself and others
- She knows not to act on these hallucinations and has enough insight to know that they are part of her mental illness and not an external voice (this is a significant improvement compared with previously)
- Her biggest concern currently is being able to fall asleep
- Trazodone (Desyrel) 25–50 mg PO at bedtime as needed for insomnia is added to help with this
- At 12 weeks postdischarge, and 2 weeks after stopping risperidone, the patient is no longer having any hallucinations
- She took a trip to Mexico over the weekend to attend a wedding – she did not have any problems and enjoyed spending time with her family
- The patient states that she wants to organize her day so she can get her homework done early on so that she can play the violin and do yoga in the afternoons
- The patient is able to fall asleep easily at 8 p.m. with the addition of the dose of trazodone at bedtime; she is waking up at 7 a.m.
- At 15 weeks postdischarge, the patient's biggest issue is weight gain
- Dietary and activity recommendations were discussed to manage weight gain

- Her psychosis has been gone for at least 3 weeks; her mother is so pleased with the progress the patient is making that she is considering going back to work full-time
- At 17 weeks postdischarge, clozapine levels are ordered
- She has a clozapine level of 28 µg/l (drawn 22.5 hours after her nightly dose)

Question

Would you increase the clozapine (Clozaril) dose to achieve typical therapeutic levels?

- Yes, in the typical treatment-resistant patient, the likelihood of response will depend on achieving trough plasma levels of at least 350 µg/l
- No, very low doses of clozapine have been shown to be beneficial in select groups of patients with schizophrenia

Attending physician's mental notes: interim follow-up visit at 17 weeks postdischarge

- The patient's clozapine (Clozaril) level is very low in comparison with what is typically required for treatment-resistant cases
- Her mother reports excellent adherence with the medication
- Clinically, the patient is without any psychosis or negative symptoms, and her old personality is back (making it almost certain that she is taking her medication as prescribed)
- The patient's symptoms are stable at this time despite a low clozapine level, which may be artificially low because the blood draw was 22.5 hours after her last clozapine dose instead of the standard 12-hour trough level
- Aside from her steady weight gain and sleeping 11–12 hours at night, she has no other side effects on the clozapine
- At 20 weeks postdischarge, weight gain continues to be her biggest complaint
- Her negative symptoms are completely absent at this point
- Her mother reports that she feels like the patient is just like her old self again
- Her mother states that her personality is back to where it was before – someone who is enthusiastic, inquisitive, and intelligent
- At 26 weeks postdischarge, the patient has put on 25 lbs compared with her baseline weight, despite attempts at dietary modification and daily pilates/yoga
- Her mother reports that the patient eats large amounts of food and seeks out carbohydrate-laden foods, often in the middle of the night

Question

How would you manage the patient's weight gain at this point?

- Continue with dietary changes
- Add metformin (Glucophage)
- Add topiramate (Topamax)
- Add a stimulant
- Add aripiprazole (Abilify)
- Increase the dose of bupropion extended-release (Aplenzin)

Attending physician's mental notes: interim follow-up visit at 17 weeks postdischarge (continued)

- The patient has gained approximately 25 lbs from her baseline
- The pharmacological agent with the most evidence to manage antipsychotic-induced weight gain is metformin (Glucophage)
- There is evidence for the other options as well, but metformin should be the first-line strategy to assist with weight gain
- Metformin can be started at 500 mg once daily for 1 week and increased thereafter

Case outcome: interim follow-up visit at 30 weeks postdischarge

- At 30 weeks postdischarge, the patient has been on metformin (Glucophage) 500 mg once daily for a week and then 500 mg twice per day thereafter
- The patient's carbohydrate cravings have become noticeably less
- The patient feels likes her focus/concentration is not quite there when it comes to doing her schoolwork from home
- Her mother reports that the patient did have problems with focus as a child but was able to still do well in school because of perseverance
- The patient enthusiastically asks whether she can physically return to school
- She reports that staying at home all day is leading to boredom
- Her biggest concern is being able to focus and be attentive to her schoolwork

Question

How should you manage the patient's focus/inattention/concentration difficulties?

- Increase bupropion extended-release (Aplenzin) from 150 mg to 300 mg
- Add atomoxetine (Strattera)

- Add a stimulant
- Add on an α_2-adrenergic agonist
- Watch and wait

Attending physician's mental notes: interim follow-up visit at 30 weeks postdischarge

- The patient appears to have some symptoms of attention-deficit/hyperactivity disorder, inattentive type, dating back to when she was younger. However, she does not appear to have had functional impairment as a youth
- The patient is likely having some element of daytime sedation secondary to her clozapine (Clozaril), which is making it harder for her to focus
- Because she has inattention as well as difficulties with weight gain, the best strategy is to add on a stimulant to help treat both
- The patient will be watched closely for emerging psychosis if a stimulant is started
- Mixed amphetamine salts, extended-release (XR) (Adderall-XR) 10 mg is chosen (although any long-acting stimulant would be okay in this situation) because of its availability on the formulary locally
- The concern for worsening psychosis with a stimulant is present, but with the psychosis fully controlled by clozapine, the benefit of treating the sedation/appetite/inattention far outweighs the risks
- The specific strategy for the patient is to stop the bupropion (Wellbutrin) for 5 days and see how she does, and then to initiate the mixed amphetamine salts XR if she remains stable after discontinuing bupropion

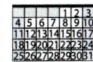

Case outcome: interim follow-up visit at 34 and 40 weeks postdischarge

- At 34 weeks postdischarge, the patient returns to school with accommodations for the first time in nearly 1 year
- The mixed amphetamine salts XR (Adderall-XR) 10 mg she is taking every morning at around 8 a.m. is wearing off by around 3 p.m.; a 2 p.m. mixed amphetamine salts immediate-release (IR) (Adderall-IR) 5 mg dose is added to her regimen to help with her afternoon inattention symptoms
- At 40 weeks postdischarge, the patient is stable on clozapine (Clozaril) 200 mg PO at bedtime, mixed amphetamine salts XR 10 mg every morning and mixed amphetamine salts IR 5 mg in the afternoon, trazodone (Desyrel) 50 mg PO at bedtime as needed for insomnia, metformin (Glucophage) 500 mg PO twice per day, and docusate (Colace) 250 mg PO twice per day

- She is continuing to flourish in school
- Weight gain remains an issue for the patient but less so than previously
- She continues to have enthusiasm and a reactive affect, and she is happy and "awakened"
- She is physically active, enjoys playing her instruments, and has fun with her dog
- Both the patient and her mother are very pleased with where she is at. She has been completely without any psychotic symptoms for the past 28 weeks

Case debrief

- The patient had an "awakening" with clozapine (Clozaril) that altered the trajectory of her life
- Despite clozapine's D_2 receptor blocking of approximately only 30%, the patient had a dramatic response, which was likely secondary to some other mechanism such as clozapine's ability to increase glutamate signaling activity in the frontal lobe
- It is believed that this increased glutamate signaling in the frontal lobe modulates the dopaminergic activity in the temporal lobe by dampening its transmission, thus causing less psychosis
- The patient had persecutory delusions along with command auditory hallucinations, a dyad of symptoms that are highly associated with psychotic violence (the patient had attempted to stab her niece with a knife)
- Clozapine is unique in that it can independently reduce violence and suicide, and likely did so in this patient

Take-home points

- Do not be afraid to use clozapine (Clozaril) in young people once they have failed two adequate trials of dose and duration of other antipsychotics or have developed significant side effects (EPS or tardive dyskinesia)
- In adolescents treated with clozapine, blood levels may not need to be in the 100s of µg/l or higher, as long as there is a robust clinical response at lower doses
- Once a patient's psychosis is fully treated with clozapine, one can relatively safely initiate a stimulant to target underlying inattentive symptoms, daytime sedation, and weight gain
- Do not forget to at least start docusate (Colace) for patients on clozapine and likely also polyethylene glycol to avoid bowel obstruction
- Intervene early with metformin (Glucophage) to help with weight gain, which can often be dramatic

Performance in practice: confessions of a psychopharmacologist

What could have been done better here?

- The introduction of metformin (Glucophage) could have been considered earlier to mitigate the weight gain

Posttest self-assessment question and answer

Which of the following is not an FDA-approved treatment for adolescent psychosis?

A. Aripiprazole (Abilify)
B. Chlorpromazine (Thorazine)
C. Olanzapine (Zyprexa)
D. Quetiapine (Seroquel)
E. Haloperidol (Haldol)
F. Perphenazine (Trilafon)
G. Lurasidone (Latuda)
H. Risperidone (Risperdal)
I. Paliperidone (Invega)
J. Clozapine (Clozaril)

Answer: J

Some atypical antipsychotics that have been FDA approved for treatment of pediatric mental health disorders are given in Figure 22.2.

Atypical Antipsychotics

	FDA-approved for pediatric use
Aripiprazole	Schizophrenia (13+); Acute mania (10+); Autism-related irritability (6-17); Tourette syndrome (6-18)
Asenapine	Acute mania (10+)
Brexpiprazole	-
Cariprazine	-
Lurasidone	Schizophrenia (13+); Bipolar depression (10+)
Olanzapine	Schizophrenia (13+); Acute mania (13+); Bipolar depression (with fluoxetine; 10+)
Quetiapine	Schizophrenia (13+); Acute mania (10+)
Risperidone	Schizophrenia (13+); Acute mania (10+); Autism-related irritability (5-16)
Ziprasidone	-

Cerullo M et al. CNS Spectrums 2013;18(4):199-208; Fountoulakis KN et al. Eur Arch Psychiatry Clin Neurosci 2012;262(suppl 1):S1-48; Fountoulakis KN et al. Int J Neuropsychopharmacol 2012;15:1015-26; Grunze H, Azorin JM. World J Biol Psychiatry 2014;15(5):355-68; Vieta E, Valenti M. J Affective Disord 2013;148:28-36; Fornaro M et al. Int J Mol Sci 2016;17(2):241. doi:10.3390/ijms17020241; Stahl SM. Prescriber's Guide. 6th ed. Cambridge University; 2017.

Figure 22.2. Atypical antipsychotics and their FDA approvals for pediatric use. The appropriate age for use is indicated. Data from Cerullo and Strakowski (2013), Fornaro et al. (2016), Fountoulakis et al. (2012a, b), Grunze and Azorin (2014), Stahl (2017), and Vieta and Valentí (2013).

References

1. Cerullo MA, Strakowski SM. A systematic review of the evidence for the treatment of acute depression in bipolar I disorder. *CNS Spectr* 2013; 18:199–208. https://doi.org/10.1017/S1092852913000102
2. Fornaro M, Stubbes B, de Berardis D, et al. Atypical antipsychotics in the treatment of acute bipolar depression with mixed features: a systematic review and exploratory meta-analysis of placebo-controlled clinical trials. *Int J Mol Sci* 2016; 17:241. https://doi.org/10.3390/ijms17020241
3. Fountoulakis KN, Kasper S, Andreassen O, et al. (2012a) Efficacy of pharmacotherapy in bipolar disorder: a report by the WPA section on pharmacopsychiatry. *Eur Arch Psychiatry Clin Neurosci.* 262 (Suppl. 1): 1–48. https://doi.org/10.1007/s00406-012-0323-x
4. Fountoulakis KN, Kontis D, Gonda X, et al. (2012b) Treatment of mixed bipolar states. *Int J Neuropsychopharmacol* 15:1015–26. https://doi.org/10.1017/S1461145711001817
5. Freudenreich, O, Brown, HE, Holt, DJ. Psychosis and Schizophrenia. In: Stern, TA, Fava, M, Wilens, TE, Rosenbaum, JF eds. Massachusetts General Hospital Comprehensive Clinical Psychiatry, 2nd ed. Elsevier, 2016; pp. 307–23
6. Grunze H, Azorin JM. Clinical decision making in the treatment of mixed states. *World J Biol Psychiatry* 2014; 15:355–68. https://doi.org/10.3109/15622975.2014.908238
7. Najjar, S, Steiner, J, Najjar, A, Bechter, K. A clinical approach to new-onset psychosis associated with immune dysregulation: the concept of autoimmune psychosis. *J Neuroinflammation* 2018; 15: 40. https://doi.org/10.1186/s12974-018-1067-y
8. Stahl, SM. *Stahl's Essential Psychopharmacology: Prescriber's Guide.* Cambridge, UK: Cambridge University Press, 2017.
9. Vieta E, Valentí M. Mixed states in DSM-5: implications for clinical care, education, and research. *J Affect Disord* 2013; 148:28–36. https://doi.org/10.1016/j.jad.2013.03.007.

Case 23: The peace keeper with a left breast mass

The Question: How can neutrophil count be monitored effectively in a patient early in clozapine (Clozaril) treatment who is also undergoing simultaneous chemotherapy?

The Psychopharmacological Dilemma: How to use the guidelines of the clozapine registration system to effectively monitor absolute neutrophil count in a patient currently taking clozapine for treatment-resistant schizophrenia while simultaneously undergoing chemotherapy?

Diem Nguyen and Brenda Jensen

Pretest self-assessment question (answer at the end of the case)

When is the risk of severe neutropenia greatest for a patient on clozapine (Clozaril) treatment?

A. Within the first week of initiating treatment
B. Within the first 18 weeks of initiating treatment
C. When there is a change in dosage
D. The risk is similar throughout clozapine treatment

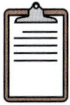

Patient evaluation on intake

- A 61-year-old woman with the chief complaint of left breast mass

Psychiatric history

- The patient had onset of paranoid symptoms in her late 20s, with her first inpatient psychiatric hospitalization at age 27
- She was diagnosed with schizophrenia at age 30
- There is a history of two episodes of sexual assault in her late 20s
- There is no history of manic episodes
- There is no history of prior suicide attempts
- She had four known prior inpatient psychiatric hospitalizations between the ages of 37 and 58. Details of her prior psychiatric history were unknown, as the patient records were limited and the patient herself is a poor historian
- The patient consistently claimed she was a top-secret translator for the United Nations due to her knowledge of multiple Arabic languages, as well as a visionary for her religious beliefs regarding prostitution rings
- She was previously in the Army Reserves, but has not worked since her early 30s
- Mental status examination revealed an obese Hispanic American female who is pleasant and cooperative. She had prolonged eye

contact and a mood congruent with her full affect. Her speech was tangential and rambling, and was rapid but not pressured. She had a disorganized thought process with flight of ideas, and varied paranoid and grandiose delusions with repeated hyper-religious and sexual themes. She endorsed positive ideas of reference and denied hallucinations but stated she "listened to the voice of God"

- Her insight was marginal but her judgment appeared intact; while she consistently refuted her diagnosis of schizophrenia, she has been compliant with psychotropic medications
- Prior psychotropic medications/combinations included ziprasidone (Geodon), valproate, risperidone (Risperdal), paliperidone palmitate long-acting injectable (Invega Sustenna), loxapine (Loxitane), and aripiprazole (Abilify) at maximum dosages with continued marked disorganized delusions and severe metabolic side effects
- The patient was started on clozapine (Clozaril) in January 2020 for treatment-resistant schizophrenia with noted improvement in positive symptoms noted by both parents and medical providers
- The patient found clozapine helpful with improvement in sleep, calmer mood, and improved relationships with family members
- The patient's vital signs were within normal limits, and her baseline echocardiogram, creatine kinase, and C-reactive protein were unremarkable. Her body mass index (BMI), hemoglobin A1c (HbA1c), and fasting lipids were documented prior to starting treatment with clozapine
- Her absolute neutrophil count (ANC) and vital signs were monitored weekly while she was on clozapine
- The clozapine caused fatigue and sedation, but the patient found these side effects manageable
- A routine mammogram in February 2020 showed an irregular left breast mass, which was later biopsied and found to be a high-grade infiltrating ductal carcinoma (estrogen receptor/progesterone receptor positive, human epidermal growth factor receptor 2 (HER-2) negative) with left maxillary lymph nodes positive for metastases
- The patient underwent a trial of tamoxifen, but this was discontinued after she developed a pulmonary embolism suspected to be related to the hormone therapy
- After the patient failed tamoxifen, her multidisciplinary team, in conjunction with her psychiatric care, decided to administer four cycles of neoadjuvant chemotherapy, specifically docetaxel (Taxotere) and cyclophosphamide

- Her clozapine dose prior to the initiation of chemotherapy was 150 mg in the morning and 200 mg at night. Her clozapine level was 477 µg/l and the metabolite norclozapine level was 308 µg/l
- Her baseline laboratory data were as follows: white blood cells 6.32 × 10³/µl, hemoglobin 13.5 g/dl, absolute lymphocyte count 2.17 × 10³/µL, ANC 3.29 × 10³/µL, and platelets 211 × 10³/µL

Social and personal history

- The patient has one prior marriage, which ended in divorce at age 31
- She has had one full-term pregnancy with a son diagnosed with neuroblastoma, who died aged 6
- She self-identifies as Catholic and states that she goes to church weekly
- She is a lifelong non-smoker
- She denies the use of alcohol or recreational drugs
- She was previously in the Army Reserves
- She previously lived with her parents for over 30 years until they moved into a retirement community; she is currently living alone with income from retirement and disability benefits and appears to be able to manage her finances independently

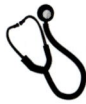

Medical history

- Morbid obesity with BMI of 47 kg/m²
- Hypertension
- Type II diabetes with HbA1c of 6.7%
- Hyperlipidemia
- Hypothyroidism
- Schizophrenia
- History of uterine fibroidectomy
- History of bilateral glaucoma surgery

Family history

- Mother with heart failure and diabetes, and a history of breast cancer
- Father with heart failure and diabetes
- Older brother with a history of lymphoma
- Son (deceased) with a history of neuroblastoma

Current medications

- Amlodipine (Norvasc) 5 mg PO daily
- Glipizide (Glucotrol) 15 mg PO twice per day

- Levothyroxine (Synthroid) 200 µg PO every morning before breakfast
- Lisinopril (Zestril) 20 mg PO daily
- Metformin (Glucophage) 1000 mg PO twice per day
- Metoprolol (Lopressor) 50 mg PO twice per day
- Simvastatin (Zocor) 20 mg PO at bedtime
- Calcium carbonate 650 mg PO daily
- Clozapine (Clozaril) 150 mg PO every morning, 200 mg PO at bedtime
- Docusate (Colace) 250 mg PO twice per day
- Sennosides 17.2 mg PO twice per day
- Polyethylene glycol 17 g PO daily as needed for constipation

Question

Based on what you have been told so far about this patient's medical and psychiatric history, and knowing the high likelihood of developing cytopenia with chemotherapy, would you continue her clozapine (Clozaril)?

- Yes, continue clozapine with the current monitoring schedule
- Yes, continue clozapine and increase ANC monitoring to three times per week
- No, discontinue clozapine and switch to another antipsychotic
- No, discontinue clozapine and monitor closely off psychotropic medications

Attending physician's mental notes: initial evaluation

- Clozapine (Clozaril) binds loosely to dopamine D_2 receptors as well as D_1, D_3, D_4, and D_5 receptors
- Sedation and fatigue are likely due to interaction at histamine H_1 receptors
- She had a history of numerous hospitalizations and continued marked psychosis despite two concurrent trials of high-dose antipsychotics prior to initiating clozapine
- The etiology of clozapine-induced neutropenia and agranulocytosis remains unclear
- Pathogenesis of clozapine-induced neutropenia and/or agranulocytosis is theorized to be mediated primarily by reactive metabolites directly and indirectly damaging myeloid precursors. Clozapine is oxidized by granulocytes to a metabolite that irreversibly binds and is toxic to neutrophils and their bone marrow precursors
- Clozapine has a 0.8–2% incidence of neutropenia, with an associated mortality of 5–10%

- The duration of clozapine use and dosage are not reliable predictors of neutropenia
- Risk factors of clozapine-induced neutropenia include older age, female, and concurrent treatment with other drugs known to cause agranulocytosis
- Both neutropenia and agranulocytosis are reversible after stopping the drug
- Clozapine-induced neutropenia often presents asymptomatically, particularly as patients are monitored for early detection
- Cessation of clozapine treatment is associated with a relapse rate up to 50%, with the further possibility of psychiatric deterioration with prominent paranoia and disorganized thought symptoms impairing her ability to comply with possibly life-saving chemotherapy
- Rechallenge after clozapine-induced neutropenia requires a latent period, and close monitoring of white blood cell count should be continued for the first 2 weeks
- 33.3% of patients with clozapine-induced neutropenia treated with olanzapine (Zyprexa) and 40% of patients with clozapine-induced neutropenia treated with quetiapine (Seroquel) showed prolonged leukopenia
- All antipsychotic medications have the potential to cause neutropenia, specifically olanzapine, which is related structurally to clozapine
- Cancer cells can infiltrate bone marrow, liver, or spleen to cause neutropenia. This is most commonly seen in leukemia, lymphoma, and multiple myeloma
- The concurrent use of chemotherapy in a patient on clozapine necessitates a higher threshold to discontinue the patient's antipsychotic, as severe cytopenia due to myelosuppressive medication is to be expected. Current guidelines recommend discontinuation of clozapine if the patient's ANC drops below 1000/µl, but patients undergoing chemotherapy often become severely neutropenic. It is unclear whether reductions in ANC are due to clozapine or chemotherapy in these patients, and strict adherence to current clozapine registration guidelines could lead to inappropriate discontinuation of a necessary antipsychotic
- Augmenting with lithium or granulocyte colony-stimulating factor (G-CSF) may promote leukocytosis and positively benefit her blood counts
- Published retrospective case reports have shown a 21% rate of repeat agranulocytosis with clozapine rechallenge alone compared with a 4% rate of repeat agranulocytosis with lithium plus clozapine rechallenge

- However, the mechanism of lithium-induced leukocytosis is poorly understood, and there are valid concerns that lithium co-use may mask impending potentially dangerous agranulocytosis
- Potential side-effect limitations of G-CSF include bone pain, allergic reactions, ruptured spleen, hemoptysis, acute respiratory distress syndrome, and a small risk of stimulation of acute myeloid leukemia in certain patients

Further investigation

Is there anything else you would especially like to know about this patient?

- Could the clozapine (Clozaril) have contributed to her development of a pulmonary embolism on tamoxifen?
  - Clozapine is known to increase platelet adhesion and aggregation, with shortened activated partial thromboplastin time
  - Clozapine-induced thromboembolism is associated with higher dosages
  - The patient has multiple known risk factors for thromboembolism including older age, obesity, inactivity, female sex, and known malignancy

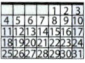

Case outcome: interim follow-up visit at week 1

- Information about the initiation of lithium was discussed with patient; however, she refused lithium because she did not like the "th" sound and felt sedated and overweight on valproate, a previously used mood stabilizer
- Moreover, the decision to start lithium was deferred due to the elevated risk of lithium neurotoxicity in conjunction with clozapine (Clozaril), possibly due to their serotonergic interactions. Although this effect is reversible, lithium has a narrow therapeutic index (0.6–1.2 mmol/l) and minor changes in plasma concentrations secondary to physiological factors can have significant clinical consequences
- The patient started the first cycle of chemotherapy in May 2020
- Pegfilgrastim injection, a PEGylated form of the G-CSF analog filgrastim but with a much longer half-life, was started prophylactically with each chemotherapy cycle to stimulate the production of neutrophils
- After a multidisciplinary discussion with psychiatry, hematology/oncology, and pharmacy, the patient was placed on a modified ANC monitoring schedule and a hold parameter for clozapine while on chemotherapy (Table 23.1)

Table 23.1 Approved modified ANC recommendations on chemotherapy

ANC level	Treatment	ANC monitoring
Mild neutropenia (ANC 1000–1499/µl)	Continue clozapine	Weekly from initiation of therapy to 6 months Every 2 weeks from 6 to 12 months Monthly after 12 months
Moderate neutropenia (ANC 500–999/µl)	Continue clozapine	Three times per week until ANC ≥1000/µl
Severe neutropenia (ANC <500/µl)	Stop clozapine	Daily until ANC ≥500/µl Three times weekly until ANC ≥1000/µl

- This monitoring schedule was modeled after the ANC monitoring guidelines of the benign ethnic neutropenia population, who have diminished myeloid progenitor cells at steady state and a smaller reserve of mature neutrophils in bone marrow and peripheral blood but with no increased frequency or severity of infections
- Benign ethnic neutropenia is seen primarily in those of African and Middle Eastern descent, and has been described in up to 25–40% of individuals of African origin
- The clozapine registry was notified of the modified ANC monitoring and a consent form was re-signed and submitted

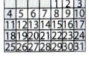

Case outcome: interim follow-up visit after 2 months

- The patient had one brief medical hospitalization in June 2020 due to leukocytosis and hypotensive dehydration, which was suspected to be secondary to a urinary tract infection and possible PICC line infection
- The patient was able to continue clozapine (Clozaril) (ultimately uptitrated to 400 mg daily) with weekly ANC monitoring while completing three out of four cycles of chemotherapy infusion until the patient's application for conversion to 14-day ANC monitoring was approved by the clozapine registry
- The patient's ANC dropped to 178/µl after the third chemotherapy cycle and clozapine had to be discontinued
- After discussion with the internal medicine service, given the historic level of the patient's baseline disorganization off clozapine and severe neutropenia in the setting of the coronavirus disease 2019 (COVID-19) pandemic, the patient was admitted to the hospital for daily ANC monitoring and neutropenic precautions
- After 8 days of inpatient hospitalization with daily ANC monitoring, her ANC increased to 1.21×10^3/µl. Clozapine was restarted at 50 mg with incremental 25 mg increased daily until the prior dosage was achieved, with weekly ANC monitoring
- The patient was discharged home and completed her last chemotherapy cycle

- One week after completing the last chemotherapy cycle, the patient was noted to have a left breast abscess with leukocytosis (white blood cell count $17 \times 10^3/\mu l$) and elevated lactate (lactate 2.3 mmol/l) with tachycardia, and was again admitted to the hospital for intravenous antibiotics with incision and drainage of abscess
- A repeat positron emission tomography/computed tomography (PET-CT) will be needed after hospital discharge to determine the status of her malignancy

Tips and pearls

- Clozapine (Clozaril) is effective in 30–60% of schizophrenic patients resistant to common neuroleptics; however, the risk of severe neutropenia remains the major limitation of clozapine treatment
- The risk of clozapine-induced neutropenia is higher in females and elderly patients
- There are no current guidelines regarding the concurrent use of clozapine and chemotherapy, and current practice is based on limited case studies
- Physicians need to have a discussion of the risks and benefits of continuing clozapine during chemotherapy with the patient and family, and to work with the clozapine registration system to monitor ANC
- The FDA has developed alternative guidelines for patients in certain ethnic groups with benign ethnic neutropenia who have lower ANCs compared with standardized baselines but no increased risk of agranulocytosis or infection
- If psychiatric benefit outweighs medical risk, clinicians can override clozapine registry rules for treatment interruptions due to neutropenia and continue clozapine treatment

Performance in practice: confessions of a psychopharmacologist

What could have been done better here?

- Was clozapine (Clozaril) initiation delayed by too many attempts at polypharmacy treatment with limited clinical evidence of effectiveness?
  - A meta-analysis study showed that clozapine can be more effective than other antipsychotics even when used as a first- or second-line treatment, and it remains the gold standard for the treatment of schizophrenia[9]

- Patient barriers include non-compliance to prolonged course of weekly blood draws, tolerating clozapine side-effect profiles, and polypharmacy
- Clinician barriers include inexperience with the clozapine registry, the known wide variety of side effects, and perception of the patient's non-compliance
- Clozapine remains a third-line treatment that is often underutilized

What are possible action items for improvement in practice?

• Get the family more involved as the patient is at high risk, given the complicated and prolonged chemotherapy course, and her parents are her major support system

• With a persistent partial response, clozapine may be augmented with electroconvulsive therapy or other antipsychotics

Posttest self-assessment question and answer

When is the risk of severe neutropenia greatest for a patient on clozapine (Clozaril) treatment?

A. Within the first week of initiating treatment
B. Within the first 18 weeks of initiating treatment
C. When there is a change in dosage
D. The risk is similar throughout clozapine treatment

Answer: B

The FDA requires patients to have a minimum ANC greater than or equal to 1500/μL prior to initiating clozapine. Peak incidence of severe neutropenia generally occurs between 1 month and 18 weeks of clozapine initiation, and 84% of agranulocytosis cases occur within the first 3 months of initiating clozapine therapy. Weekly ANC monitoring is required for all patients during the first 6 months of treatment. Clozapine-induced neutropenia is not dose dependent based on logistic-regression analysis. The cumulative incidence of clozapine-induced neutropenia at more than 1 year of treatment is less than 1%.

References

1. Aydin M, Ilhan BC, Calisir S, et al. Continuing clozapine treatment with lithium in schizophrenic patients with neutropenia or leukopenia: brief review of literature with case reports. *Ther Adv Psychopharmacol* 2016; 6: 33–8. https://doi.org/10.1177/2045125315624063

2. Barreto JN, Leung JG, Philbrick KL, et al. Clozapine therapy throughout myelosuppressive chemotherapy: regulations without standardization. *Psychooncology* 2015; 24:1581–5. https://doi.org/10.1002/pon.3779

3. Clozapine REMS Program. 2020. Available from https://www
   .clozapinerems.com/CpmgClozapineUI/home.u (accessed March
   26, 2021).
4. Coşar B, Taner ME, Eser HY, et al. Does switching to
   another antipsychotic in patients with clozapine-associated
   granulocytopenia solve the problem? Case series of 18 patients. *J
   Clin Psychopharmacol* 2011; 31:169–73. https://doi.org/10.1097/
   JCP.0b013e31820e3d9d
5. de Berardis D, Rapini G, Olivieri L, et al. Safety of antipsychotics
   for the treatment of schizophrenia: a focus on the adverse effects
   of clozapine. *Ther Adv Drug Saf* 2018; 9: 237–56. https://doi
   .org/10.1177/2042098618756261
6. Ghaznavi S, Nakic M, Rao P, et al. Rechallenging with clozapine
   following neutropenia: treatment options for refractory
   schizophrenia. *Am J Psychiatry* 2008; 165:813–18. https://doi
   .org/10.1176/appi.ajp.2008.07111823
7. Grainger BT, Arcasoy MO, Kenedi CA. Feasibility of
   myelosuppressive chemotherapy in psychiatric patients on
   clozapine: a systematic review of the literature. *Eur J Haematol*
   2019; 103:277–86. https://doi.org/10.1111/ejh.13285
8. Lally J, Malik S, Whiskey E, et al. Clozapine-associated
   agranulocytosis treatment with granulocyte colony-stimulating
   factor/granulocyte-macrophage colony-stimulating factor: a
   systematic review. *J Clin Psychopharmacol* 2017; 37:441–6.
   https://doi.org/10.1097/JCP.0000000000000715
9. Masuda T, Misawa F, Takase M, et al. Association with
   hospitalization and all-cause discontinuation among patients
   with schizophrenia on clozapine vs other oral second-generation
   antipsychotics: a systematic review and meta-analysis of cohort
   studies. *JAMA Psychiatry* 2019; 76:1052–62. https://doi
   .org/10.1001/jamapsychiatry.2019.1702
10. Meyer J, Stahl SM. *Clozapine Handbook*. New York, NY: Cambridge
   University Press, 2019.

Case 24: The girl who slept with problems

The Question: What is a treatment approach for insomnia in children with trauma and comorbid psychiatric conditions?

The Psychopharmacological Dilemma: There is limited data regarding the safety and efficacy of medications for sleep promotion in children and adolescents, especially those with trauma

Joseph Yasmeh and Ijeoma Ijeaku

Pretest self-assessment question (answer at the end of the case)

Which of the following medications may most benefit a child with attention-deficit/hyperactivity disorder (ADHD) and trauma-related difficulty in sleep initiation and maintenance?

A. Clonidine (Catapres) 0.1 mg

B. Eszopiclone (Lunesta) 1 mg

C. Doxepin (Sinequan) 3 mg

D. Doxylamine (Unisom) 25 mg

E. Melatonin 5 mg

Patient evaluation on intake

- A 13-year-old girl with the chief complaints of "insomnia and depression"
- She is essentially physically healthy, is about to start 8th grade, and lives in a group home

Psychiatric history

- The patient started receiving mental health services at age 8 due to ongoing depressive symptoms secondary to extensive abuse issues
- She has a history of self-injurious behaviors (cutting) starting at age 11, and this is reportedly for stress relief, with the most recent episode a few days before presentation
- She is reportedly aggressive when triggered
- There is a history of three suicide attempts by overdose and requiring psychiatric admissions for each of the episodes (2, 4, and 6 months prior to this initial evaluation)
- She has been admitted to the psychiatric hospital five times for being a danger to self; all of these have been within the last year

Substance use history

- The patient started using marijuana at age 9. She reports that it "is relaxing" and "helps me forget and have fun." The last use was 3 months ago

- She started drinking alcohol at age 9 due to peer pressure. She did not really like it ("Other people made me drink – it was not my thing") and her last drink was a year ago
- Her "boyfriend" forced methamphetamine on her once 3 months ago but she hated it and she states that she has not used it again
- She admits to using alprazolam (Xanax) once to feel "high"
- She denies the use of other drugs

Medication history

- The patient reportedly started on psychotropic medications at age 8 and was last on psychotropic medications 6 months prior to this initial evaluation
- She has been on various psychotropic medications including methylphenidate ER (Concerta), risperidone (Risperdal), and sertraline (Zoloft)
- It is unclear how long she was on her most recent medication regimen but she had been off the regimen when she came to the group home
- The patient was unable to state why she stopped taking the medications at the time that she did

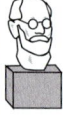

Psychotherapy history

- She reports that she has been in therapy for the most part since the age of 8 due to ongoing depressive symptoms secondary to extensive abuse issues

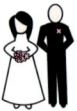

Social and personal history

- She is the oldest of five children. She reportedly lived with both parents until she was almost 6 years old, when she and her siblings were removed from her parents' custody due to concerns for negligence secondary to her parents' drug use as well as sexual abuse by male relatives/family friends
- The patient and siblings were placed with her maternal grandmother who later became her legal guardian after her parents lost their parental rights due to their inability to satisfy court orders
- Her biological mother had an inappropriate relationship with her and reportedly committed suicide 2 months prior to this initial evaluation. She reported that she and her mother would use drugs together and then quarrel later like they were contemporaries ("We'd call each other sluts")
- She reports that she does not like her father's girlfriend and this affects her relationship with her father

Sexual history

- She reports that her maternal grandmother had walked in on her having sex with an adult male in his late 20s who gave her methamphetamine. The maternal grandmother did not do anything about it. She states that her maternal grandmother had ended up having a sexual relationship with "my guy" and "that's why I don't wanna have anything to do with her!"
- She has had sexual experiences with three older males (these constitute statutory rapes based on age; all three were 18 and above, and this minor is unable to give consent to sex)
- She has also been sexually active with both boys and girls within her developmental age and stage
- Child Protective Services (CPS) was informed of rape by the patient's younger brother during a routine check on their home, leading to the removal of this patient from her legal guardian's custody
- During this initial encounter with the patient, she appeared to be most engaged in the evaluation process when she discussed her sexual relationships. Her eagerness to share her "body counts" was a red flag about possible abuse and led to thorough questioning to ascertain who she has slept with, how old these individuals are, and why she slept with them
- She had a certain gleefulness while discussing her sexual experiences, suggesting that this might be an unhealthy coping pattern: the use of sex as a means, albeit an unhealthy one, to attempt to connect to others
- While the eagerness and gleefulness exhibited by this patient might be misleading, it is important to note that child abuse does not always mean that the child will recount the experience as painful or traumatic. The examiner has to explore a patient's sexual activities and experiences with the goal of ascertaining what might constitute rape (to inform the CPS and the appropriate law enforcement agency) as well as abnormal patterns related to sex (to inform adequate and appropriate treatment)

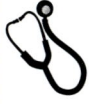

Medical history

- The patient denies any acute medical issues
- She denies any history of any cardiac issues or early cardiac deaths in her family
- Her vitals and body mass index are within normal limits
- There was possible *in utero* exposure to cocaine and nicotine, as her mother struggled with drug addiction, but it is unclear if this was during pregnancy as well

Family history

- Her mother struggled with drug addiction and depression, and committed suicide 2 months before the patient's presentation
- She claims that there is bipolar disorder in multiple maternal relatives

Patient evaluation on initial visit

- The patient has had difficulty with sleep onset and maintenance for over 3 months
- She usually goes to bed at 9 p.m. and falls asleep at 12 a.m.
- She wakes in 4 hours and has difficulty falling back asleep
- The patient is tired throughout the day and was observed yawning multiple times during the interview
- She reports depressed mood, anhedonia, low energy, and feelings of hopelessness
- She also reports irritability, being easily agitated, and poor concentration
- She denies nightmares or auditory/visual hallucinations
- She currently denies suicidal ideation, but concedes that she may attempt again in the future "if things get bad"
- Additional history obtained reveals dissociative tendencies
- She meets the criteria for major depressive disorder (MDD) and posttraumatic stress disorder (PTSD)
- ADHD should be ruled out
- The patient will benefit from a trial of clonidine (Catapres) 0.05 mg at bedtime, given its anxiolytic and sedative effects, as well as indications in ADHD
- Given her history of neglect and trauma, she may also benefit from strength-based therapy
  - Point out positive attributes to the patient and challenge negative perceptions of self, promoting resiliency and improved self-esteem
  - Remind the patient of what is already working well in her life, rather than focusing purely on her deficits

Attending physician's mental notes: initial evaluation

- A diagnosis of insomnia disorder requires that the symptoms cannot be explained by coexisting mental disorders, medical conditions, or substance use
- Screen for primary sleep disorders such as obstructive sleep apnea, narcolepsy, and restless leg syndrome

- In addition to treating the underlying cause, promoting sleep hygiene may be a first-line intervention
  - Use the bedroom for sleep only
  - Maintain a regular sleep/wake cycle and avoid daytime naps
  - Avoid screen use 2 hours before bedtime, including TVs, computers, and phones
  - Limit caffeine, tobacco, and alcohol intake
- Pharmacological interventions include:
  - Melatonin
    - Improves sleep-onset latency but not sleep maintenance
    - Side effects are infrequent but include hypotension, bradycardia, and a slightly increased or decreased seizure threshold
    - The safety of long-term use in children is unknown
    - It may be more effective in children with ADHD or autism spectrum disorder (ASD), given that some have a circadian-mediated phase delay
    - A maximum dose of 3 mg for children or 5 mg for adolescents has been suggested, with up to 10 mg in those with ASD
    - Combine with morning light to treat phase delay common both in normal adolescents and in those with MDD
  - Trazodone (Desyrel)
    - Like several other antidepressants (e.g. mirtazapine (Remeron)), it can be used off label for insomnia
    - It may be preferred for comorbid mood or anxiety disorders
    - Evidence is weak and therefore it is not a first-line treatment
  - Clonidine (Catapres)
    - It may be preferred in comorbid ADHD
    - Given the narrow therapeutic index, educate parents on the importance of giving the medication as prescribed, and not increasing the dose in an attempt to control symptoms
    - Although guanfacine (Tenex) is in the same class, one study showed that it decreased total sleep time in children with ADHD[14]
    - If the patient is taking a stimulant for ADHD, a low dose (e.g. 2.5–5 mg methylphenidate (Concerta)) prior to bedtime may help improve sleep; adjusting the dosage and timing of stimulant administration should also be considered
  - Hydroxyzine (Vistaril)
    - It may improve sleep-onset latency and maintenance
    - The efficacy evidence for diphenhydramine (Benadryl), another antihistamine, is mixed

- ° There is the potential for tolerance
- ° Consider for short-term use, especially with comorbid atopic disease
  - – Zolpidem (Ambien)
    - ° It improves sleep-onset latency and maintenance, but evidence is lacking for use in children
    - ° It may require higher weight-based dosing (per kg) than adults due to metabolism differences
    - ° Zaleplon (Sonata) is a similar alternative
    - ° There is potential for abuse and overdose
- Some prescribe second-generation antipsychotics (i.e. olanzapine (Zyprexa), quetiapine (Seroquel), or risperidone (Risperdal)) for off-label treatment of insomnia, but this should be limited to those cases in youth when the patient has another indication such as bipolar disorder
- The safety of benzodiazepines such as temazepam (Restoril) in those younger than 18 years has not been established and thus its use is not recommended
- Set realistic treatment goals with the family – such as improvement rather than elimination of sleep problems – and milestones for termination of medication

Case outcome: initial evaluation

- Start clonidine (Catapres) 0.05 mg PO at bedtime
- Continue with therapy at the group home; recommend trauma-informed therapy
- Consider using Therapeutic Behavioral Services
- Return in 1 week or sooner if needed

Attending physician's mental notes: initial evaluation (continued)

- Besides trauma during adulthood, adverse childhood events (ACEs) are particularly common in those seeking mental health services
  - – ACEs are associated with lifelong physical and mental conditions, in addition to neurobiological changes in brain development
- Trauma-informed care is sensitive to the potential for trauma-related issues to contribute to a patient's conditions and behaviors
  - – This perspective is applied to all patients, even if the patient's symptoms are not clearly related to trauma at first glance
  - – For example, a child may become excessively distraught during an attempt to hold her arm down to administer a vaccine; if this child has a history of physical abuse, the response may be an adaptive coping mechanism due to retraumatization

- Principles that guide this framework include:
  - Safety: be mindful of how clinical spaces and procedures may impact feelings of physical and emotional safety
    - For example, touching without permission or entering a room without knocking may violate patient boundaries
  - Collaboration: encourage patient choice and control over treatment where possible
    - Sharing power may reduce feelings of being controlled by an authority figure, which may recapitulate the experience of trauma
  - Empowerment: use a strength-based model to reinforce a patient's positive attributes
    - If a patient interaction is focused only on discussing patient deficits, it may reinforce a message that a patient is defective and hopeless

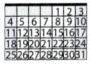

Case outcome: first interim follow-up visit 1 week later

- The patient reports improvement in insomnia
- The group home nurse reports issues with aggression and irritability when dealing with peers
- The patient reports that she has started cutting again to cope with her emotions
- Start sertraline (Zoloft) 50 mg PO every morning
- Continue clonidine (Catapres) 0.05 mg PO at bedtime
- Consider methylphenidate (Concerta)
- Continue trauma-informed care/therapy at the group home
- Continue the ongoing psychoeducation

Attending physician's mental notes: first interim follow-up visit 1 week later

- It is apparent from the discussion with the patient during this visit that she is avoidant and has no way of dealing with stressors. She lacks the tools to deal with interpersonal conflict
- This contributes to her preference to only have male peers and avoid "girl drama," as males do not engage her emotionally and treat her as a sex object
- When forced to interact with female peers in a group home, the patient becomes so emotionally dysregulated and overwhelmed that she engages in cutting to deal with her mood
- This is complicated by her inability to identify with and describe her own emotions (alexithymia). She is unable to take responsibility for her own reactions as she is unable to identify emotions within herself

- Psychoeducation can help develop this awareness
- For example, when asked why she cuts, the patient responds that it is because of "girl drama," so the interviewer challenged the patient to consider why everyone else does not cut in response to "girl drama"
- An underlying cause of these problems is negligence and the absence of a stable caregiver who could have role modeled appropriate emotion regulation

Case outcome: second interim follow-up visit 1 week later

- During the follow-up 2 weeks after the initial evaluation, the patient reports improvement in insomnia and her mood
- The group home nurse reports issues with her "being all over the place"
- Start clonidine (Catapres) 0.05 mg PO every morning
- Continue clonidine 0.05 mg PO at bedtime
- Continue sertraline (Zoloft) 50 mg PO every morning
- Continue trauma-informed care/therapy at the group home
- Continue the ongoing psychoeducation

Performance in practice: confessions of a psychopharmacologist

What could have been done better here?

If just treating the patient's presenting symptoms of trauma with biopsychosocial or medical models, there is a risk of ignoring big-picture systems that may lead to patient morbidity and mortality

What are possible action items for improvement in practice?

- Other than treating the patient's presenting symptoms, the clinician should keep in mind the long-term health risks for this patient
  - Suicide
    - ° This should considered given the patient's past attempts and completed suicides in the family
    - ° Ensure safety by inquiring about ideation or plans for suicide
  - Teen pregnancy and sexual health
    - ° Consider the need for long-term contraception (e.g. etonogestrel implant or an intrauterine device) and sexually transmitted infection screening
  - Unsafe home environment
    - ° The long-term goal is to transition from the group home to a stable caregiver's home
    - ° Safety under the current caregiver is questionable, given the failure to report the patient's sexual abuse

- Development of borderline personality disorder
  ∘ This is a possibility given her early trauma history
  ∘ One of the benefits of a trauma-informed treatment approach early enough in the child's or adolescent's life is the ability to address the specific trauma and hopefully provide the individual with the tools to change the trajectory

Take-home points

- In treating childhood insomnia, consider the underlying cause and also promote sleep hygiene
- If using a pharmacological agent, aim to choose one that also treats a comorbid condition
- Distinguish sleep-onset latency insomnia from sleep-maintenance insomnia, and choose a drug that therefore treats the symptoms appropriately
- In children presenting with trauma, create a treatment plan that addresses the big-picture risks to future health, in addition to the patient's presenting symptoms
- A strength-based approach can promote resiliency and improved self-esteem
- Trauma-informed care can help conceptualize and address patient symptoms and problems, while preventing retraumatization from clinical settings

Posttest self-assessment question and answer

Which of the following medications may most benefit a child with ADHD and trauma-related difficulty in sleep initiation and maintenance?

A. Clonidine (Catapres) 0.1 mg
B. Eszopiclone (Lunesta) 1 mg
C. Doxepin (Sinequan) 3 mg
D. Doxylamine (Unisom) 25 mg
E. Melatonin 5 mg

Answer: A

As a centrally acting α_2-adrenergic agonist, clonidine (Catapres) can help with impulsivity and other ADHD symptoms, as well as providing sedation. The non-benzodiazepine hypnotic eszopiclone (Lunesta) is not approved for use in children and in one trial, it failed to treat insomnia associated with ADHD.[15] While there is some evidence that the tricyclic amine doxepin (Sinequan) may help treat insomnia in ADHD, clonidine may be a better choice in this scenario as it also treats the patient's impulsivity. The antihistamine doxylamine (Unisom) would be a first-line treatment for pregnancy-related insomnia but not for other patient populations. Although up to 5 mg of melatonin is safe in adolescents, its indication is specifically for improving sleep-onset latency and it has no role in sleep-maintenance insomnia.

References

1. Babineu S, Goodwin C, Walker B. Medications for insomnia treatment in children. *Am Fam Physician* 2008; 77: 358–9.
2. Badin E, Haddad C, Shatkin JP. Insomnia: the sleeping giant of pediatric public health. *Curr Psychiatry Rep* 201618: 47. https://doi.org/10.1007/s11920-016-0687-0
3. Blumer JL, Findling RL, Shih WJ, et al. Controlled clinical trial of zolpidem for the treatment of insomnia associated with attention-deficit/hyperactivity disorder in children 6 to 17 years of age. *Pediatrics* 2009; 123:e770–6. https://doi.org/10.1542/peds.2008-2945
4. Bruni O, Alonso-Alconada D, Besag F, et al. Current role of melatonin in pediatric neurology: clinical recommendations. *Eur J Paediatr Neurol* 201519:122–33. https://doi.org/10.1016/j.ejpn.2014.12.007
5. Buckley AW, Hirtz D, Oskoui M, et al. Practice guideline: treatment for insomnia and disrupted sleep behavior in children and adolescents with autism spectrum disorder: report of the Guideline Development, Dissemination, and Implementation Subcommittee of the American Academy of Neurology. *Neurology* 2020; 94:392–404. https://doi.org/10.1212/WNL.0000000000009033
6. Butler LD, Critelli FM, Rinfrette ES. Trauma-informed care and mental health. *Dir Psychiatry* 2011; 31:197–212.
7. Chen Y, Baram TZ. Toward understanding how early-life stress reprograms cognitive and emotional brain networks. *Neuropsychopharmacology* 2016; 41:197–206. https://doi.org/10.1038/npp.2015.181
8. Felitti VJ, Anda RF, Nordenberg D, et al. (1998). Relationship of childhood abuse and household dysfunction to many of the leading causes of death in adults: the Adverse Childhood Experiences (ACE) Study. *Am J Prev Med* 14:245–58. https://doi.org/10.1016/s0749-3797(98)00017-8
9. Felt BT, Chervin RD. Medications for sleep disturbances in children. *Neurol Clin Pract* 2014; 4:82–7. https://doi.org/10.1212/01.CPJ.0000442521.30233.ef

10. Kezelman C, Stavropoulos P. *Practice Guidelines for Treatment of Complex Trauma and Trauma Informed Care and Service Delivery.* Sydney: Adults Surviving Child Abuse, 2012.

11. Matheson E, Hainer BL. Insomnia: pharmacologic therapy. *Am Fam Physician* 2017; 96:29–35.

12. Oral, R, Ramirez, M, Coohey, C, et al. Adverse childhood experiences and trauma informed care: the future of health care. *Pediatr Res* 2016; 79:227–33. https://doi.org/10.1038/pr.2015.197

13. Owens, JA, Moturi, S. Pharmacologic treatment of pediatric insomnia. *Child Adolesc Psychiatr Clin N Am* 2009; 18:1001–16. https://doi.org/10.1016/j.chc.2009.04.009

14. Rugino TA. Effect on primary sleep disorders when children with ADHD are administered guanfacine extended release. *J Atten Disord* 2018; 22:14–24. https://doi.org/10.1177/1087054714554932

15. Sangal RB, Blumer JL, Lankford DA, et al. Eszopiclone for insomnia associated with attention-deficit/hyperactivity disorder. *Pediatrics* 2014; 134:e1095–103. https://doi.org/10.1542/peds.2013-4221

16. Shah YD, Stringel V, Pavkovic I, Kothare SV. Doxepin in children and adolescents with symptoms of insomnia: a single-center experience. *J Clin Sleep Med* 2020; 16:743–7. https://doi.org/10.5664/jcsm.8338

17. Smith EJ. The strength-based counseling model. *Couns Psychol* 2006; 34:13–79. https://doi.org/10.1177/0011000005277018

18. Stahl SM. *Stahl's Essential Psychopharmacology*, 4th edn. New York, NY: Cambridge University Press, 2013.

Case 25: Not all child's play: a path to pediatric stability

The Question: What can you do to manage symptoms and achieve long-term stability in a pediatric patient with multiple psychiatric conditions?

The Psychopharmacological Dilemma: Finding an effective medication regimen for a complex pediatric patient with multiple diagnoses and previous hospitalizations

Joseph Wong, Justine Ku, and Takesha Cooper

Pretest self-assessment question (answer at the end of the case)

Which of the following is/are an approved treatment for pediatric bipolar I disorder?

A. Lithium
B. Valproic acid (Depakote)
C. Olanzapine (Zyprexa)
D. Quetiapine (Seroquel)
E. Risperidone (Risperdal)
F. Lurasidone (Latuda)
G. Ziprasidone (Geodon)
H. Aripiprazole (Abilify)
I. Carbamazepine (Equetro)
J. Asenapine (Saphris)

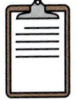

Patient evaluation on intake

- A 12-year-old female with prior diagnoses of bipolar I disorder diagnosed at age 7, attention-deficit/hyperactivity disorder (ADHD), oppositional defiant disorder, intermittent explosive disorder, and anxiety with extensive psychiatric history including multiple hospitalizations for danger to self/danger to others. She is tolerating her current regimen with side effects of sedation
- Her mother, who brought the patient in along with her biological father, has taken her daughter to many psychiatrists and accompanied her to numerous hospitalizations, but is concerned that her daughter is still not stable

Psychiatric history

- The mother recounts that, as a toddler, the patient would have 3-hour "meltdowns" if she did not have her way
- She was suspended from kindergarten for severe hyperactivity, restlessness, inattentiveness, and temperamental behavior

- In school, the patient would easily become annoyed, blaming others. She fought with teachers and classmates and would have to be restrained once or twice daily due to aggression
- The patient has had numerous depressive episodes: excessive sadness, hypersomnia, fatigue, decreased concentration at school, and worthlessness (e.g. wanting to die, wishing she was not born, thinking everyone hates her)
- She has a history of manic episodes, which involved staying up late, only requiring 4 hours of sleep, being hyperverbal, and having racing thoughts. The patient demanded her mother buy her art supplies with grandiose thoughts of becoming a famous artist. Beginning in 7th grade, the patient began running away from home when manic
- The patient also admitted to years of auditory hallucinations; it is unclear whether the patient only heard them during manic episodes. The patient described them as beeping sounds or voices. She has had occasional command auditory hallucinations of voices telling her to harm herself or others, or else someone will harm her family
- She had visual hallucinations on one occasion while hospitalized
- The patient also has persistent paranoia that something bad will happen to her mother
- Her history also includes more than 10 hospitalizations and suicide attempts. Some events included:
  - Age 11: an overdose of pills; she was in the intensive care unit for 7 days and then remained in the local hospital for 2 weeks
  - Age 11: she went missing from school with a 16-year-old boy and was hospitalized for 2 days after being aggressive with the police
  - Age 13: episodes of self-injury and hospitalization for running away from school, belligerent behavior, and threatening to self-harm
- The patient was referred for psychoeducational testing by her school one year prior to initial intake and was found to have no learning disorders or developmental delays

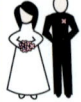

Social and personal history

- The patient lives with her mother. Her father lives locally, and has only been active in the patient's life for the past 8 months
- The patient's developmental history was within normal limits with no complications, abuse, or trauma
- The patient has an Individualized Education Plan (IEP) and attends a school that provides special education services; she attends individual and group therapy at school. According to her teachers, the patient is very smart, but her academic functioning varies

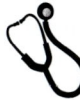

PATIENT FILE

Medical history

- There is no significant medical history besides being overweight, with a body mass index of 26.1 kg/m^2
- Her laboratory results are within normal limits

Family history

- Paternal side
  - Father with bipolar disorder and ADHD
  - Uncle with ADHD
  - Father, great aunt, and great grandfather with substance use
- Maternal side
  - Aunt, uncle, grandmother, and great grandparents with substance use

Current medications

- Lurasidone (Latuda) 40 mg in the morning and 80 mg at night
- Clonidine (Catapres) 0.1 mg twice per day
- Hydroxyzine (Vistaril) 50 mg twice per day

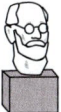

Psychotherapy history

- Individual and group therapy within therapeutic school setting
- The patient had intensive in-home therapy (Therapeutic Behavioral Services) and has been seeing the same therapist since the age of 8

Questions

Based on what you know about this patient's history and symptoms, do you agree with her prior diagnoses?

- Yes
- No

Would you continue her current medications?

- Yes
- No

Attending physician's mental notes: patient evaluation on initial intake

- The lifetime risk for bipolar disorder is 15–30% in individuals with one first-degree relative with bipolar disorder and up to 75% in those with two affected first-degree relatives
- Due to this patient's early symptom onset and a father with adult-onset bipolar disorder, her outcome is expected to be worse (genetic anticipation)

- Psychologically, the patient struggles with feelings of abandonment by other caregivers
- Socially, she struggles with difficulty maintaining relationships due to her explosive behavior
- On mental status examination, the patient is casually dressed, well groomed, and overweight. Her speech is loud and pressured. Her motor activity is restless. Her affect is labile and irritable
- This 12-year-old female meets the criteria for bipolar I disorder and ADHD, with her extensive psychiatric history including hospitalizations, seclusion and restraint with multiple medication trials; she is currently stable on a medication regimen with the side effect of sedation
- Due to her mother's concern for sedation, clonidine (Catapres) 0.1 mg twice per day will be changed to 0.1 mg half-tablet every morning, half-tablet at 3 p.m. and one tablet at bedtime. Other medications will be continued as is

Further investigation

Is there anything else you would especially like to know about this patient?

- What about details concerning past medication treatments?
  - The patient has experienced adverse effects from previous medication trials including:
    - Haloperidol (Haldol): the patient experienced excessive sedation
    - Risperidone (Risperdal): although effective, the patient gained 30 lbs in less than 1 month; she was also drooling more
    - Amphetamine/dextroamphetamine, melthyphenidate: the patient had racing thoughts, which "made her almost psychotic" according to the mother. According to the patient, "It feels like my mind is on fire, my mind won't stop"

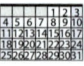

Case outcome: interim follow-up visit at 2 months

- The patient's mother reports that the change in clonidine (Catapres) dosing has helped reduce sedation; however the patient continues to be hyperactive during school (worse in afternoon). The police were called after she hit a teacher
- The patient is currently taking clonidine 0.1 mg half-tablet every morning, half-tablet at 3 p.m. and one tablet at bedtime. After this visit, the late afternoon dose is moved to 11 a.m. Other medications and therapy are continued as usual

Attending physician's mental notes: interim follow-up visit at 2 months

- Clonidine (Catapres) is typically dosed three to four times daily Moving the afternoon dose to earlier should help reduce the symptoms of hyperactivity when most needed
- Caution must be taken for the risk of hypotension with clonidine, and if a dose reduction is needed, this should be done gradually to reduce the risk of rebound hypertension

Question

In addition to the adjustments made to her medications, what other changes would you make to further help this patient?

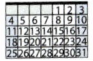

Case outcome: interim follow-up visit at 9 months

- Her mother reports that the patient has been anxious recently since her IEP review last month. Last year around this time, she had to change schools and was anxious, hyperactive, and got very little sleep. Although her mother felt this year's IEP review went well, the patient continued to be irritable, rude, agitated, impulsive, and argumentative at school. While a peer was drinking from a water fountain, she hit the child on the back of the head; the patient had to be restrained
- At home, the patient had a week of feeling anxious and agitated, was hyperverbal, and was staying up throughout the night. After arguments with her mother, she would make a mess with soaps and shampoos and respond with profanity when asked to clean it up. The patient had another incident where she walked away from home, which resulted in the police being called
- In the office, the patient denied suicidal ideation, and auditory or visual hallucinations
- She is currently taking lurasidone (Latuda) 40 mg in the morning and 80 mg at night. The morning dosage was raised to 60 mg to target the manic state. Other medications and therapy are continued as usual

Attending physician's mental notes: interim follow-up visit at 9 months

- The patient presented as loud and defiant and then abruptly refused to speak, but communicated by writing instead
- It is hoped that increasing lurasidone (Latuda) from 40 mg in the morning to 60 mg will target the manic symptoms reported by the mother and exhibited during the office visit

- Lurasidone is a second-generation antipsychotic that has been shown to be safe and effective in the treatment of pediatric bipolar disorder depression, but almost all atypical antipsychotics have proven effective in acute treatment of mania as well
- Clinically, lurasidone, compared with other second-generation antipsychotics, has not been associated with significant prolactin elevation, weight gain, dyslipidemia, or corrected QT interval (QTc) prolongation
- Her mother was reminded that lurasidone was to be taken with meals of at least 350 calories in order to increase absorption
- For treating pediatric bipolar disorder depression, the recommended starting dosage is 20 mg daily with a maximum dosage of up to 80 mg daily
  - The adult starting dosage for schizophrenia is 40 mg with a maximum dosage of up to 160 mg
- This patient is currently on lurasidone due to its favorable side-effect profile (e.g. not generally associated with sedation or metabolic syndrome) and is on the adult dosage of 140 mg due to the severity of her symptoms

Mechanism of action moment

- Lurasidone (Latuda) lacks potent histamine H_1, dopamine D_1 or muscarinic M_1 receptor affinity leading to less weight gain, sedation, and cognitive impairment
- Lurasidone's D_2 antagonism contributes to its antipsychotic effect
- Lurasidone's serotonin 5-HT_{2A} receptor antagonism contributes to lower extrapyramidal symptoms compared with typical antipsychotics, which is one of the distinguishing factors that makes second-generation antipsychotic "atypical"
- Lurasidone's 5-HT_{1A} receptor partial agonism, and 5-HT_7 and α_2-adrenergic antagonism contributes to its antidepressant and pro-cognitive effects

Question

How might this patient's manic symptoms be better managed?

- Switch lurasidone (Latuda) to another antipsychotic
- Augment lurasidone with an anticonvulsant
- Raise the dosage of lurasidone to the adult maximum dosage for schizophrenia of 160 mg daily
- Discontinue lurasidone and start lithium

Case outcome: interim follow-up visit at 14 months

- During this visit, the patient was emotionally labile, tearful, and bawling
- Over the past 5 months, the patient has undergone several medication adjustments to address sedation (which has been more prominent in the morning), and her aggressive, hyperactive, and impulsive symptoms. The medication adjustments included:
  - Adjusting lurasidone (Latuda) 60 mg every morning and 80 mg at bedtime to 40 mg every morning and 100 mg at bedtime
  - Discontinuing the morning hydroxyzine (Vistaril), continuing only 50 mg at bedtime
  - She tried to discontinue clonidine 0.1 mg half-tablet in the morning; however, her mother noted that the patient became more hyperactive and impulsive without it, so the patient resumed this medication
- During the past month, the patient was hospitalized twice for belligerent behavior, running away from school, and threatening to harm herself
- The patient is medication adherent but skips lunch
- Start lamotrigine (Lamictal) 25 mg daily for 14 days, 50 mg daily for 14 days, and then 100 mg as tolerated
- Her mother was afraid to change from lurasidone, given previous failed medicine trials. Therefore, the morning lurasidone is increased back to 60 mg every morning and she will continue the 100 mg at bedtime
- Her mother was worried about the patient's agitation, so was advised to give lurasidone 20 mg as needed if the patient's agitation becomes overwhelming

Attending physician's mental notes: interim follow-up visit at 14 months

- The dosing of the lurasidone (Latuda) was adjusted so that although the dosage is the same at 140 mg, more of it would be at night to reduce the patient's daytime sedation
- Hydroxyzine (Vistaril) 50 mg every morning was discontinued to also address the patient's morning sedation
- As lurasidone is better absorbed with food, the patient skipping meals may explain her outbursts. The patient's dosage of lurasidone was increased to 160 mg, the maximum adult dosage, as her symptoms still have room for improvement
- As the patient was still not stable on antipsychotic monotherapy, lamotrigine (Lamictal), an anticonvulsant and mood stabilizer, was

added to the patient's medication regimen due to its efficacy in maintenance of bipolar I disorder
- The mechanism of action of lamotrigine is currently understood to involve reducing the release of the excitatory neurotransmitter glutamate; however, this mechanism has yet to be fully explored
- Lamotrigine is generally well tolerated, with minimal risk for metabolic syndrome and weight gain. Of its side effects, its dermatological side effects are the most concerning. While most patients who do develop a rash develop a benign rash, there is a risk for Stevens–Johnson syndrome/toxic epidermal necrolysis, which can be potentially fatal. This risk can be reduced by:
  - Slowly titrating lamotrigine
  - Avoiding drug–drug interactions such as co-administration of lamotrigine with valproic acid (Depakote), which increases the level of lamotrigine by decreasing its clearance
- For this patient, lamotrigine can address mood lability. One study showed that lamotrigine was effective for rapid cycling, which would be helpful for this patient[14]

Question

As an alternative to lamotrigine (Lamictal), what other anticonvulsants would you consider?

- Carbamazepine (Equetro)
- Valproic acid (Depakote)
- Topiramate (Topamax)
- Gabapentin (Neurontin)
- Lithium

Case outcome: interim follow-up visit at 15 months

- The patient was initially stable on her new medication regimen for a couple of weeks, but her mother called to report that the patient had begun to hear voices and was becoming more paranoid. She also pulled the fire alarm and walked out of school
- A trial of asenapine (Saphris) 2.5 mg twice per day for 3 days followed by 5 mg twice per day thereafter was recommended and started. Lurasidone (Latuda) was tapered to 40 mg at bedtime for 3 days when asenapine was started and then discontinued. Other medications were continued as usual

- The patient stopped asenapine after 2 weeks because she did not like the taste of the medication and continued to hear voices; she is unwilling to disclose what she heard
- Olanzapine (Zyprexa) 5 mg at bedtime was then started. Other medications were continued as usual

Attending physician's mental notes: interim follow-up visit at 15 months

- A trial of asenapine was considered after a literature review in order to target the patient's mood lability and also to reduce the risk of hospitalization
- Asenapine (Saphris) is a newer addition to the class of atypical antipsychotics that has been shown to be efficacious in treating pediatric bipolar with manic or mixed symptoms
- Theoretically, asenapine's antidepressant effects are thought to be due to its activity on numerous serotonergic receptors including 5-HT_7 and 5-HT_{2C} antagonism
- Unlike other second-generation antipsychotics, asenapine is taken sublingually because, if taken orally, it has poor bioavailability due to high first-pass metabolism

  - The patient and mother were reminded not to eat or drink within 10 minutes of taking the medication to decrease the risk of reduced asenapine exposure
- Common side effects of asenapine include sedation and dizziness

Case outcome: interim follow-up visits at 20 and 24 months

- At 20 months, the patient's mood has become steadier and happier according to the patient and her mother since she started on olanzapine (Zyprexa) 5 mg at bedtime. Her mother has noted a mild increase in appetite and a 5 lb weight gain since starting olanzapine. The mother and patient were counseled on the importance of exercise and a healthy diet while on olanzapine. They have both started going to the gym four times a week
- At 24 months, olanzapine was increased to 7.5 mg at bedtime
- She started metformin (Glucophage) 500 mg every morning for 14 days, and then the dosage was increased to 1000 mg every morning to reduce weight gain
- The patient's mood lability has stabilized tremendously according to the patient and her mother. The patient has only had small behavioral problems at school and has had to be restrained only once in the last 3 months. The patient feels well and has begun to raise a pig and plans to enter her into shows

PATIENT FILE

Attending physician's mental notes: interim follow-up visits at 20 and 24 months

- At 20 months, although the patient was starting to gain weight on olanzapine (Zyprexa), the benefits of olanzapine outweigh the risks of decompensation and hospitalization
- The patient's weight gain and subsequent lifestyle changes were first observed for a few visits before metformin (Glucophage) was added in order to see how the patient responded to olanzapine and to reduce unnecessary addition of medication if possible
- At 24 months, the patient was initially started on olanzapine 5 mg at bedtime but this was soon increased to 7.5 mg at bedtime due to continued symptoms

Question

Would you have added metformin (Glucophage) to this patient's medication regimen earlier?

- Yes, it would have prevented the patient's weight gain and its addition should not be a cause of concern since its side-effect profile is quite favorable
- No, although the patient did eventually gain weight on olanzapine, it was appropriate to observe the patient's situation in order to avoid prescribing unnecessary medications

Case debrief

- Many children with bipolar disorder have their symptoms attributed to ADHD, which has a high comorbidity with pediatric bipolar disorder
- While the manic symptoms of bipolar disorder may overlap with the impulsive and hyperactive symptoms of ADHD, bipolar disorder is distinguished from ADHD by its cyclical pattern while the symptoms of ADHD are more persistent and constant
- Patients with ADHD also tend to not have the grandiosity and decreased need for sleep associated with bipolar disorder, although a side effect of ADHD treatment with stimulants can lead to insomnia
- For complicated pediatric patients with multiple diagnoses, first carefully assess to ensure an accurate diagnosis. Finding an effective medication regimen is a difficult task and can require many medication trials
- For this patient's ADHD, she was eventually put on clonidine (Catapres) after unsuccessful trials of stimulants (i.e. amphetamine/

dextroamphetamine, methylphenidate (Concerta)) in addition to hydroxyzine (Vistaril) as needed for agitation
  - Stimulants tend to worsen mania in bipolar patients, as in this case
- For this patient's bipolar disorder, multiple trials of antipsychotics were tried including risperidone (Risperdal), lurasidone (Latuda), and asenapine (Saphris) with varying success until the patient was put on lamotrigine (Lamictal) and olanzapine (Zyprexa) and was finally stable.

Take-home points

- Adjusting medications to reach stability is a process of patience, as shown in this case, which took over 2 years from the initial visit to reach a point where the patient's symptoms were well managed with few to no adverse side effects
- An important lesson learned during this process is that when working together with patients and their family members who have gone through a lot of difficulties, the key for the entire treatment process is to build trust through communication and understanding of their situation

Performance in practice: confessions of a psychopharmacologist

What could have been done better here?
- Should lithium have been added sooner rather than trying more trials of atypical antipsychotic monotherapy?

What are possible action items for improvement in practice?
- Lithium should have been added to augment as a mood stabilizer after lurasidone monotherapy approached maximum dosage and before other anticonvulsants were added, such as lamotrigine
  - Not only is lithium the first-line medication for mood stabilization, it also has remarkable effects in reducing the risk of suicidality by up to fivefold, which is extremely beneficial in the case of this patient

Tips and pearls

- Children with early onset of symptoms and a positive family history may necessitate observation over a longer period of time in order to come up with a proper diagnosis
- As there are no diagnostic criteria for pediatric bipolar disorder in DSM-5, the diagnostic criteria is based on the adult diagnostic criteria and thus clinician experience and expertise play a large role in dissecting out the symptoms of bipolar disorder from other commonly comorbid conditions (i.e. ADHD)

Mechanism of action moment

- Olanzapine (Zyprexa) is an atypical antipsychotic that has been shown to be efficacious in treating pediatric bipolar disorder mania and mixed episodes
- Among the atypical antipsychotics, olanzapine is perhaps most well known for having the greatest risk for cardiometabolic side effects including increased insulin resistance, increasing fasting glucose, increased fasting cholesterol, increased fasting low-density lipoproteins, increased fasting triglyceride levels, and weight gain
  - The mechanism behind these side effects include olanzapine's H_1 and 5-HT_{2C} receptor antagonism
- In terms of other side effects, olanzapine has a low risk for extrapyramidal symptoms compared with other atypicals (i.e. risperidone (Risperdal) and lurasidone (Latuda)), but does carry a greater risk for prolonged QTc compared with aripiprazole (Abilify) and lurasidone, although this is not as significant as ziprasidone (Geodon)
- Compared with adults on olanzapine, olanzapine usage in the pediatric population has been associated with elevated prolactin
- In order to reduce the cardiometabolic side effects of olanzapine, consider adding metformin (Glucophage) to reduce weight gain and increase insulin sensitivity

Posttest self-assessment question and answer

Which of the following is/are an FDA-approved treatment for pediatric bipolar I disorder?

A. Lithium
B. Valproic acid (Depakote)
C. Olanzapine (Zyprexa)
D. Quetiapine (Seroquel)
E. Risperidone (Risperdal)
F. Lurasidone (Latuda)
G. Ziprasidone (Geodon)
H. Aripiprazole (Abilify)
I. Carbamazepine (Equetro)
J. Asenapine (Saphris)

Answer: See Figure 25.1 and Figure 22.2 in Chapter 22 for details of FDA-approved medicines for pediatric bipolar disorder

In addition to the above, olanzapine-fluoxetine (Symbyax) is approved for pediatric bipolar depression in children 10 years and up. Also, a combination of samidorphan-olanzapine was recently approved by the FDA for treatment of schizophrenia and bipolar I disorder in adults and has the potential of reducing weight gain associated with olanzapine.

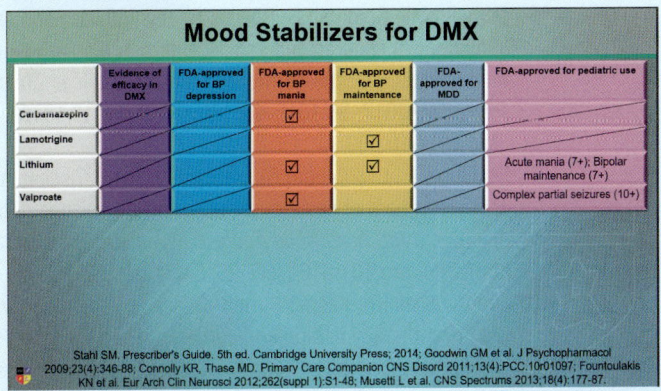

Figure 25.1. Mood stabilizers for depressive mixed state (DMX). BP, bipolar disorder; MDD, major depressive disorder. Data from Stahl (2014), Goodwin et al. (2009), Connolly and Thase (2011), Fountoulakis et al. (2012), Musetti et al. 2013).

References

1. de Miranda AS, de Miranda AS, Teixeira AL. Lamotrigine as a mood stabilizer: insights from the pre-clinical evidence. *Expert Opinion on Drug Discovery* 2019; 14:179–90, https://doi.org/10.1080/1746 0441.2019.1553951

2. Anon. Drugs for ADHD. *Med Lett Drugs Ther* 2020; 62:9–15.

3. Biederman J, Mick E, Hammerness P, et al. Open-label, 8-week trial of olanzapine and risperidone for the treatment of bipolar disorder in preschool-age children. *Biol Psychiatry* 2005; 58: 589–94. https://doi.org/10.1016/j.biopsych.2005.03.019

4. Biederman J, Joshi G, Mick E, et al. A prospective open-label trial of lamotrigine monotherapy in children and adolescents with bipolar disorder. *CNS Neurosci Ther* 2010; 16:91–102. https://doi .org/10.1111/j.1755-5949.2009.00121.x

5. Carandang C, Robbins D, Mullany E, et al. Lamotrigine in adolescent mood disorders: a retrospective chart review.*J Can Acad Child Adolesc Psychiatry* 2007; 16:1–8.

6. Cerullo, MA, Strakowski, SM. A systematic review of the evidence for the treatment of acute depression in bipolar I disorder. *CNS Spectr* 2013; 18:199–208. https://doi.org/10.1017/ S1092852913000102

7. Connolly KR, Thase MD. The clinical management of bipolar disorder: a review of evidence-based guidelines. *Prim Care Companion CNS Disord* 2011; 13:PCC.10r0109. https://doi .org/10.4088/PCC.10r01097

8. DelBello MP, Goldman R, Phillips D, et al. Efficacy and safety of lurasidone in children and adolescents with bipolar I depression: a double-blind, placebo-controlled study. *J Am Acad Child Adolesc Psychiatry* 2017; 56:1015–25. https://doi.org/10.1016/j.jaac.2017.10.006

9. Findling RL., Landbloom RL., Szegedi A., et al. Asenapine for the acute treatment of pediatric manic or mixed episode of bipolar I disorder. *J Am Acad Child Adolesc Psychiatry* 2015; 54:1032–41. https://doi.org/10.1016/j.jaac.2015.09.007

10. Fountoulakis KN, Kasper S, Andreassen O, et al. Efficacy of pharmacotherapy in bipolar disorder: a report by the WPA section on pharmacopsychiatry. *Eur Arch Psychiatry Clin Neurosci.* 2012; 262 (Suppl. 1): 1–48. https://doi.org/10.1007/s00406-012-0323-x

11. Fountoulakis KN, Kontis D, Gonda X, et al. Treatment of mixed bipolar states. *Int J Neuropsychopharmacol.* 2012; 15:1015–26. https://doi.org/10.1017/S1461145711001817

12. Frazier JA, Biederman J, Tohen M, et al. A prospective open-label treatment trial of olanzapine monotherapy in children and adolescents with bipolar disorder. *J Child Adolesc Psychopharmacol* 2001; 11:239–50. https://doi.org/10.1089/10445460152595568

13. Fusar-Poli P, Howes O, Bechdolf A, Borgwardt S. Mapping vulnerability to bipolar disorder: a systematic review and meta-analysis of neuroimaging studies. *J Psychiatry Neurosci* 2012; 37:170–84. https://doi.org/10.1503/jpn.110061

14. Goldberg JF Bowden CL Calabrese JR et al. Six-month prospective life charting of mood symptoms with lamotrigine monotherapy versus placebo in rapid cycling bipolar disorder. *Biol Psychiatry* 2008; 63:125–30. https://doi.org/10.1016/j.biopsych.2006.12.031

15. Goodwin GM, Consensus Group of the British Association for Psychopharmacology. Evidence-based guidelines for treating bipolar disorder: revised second edition--recommendations from the British Association for Psychopharmacology. *J Psychopharmacol* 2009; 23:346–88. https://doi.org/10.1177/0269881109102919

16. Lewitzka U, Severus E, Bauer R, et al. The suicide prevention effect of lithium: more than 20 years of evidence – a narrative review. *Int J Bipolar Disord* 2015; 3:32. https://doi.org/10.1186/s40345-015-0032-2

17. Musetti L, Del Grande C, Marazziti D, Dell'Osso L. Treatment of bipolar depression. *CNS Spectr* 2013; 18:177–87. https://doi.org/10.1017/S1092852912001009

18. Pavuluri MN, Henry DB, Moss M, et al. Effectiveness of lamotrigine in maintaining symptom control in pediatric bipolar disorder. *J Child Adolesc Psychopharmacol* 2009; 19:75–82. https://doi .org/10.1089/cap.2008.0107

19. Praharaj SK, Jana AK, Goyal N, Sinha VK. Metformin for olanzapine-induced weight gain: a systematic review and meta-analysis. *Br J Clin Pharmacol* 2011; 71:377–82. https://doi .org/10.1111/j.1365-2125.2010.03783.x

20. Stahl SM. *Stahl's Essential Psychopharmacology: Neuroscientific Basis and Practical Applications*, 4th edn. New York, NY: Cambridge University Press, 2013.

21. Stahl SM. *Stahl's Essential Psychopharmacology: Prescriber's Guide*, 5th edn. New York, NY: Cambridge University Press, 2014.

22. Tohen M, Kryzhanovskaya L, Carlson G, et al. Olanzapine versus placebo in the treatment of adolescents with bipolar mania. *Am J Psychiatry* 2007; 164:1547–56. https://doi.org/10.1176/appi .ajp.2007.06111932

23. Vázquez M, Maldonado C, Guevara N, et al. Lamotrigine–valproic acid interaction leading to Stevens–Johnson syndrome. *Case Rep Med* 2018; 2018:5371854. https://doi.org/10.1155/2018/5371854

Case 26: The young woman who was "nothing but skin and bones"

The Question: What is the most likely diagnosis?

The Psychopharmacological Dilemma: How to distinguish anorexia nervosa from other possible diagnoses and formulate a plan of treatment

Kayla L. Fisher and Michelle Tom

Pretest self-assessment question (answer at the end of the case)

Which of the following is not a complication of anorexia nervosa?

A. Osteopenia
B. Leukocytosis
C. Hypophosphatemia
D. Cerebral atrophy
E. Arrhythmias

Patient evaluation on intake

- An 18-year-old woman presents to the clinic at the request of her parents, who have told her that she is "too thin." Her father, who is a pharmacist, has told her she needs to see a psychiatrist
- The patient has lost 30 lbs over the past 3 months

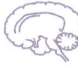

Psychiatric history

- The patient has no history of psychiatric treatment and denies any history consistent with major depression, mania, or psychosis
- She denied difficulties carrying out daily life functions
- She reported increased anxiety starting about 3 months ago
- She denies difficulties with sleep
- She reports her energy as good, allowing her to maintain a daily vigorous exercise routine
- Her appetite is poor. She reports eating approximately 50% of the food that she ate 3 months ago, but states that she just is not hungry
- The patient reports starting a diet approximately 3 months ago after she overheard peers talking about her shirt being too tight. She reports that she researched weight loss and found that she could lose weight easily. She does not believe she is too thin, but came for the appointment to please her parents
- She denies any history of wanting to harm herself or end her life
- She denies any history of wanting to harm others

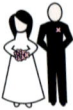

Social and personal history

- There is no history of tobacco or alcohol use
- There is no history of recreational drug use
- She denies any history of sexual, physical, or mental abuse
- She was valedictorian of her high school and is currently a full-time freshman at a highly ranked private university. Her grades have been slipping over the past few weeks, but previously were all straight As
- She is an only child. She characterizes her relationship with her parents as good until recently. Now, they disagree over how much she should eat and what she should weigh
- She plays the violin in the university orchestra and teaches violin lessons for extra spending money. She states that her anxiety over the past month has caused her to take a leave of absence from playing in the orchestra

Family history

- Her father works as a pharmacist
- Her mother does interior designing, part-time
- Her mother had mild postpartem depression that did not require treatment. Otherwise, there is no psychiatric history in the family

Medical history

- There is no significant medical history
- She is not taking any prescription medications
- She takes a daily multivitamin but no supplements
- Her general appearance is very thin and well groomed, with no signs of distress
- Her weight as of 3 months ago was 132 lbs; her current weight is 102 lbs
- Her height is 5'5" and her body mass index (BMI) is 16.97 kg/m^2
- Vital signs: blood pressure 102/65 mmHg, heart rate 64 bpm, respiration rate 18/minute, temperature 98.2°F
- She has had no menses for the past 2 months
- Otherwise her physical and neurological examination is normal

Two-minute tutorial

From the information given, what is the most likely diagnosis?

- The most common cause of significant weight loss in young women in Western countries is anorexia nervosa

What are other general medical causes of substantive weight loss in young women?

- Malignancies
- Chronic infections such as tuberculosis or acquired immunodeficiency syndrome
- Uncontrolled diabetes mellitus
- Hyperthyroidism
- Malabsorption syndromes such as Celiac disease
- Inflammatory bowel disease such as Crohn's disease

This patient did not present with symptoms suggestive of one of the above diagnoses, although workup laboratory results and other studies may suggest otherwise. Is there anything we already know about this patient that points toward anorexia nervosa rather than one of these other etiologies?

- This patient is not concerned about her weight loss. In fact, she does not believe she is too thin, despite having a BMI under 17 kg/m^2. When weight loss is due to other medical conditions, patients typically express concern about this loss and would like to restore their weight to a healthy range

What are other possible psychiatric causes of substantive weight loss in young women?

- Major depressive disorder: although severe weight loss may occur in patients with major depressive disorder, these patients do not desire excessive weight loss and do not have an intense fear of gaining weight
- Psychotic disorder: patients with schizophrenia and other psychotic disorders may experience weight loss and may have delusions about eating some foods. They rarely, however, have the intense fear of gaining weight and the distorted body image required for anorexia nervosa
- Substance use disorder: substances such as cocaine and other stimulants can lead to significant weight loss. Other substance use disorders can lead to weight loss through poor nutritional intake. However, patients with substance use disorder do not have an intense fear of gaining the weight back and do not have the distorted body image seen in anorexia nervosa
- Social anxiety disorder: patients with anorexia nervosa may have anxiety about their weight, body image, or obtaining the food that can best help them avoid gaining weight. These anxieties alone would not constitute the need for an additional diagnosis. In social anxiety disorder, the patient may have anxiety about eating in public, but does not exhibit the other aspects of anorexia nervosa
- Obsessive–compulsive disorder: patients with anorexia nervosa may have obsessions and compulsions related to food, but these

would not warrant a separate diagnosis unless the patient also had obsessions and compulsions unrelated to the anorexia nervosa

- Bulimia nervosa: bulimia nervosa and anorexia nervosa of the binge-eating/purging type are similar in that both disorders involve binge eating and self-induced vomiting to avoid weight gain. In bulimia nervosa, however, the weight is normal or above normal
- Avoidant/restrictive food intake disorder: patients with this disorder can lose significant amounts of weight and have significant nutritional deficiencies. These patients, however, do not have an intense fear of gaining weight or the perceptual body distortions seen in anorexia nervosa
- Body dysmorphic disorder: while patients with anorexia nervosa often have beliefs that they look fat when they are very thin, these perceptual body distortions do not warrant a separate diagnosis of body dysmorphic disorder unless they also have body distortions unrelated to weight, size, and body shape

Question

What steps should be taken to rule out other psychiatric causes?

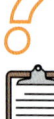

Patient evaluation on initial visit

- The patient was alert and oriented to person, place, time, and situation
- The patient appeared her stated age of 18. She was well groomed and dressed stylishly in a manner consistent with her age
- Eye contact was acceptable, but the patient often looked down before answering questions related to appetite, exercise, or weight
- The patient had fluid movements, and nervously bounced her legs up and down intermittently while answering questions
- Her speech was normal
- She described her mood as "fine." Her affect was mildly restricted
- When asked about anxiety, she said she had felt increased anxiety over the past several months. Upon questioning, the patient said that she was constantly battling with her parents about how much she was eating and her weight. She felt anxious that they would force her to eat more food that she wanted to. Her anxiety focused around her food and how much she would be forced to eat. She said she was fearful that she would end up gaining the weight that she had lost. She felt much better at her current weight and wanted to do everything she could to prevent herself from gaining weight
- The patient said her sleep was generally good, as was her energy

- Upon questioning about exercise, the patient reported that approximately 3 months ago she began to increase the amount she was exercising to at least 1 hour every day
- The patient reported that her appetite had diminished over the past couple of months and estimated that she was eating approximately 50% of what she had been previously
- Upon questioning, the patient reported that she was very careful about what she ate. She had been limiting her diet to mostly fresh vegetables and a few fruits. She would carefully measure her food and had become very knowledgeable about the calorie content of various foods
- The patient reported normal menses until approximately 3 months ago. Now, she has been amenorrheic for the past 2 months
- The patient stated she had never made herself vomit to try to keep her intake down and had never used laxatives
- She reported a recent practice of weighing herself at least four times a day. If her weight was higher than she wanted it to be, she compensated by exercising longer that day, so she would not "get fat"
- Her thought process was linear and goal directed
- She said that she had never had any experience of hearing or seeing things that she believed that others could not. There was no evidence of attending to internal stimuli
- She said she did not hold any unusual beliefs not held by others. When asked if others thought that she was too thin, she said that her parents believed she was too thin, but she believed she still needed to lose weight
- The patient said she had never used recreational drugs or consumed alcohol. She said that she had recently turned 18 and was looking forward to having a glass of wine at the next family celebration
- She reported that she was not having any thoughts of self-harm or suicide and had never considered or engaged in self-harm or suicide in the past
- She reported that she was not angry with anyone to the point of thinking about harming or killing them, and had never considered or engaged in harming or killing anyone in the past
- Her short-term memory was intact because after she learned what her BMI was, she easily remembered this value after 3 minutes
- Her insight into the fact that her own perceptions of her body were incongruent with her actual weight and others' perceptions of her body was poor
- The patient's judgment regarding the next steps in her workup and treatment is poor because, although she came for this evaluation at the urging of her parents, she is resisting information regarding her need for treatment

Attending physician's mental notes: initial visit

- A distorted body image is also seen with body dysmorphic disorder
- The patient has anxiety about her food and her weight, but no elevated anxiety otherwise
- She has been amenorrheic for 2 months– is the patient pregnant?
- Fear of gaining weight would point to anorexia nervosa rather than body dysmorphic disorder or other psychiatric disorders as etiologies
- Compensatory exercise is reported. Are there other compensatory behaviors?
- A BMI of 16.97 would be associated with moderate severity of anorexia nervosa
- The diagnostic criteria for anorexia nervosa may have been met. The patient is restricting intake, believes she still needs to lose weight even though she is very thin, and fears gaining weight
- Nothing in the patient's history or evaluation to date points to a general medical illness as the etiology of the weight loss. Additionally, the patient here is restricting her intake and fears gaining weight. Those with general medical etiologies of weight loss typically desire gaining their weight back

Questions

Is amenorrhea required for a diagnosis of anorexia nervosa?

- A review of the DSM-5 diagnostic criteria indicates that DSM-5, unlike DSM-4, does not include amenorrhea as a diagnostic criterion for anorexia nervosa
- The DSM-5 diagnostic criteria for anorexia nervosa are:
  - Restriction of energy intake relative to requirements, leading to a significantly low body weight in the context of age, sex, developmental trajectory, and physical health. Significantly low weight is defined as a weight that is less than minimally normal or, for children and adolescents, less than that minimally expected
  - An intense fear of gaining weight or of becoming fat, or persistent behavior that interferes with weight gain, even though at a significantly low weight
  - Disturbance in the way in which one's body weight or shape is experienced, undue influence of body weight or shape on self-evaluation, or persistent lack of recognition of the seriousness of the current low body weight

- Specify whether:
  - F50.01: Restricting type. During the last 3 months, the individual has not engaged in recurrent episodes of binge eating or purging behavior (i.e. self-induced vomiting or the misuse of laxatives, diuretics, or enemas). This subtype describes presentations in which weight loss is accomplished primarily through dieting, fasting, and/or excessive exercise
  - F50.02: Binge-eating/purging type. During the last 3 months, the individual has engaged in recurrent episodes of binge eating or purging behavior (i.e. self-induced vomiting or the misuse of laxatives, diuretics, or enemas)
- Specify if:
  - In partial remission. After full criteria for anorexia nervosa were previously met, Criterion A (low body weight) has not been met for a sustained period, but either Criterion B (intense fear of gaining weight or becoming fat or behavior that interferes with weight gain) or Criterion C (disturbances in self-perception of weight and shape) is still met
  - In full remission. After full criteria for anorexia nervosa were previously met, none of the criteria has been met for a sustained period of time
- Specify current severity:
  The minimum level of severity is based, for adults, on current BMI (see below) or, for children and adolescents, on BMI percentile. The ranges below are derived from World Health Organization categories for thinness in adults; for children and adolescents, corresponding BMI percentiles should be used. The level of severity may be increased to reflect clinical symptoms, the degree of functional disability, and the need for supervision
    - Mild: BMI ≥ 17 kg/m^2
    - Moderate: BMI 16–16.99 kg/m^2
    - Severe: BMI 15–15.99 kg/m^2
    - Extreme: BMI <15 kg/m^2

Which studies are useful in a patient with anorexia nervosa and why?
- Complete blood count: malnutrition can lead to leukopenia, thrombocytopenia, and mild anemia. The leukopenia typically includes a loss of all cell types, with apparent lymphocytosis. Bleeding problems are rare
- Comprehensive metabolic panel:
  - Glucose: hypoglycemia is seen with a lack of glucose precursors in the diet or low glycogen stores
  - Total protein: malnutrition can cause low total protein

- Albumin: malnutrition can cause hypoalbuminemia, while dehydration can cause hyperalbuminemia
- Total calcium: dehydration can be a cause of hypercalcemia. However, low protein, low magnesium, or vitamin D deficiency are all causes of hypocalcemia. If the albumin level is low, order an "ionized calcium" level
- Sodium: dehydration leads to hypernatremia, while overhydration leads to hyponatremia. Diuretic use can also lead to hyponatremia
- Potassium: dehydration can lead to hyperkalemia. Vomiting and diuretic and laxative use can lead to hypokalemia
- Bicarbonate: vomiting can lead to metabolic alkalosis. Low bicarbonate can be seen in metabolic acidosis. Laxative abuse can cause metabolic acidosis
- Chloride: vomiting and diuretic use can lead to hypochloremia
- Blood urea nitrogen (BUN): dehydration elevates BUN levels. Malnutrition, overhydration, and a very low-protein diet can lead to lower BUN levels
- Creatinine: dehydration causes creatinine levels to increase
- Liver enzymes: a low BMI and low body fat are correlated with increased liver enzymes. Refeeding can occasionally cause liver enzymes to temporarily elevate. Thus, alkaline phosphatase, alanine amino transferase (ALT/SGPT), and aspartate amino transferase (AST/SGOT) may be elevated in malnutrition. These elevations can signal resultant inflammation or liver damage

• Serum iron: malnutrition can cause low iron levels and iron-deficiency anemia

• Amylase: this is increased in chronic vomiting

• Serum phosphorous: low calcium levels and the use of phosphate-containing laxatives can result in hyperphosphatemia. Malnutrition, diuretic use, and chronic antacid use can lead to hypophosphatemia. This needs to be monitored closely in refeeding, as the hallmark biochemical feature of refeeding syndrome is hypophosphatemia

• Serum magnesium: dehydration and the use of magnesium-containing laxatives cause levels to elevate. Diuretics, malnutrition, and the use of non-magnesium laxatives can result in hypomagnesemia. This needs to be monitored closely in refeeding, as hypomagnesemia may be seen

• Thyroid panel: hyperthyroidism may contribute to weight loss.
  ◦ Thyroid-stimulating hormone (TSH): this is high in hypothyroidism and low in hyperthyroidism

- ○ Triiodothyronine (T3): this is high in hyperthyroidism and low in hypothyroidism; in malnutrition, T3 is decreased and reverse T3 is elevated
- ○ Thyroxine (T4); this is high in hyperthyroidism and low in hypothyroidism, and is in the low normal range in malnutrition
- Transthyretin (prealbumin): this is low in malnutrition and hyperthyroidism
- Lipid profile: patients acutely ill with anorexia nervosa have higher lipid values than normal controls, and some of these elevations persist after weight restoration. However, these elevations are typically still within the normal value ranges
- Vitamin D: low levels can be associated with osteopenia or osteoporosis
- Urinalysis: assess renal function
- Pregnancy test: this is needed for all women of child-bearing age
- Electrocardiography: cardiovascular complications account for much of the morbidity and mortality in anorexia nervosa. Sinus bradycardia is common. Prolongation of the QT interval can indicate that the patient is at risk of sudden arrhythmia and death

Are there any additional studies to consider?

- Serum estrogen (females): this is low in malnutrition
- Serum testosterone (males): this is low in malnutrition
- Bone mass study: often a low bone mineral density is seen along with areas of osteopenia and/or osteoporosis
- Electroencephalography: when significant fluid and electrolyte disturbances are present, an EEG can reflect a metabolic encephalopathy with diffuse abnormalities
- Cortisol level: this is increased in anorexia nervosa. Cortisol, which is associated with stress and anxiety, may further suppress eating
- Magnetic resonance imaging of the brain: consider this when cognitive impairments are present or there is an atypical or unremitting course. Cerebral atrophy may be seen with reductions in gray and white matter volume, ventriculomegaly, enlarged cortical sulci and interhemispheric fissure, and cerebellar atrophy

Further investigation

Is there anything else you would like to know?

- Explore whether patient is engaging in binge eating. Recall that she stated she is not purging (see mental status examination)
- Ask the patient about compensatory use of diuretics. Recall that she stated she is not using laxatives (see mental status examination)

Two-minute tutorial

- Anorexia nervosa has one of the highest mortality rates of any mental illness
- Extreme weight loss induces protein and fat catabolism
- Complications result from atrophy of the heart, brain, liver, intestines, kidneys, and muscles
- Arrhythmias can result in sudden death
- Hypothalamic–pituitary abnormalities contribute to osteopenia
- Renal and electrolyte complications may include hypokalemia, and depletion of magnesium and phosphate
- Hematological complications include anemia, leukopenia, and thrombocytopenia
- Neurological complications include cerebral atrophy with a reduction in gray and white matter volume, peripheral neuropathy, seizures, and cognitive impairment

Patient evaluation on initial visit (continued)

- Upon questioning, the patient states that she has not engaged in binge eating and has not used diuretics
- She is advised that although her heart rate is in the lower normal range at 64 bpm, her ECG is normal at this time
- As the working diagnosis of anorexia nervosa, restricting type, is discussed with the patient, she is receptive to learning about the disorder and manifests a degree of acceptance of the diagnosis and risks involved if weight loss is not halted and restored to a normal range
- The patient is not interested in discussing treatment options at this time. She agrees to try to gain 1 lb by the follow-up visit in 1 week. Laboratory results and treatment options will be discussed at that time
- The patient signs a consent for you to speak with her parents

Attending physician's mental notes: initial visit (continued)

- With a BMI of 16.97 kg/m², the specifier 'moderate' should be added to the diagnosis of anorexia nervosa
- Suicide-related ideation and behaviors should be assessed, as well as risk factors, on each visit because suicide risk is elevated in anorexia nervosa
- The patient's acceptance of her diagnosis and the associated risks is a positive sign
- Evidence of perfectionistic traits, often seen in anorexia nervosa, exists in this case. Note that the patient stated she began losing

weight when she overheard peers commenting on her shirt being too tight. The patient was valedictorian of her high school and maintained straight As in college until the past few weeks. The patient has never used alcohol, tobacco, or drug products, and stated that she came to the appointment on the request of her parents. Is the patient's expressed receptive attitude toward the diagnosis and associated risks explained by her perfectionistic traits?

- Prognosis is best in young patients whose illness is identified early and treated quickly. Hopefully, this patient will recover quickly and not have additional episodes

Question

What treatment options should be considered?

- The initial treatment of anorexia nervosa must focus on nutrition and weight restoration. When the brain is in starvation mode, treatments such as cognitive behavioral therapy are not likely to work
- If the patient is medically unstable, inpatient hospitalization is needed unless treatment can be safely provided at a lower level of care
- While there are currently no medications approved by the FDA for treating anorexia nervosa, olanzapine is an off-label treatment that has shown promise in some recent studies. Olanzapine (Zyprexa) is believed to assist with weight restoration through its histamine H_1 receptor blockade in the brain
- As the patient still lives with her parents, a family-based treatment approach should be considered

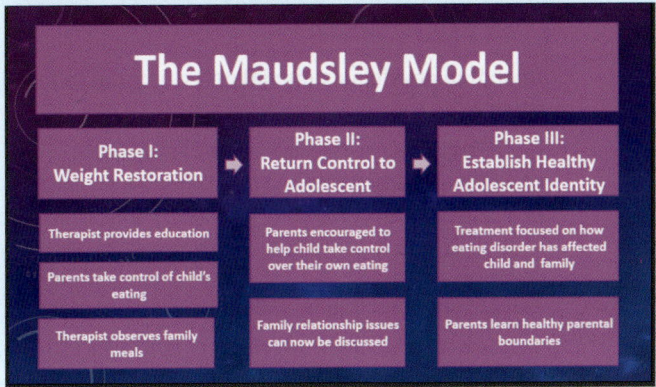

Figure 26.1. The Maudsley Model for treatment of anorexia nervosa.

- The Maudsley Model, a three-phased series of family therapy sessions over a period of 6–12 months, is an outpatient treatment program that has been shown to be efficacious in the treatment of adolescents with anorexia nervosa (Figure 26.1). Phase I focuses on weight restoration and family takes over responsibility of meals. Phase II returns control over eating to the patient. Phase III focuses on establishing a healthy identity.

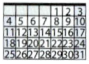

Case outcome: interim follow-up visit at week 1

- The patient arrives to the appointment with her parents. The patient explains that she knows she needs their help with this disease but states that sometimes she wants to leave home so that she can continue to lose weight
- You review with them that all studies are normal at this point
- The patient has gained 1 lb. She describes how her fear of gaining "too much weight" remains, but she is also afraid of the possible complications of anorexia nervosa
- Her weight is 103 lbs, height 5'5", and BMI 17.14 kg/m²
- Vital signs: blood pressure 104/68 mmHg, heart rate 64 bpm, respiration rate 18/minute, temperature 98.4°F
- The patient is not orthostatic
- The patient is anxious about gaining weight but has no other anxieties outside of her anorexia nervosa disorder
- The patient denies thoughts of suicide. She has not engaged in self-harming behaviors
- The patient continues to exercise for at least 1 hour a day. She agreed to limit her exercise to no more than 50 minutes each day
- When treatment options are reviewed with the patient and her parents, the patient agrees to try a low dose of olanzapine (Zyprexa) 2.5 mg at bedtime along with family-based therapy

Attending physician's mental notes: interim follow-up visit at week 1

- The patient is weighed and her BMI is checked
- Her blood sugar, lipids, and blood pressure are checked
- A baseline history (personal and family) is obtain for diabetes, dyslipidemia, hypertension, cardiovascular disease, and obesity

Mechanism of action moment

What are some common side effects of olanzapine (Zyprexa)?

- Weight gain: olanzapine blocks H_1 receptors in the brain and possibly pancreatic muscarinic M_3 receptors, which causes most

patients to experience weight gain. This tends to occur more with olanzapine than with other antipsychotics
- Sedation: olanzapine blocks multiple receptors, which can contribute to the side effect of sedation (H1, α_1-adrenergic, and M_1 receptors). The sedation tends to be transient
- Constipation: olanzapine blocks M_1 receptors, which can cause constipation

What are some possible serious side effects of olanzapine?
- Hyperglycemia: this can be associated with ketoacidosis, hyperosmolar coma, and/or death
- There is a rare risk of neuroleptic malignant syndrome
- There is a rare risk of seizures.
- Falls from orthostatic hypotension: these typically occur during initial dose titration
- Rare risk of DRESS (drug reaction with eosinophilia and systemic symptoms). This begins as a rash and spreads. It can include fever, enlarged lymph nodes, facial swelling, organ inflammation, eosinophilia, and death
- Although not an issue with this patient, in elderly patients with dementia-related psychosis, olanzapine carries an increased risk of death and cerebrovascular events
- For more information on olanzapine, see *Stahl's Essential Psychopharmacology Prescriber's Guide*, 6th edn[20]

Attending physician's mental notes: interim follow-up visit at week 1 (continued)
- Patients with anorexia nervosa typically struggle to accept their diagnosis as they continue to see themselves as too fat, even at the point of starvation. This patient's younger age and shorter duration of illness may provide her with a better prognosis
- The patient has gained 1 lb. While that sounds encouraging, the patient must still be followed closely as she is still considerably underweight. Hopefully, the patient did not try to boost weight by extra water intake just prior to her appointment. Some anorexics even sew small weights in their undergarments to "weigh in" at a higher weight. If this becomes a concern, the patient will be asked to weigh wearing only a paper gown at each visit
- Her parents are supportive and motivated to help their daughter. Although the patient is at the upper age limit for using the Maudsley Model, it is a reasonable choice and has been shown to be efficacious

Case outcome: interim follow-up visit at 8 months

- The patient is now on phase III of the Maudsley Model and is focused on establishing a healthy identity
- Her weight is 118 lbs on a 5'5" frame. Her BMI is now 19.64, in the lower end of the normal range
- After 8 months of amenorrhea, the patient began menstruating 2 months ago
- The patient reports that her anxiety around eating and weight is very mild
- The patient recently started cognitive behavioral therapy with an individual therapist
- Her laboratory results are normal
- The patient asks whether she can stop taking olanzapine (Zyprexa) 2.5 mg at bedtime. Although she has not had any side effects, she does not think she needs it anymore
- The patient asks whether, if she has children, if they will be more likely to have anorexia nervosa
- She has noticed that she is no longer fearful about gaining weight as she once was and is curious whether there is any scientific explanation

Tips and pearls

Is anorexia nervosa exclusively environmental?

- Family and twin studies have demonstrated a significant genetic component for anorexia nervosa, suggesting that there may be a genetic component of the illness
- Studies utilizing functional brain imaging find that those with anorexia nervosa undergo altered brain reward circuits. They found that the more severe the dopamine reward pathways were altered, the more difficult it was for patients to gain weight in treatment
- Genome-wide association studies have identified one locus on chromosome 12 that reached genome-wide specific association with anorexia nervosa[22]
- Researchers report that positive genetic correlations were found between anorexia nervosa, neuroticism, and schizophrenia

What is the heritability of anorexia nervosa?

- Twin studies have consistently supported a genetic basis, with heritability estimates for anorexia nervosa in the range of 48–74%

Why is it so difficult for those with anorexia nervosa to gain weight?

- Self-induced starvation may cause alterations in the brain that result in food avoidance and perpetuate anorexia nervosa

- One of the ways anorexia nervosa changes the brain can be seen in the insula, which processes taste along with processing self-awareness
- Recent findings suggest that those with anorexia nervosa are negatively conditioned to sweet taste. This correlates with harm avoidance, body dissatisfaction, and a drive to thinness
- A recent study found that neural reward circuits of patients with anorexia nervosa respond differently from controls to receipt or deprivation of taste rewards. This strengthens the idea that starvation greatly changes the brain's dopamine-linked reward system. The greater the alteration of these dopamine systems, the more difficult it is to gain weight
- The increased cortisol levels often seen with anorexia nervosa are also associated with stress and anxiety, which can suppress eating
- For the reasons above, weight loss in anorexia nervosa can become a downward spiral – the more weight is lost, the harder it is to regain the weight

Take-home points

- The most common cause of significant weight loss in young women in Western countries is anorexia nervosa
- Anorexia nervosa differs from other general medical and psychiatric diagnoses that result in significant low weight in that with anorexia nervosa the patient is fearful of gaining weight or becoming fat and the patient does not recognize that they are underweight and the associated risks of their condition
- Patients with anorexia nervosa may have anxiety about their weight, body image, or obtaining the food that can best help them avoid gaining weight. These anxieties alone would not constitute the need for an additional diagnosis of an anxiety disorder
- Patients with anorexia nervosa may have obsessions and compulsions related to food, but these would not warrant a separate diagnosis unless the patient also had obsessions and compulsions unrelated to the anorexia nervosa
- DSM-5, unlike DSM-4, does not include amenorrhea as a diagnostic criterion for anorexia nervosa
- Anorexia nervosa has been associated with genetic variations on chromosome 12
- Studies have shown higher cortisol levels in patients with anorexia nervosa, with may perpetuate stress and anxiety around eating
- Self-induced starvation may cause alterations in the brain that result in food avoidance and perpetuate anorexia nervosa
- The initial treatment of anorexia nervosa must focus on nutrition and weight restoration

- While there are currently no medications approved by the FDA for treating anorexia nervosa, olanzapine (Zyprexa) is an off-label treatment that has shown promise in some recent studies
- When the patient lives at home, a family-based treatment approach should be considered
- Medical complications from anorexia nervosa include hypotension, bradycardia, hypothermia, amenorrhea, and osteopenia/osteoporosis
- Complications result from atrophy of the heart, brain, liver, intestines, kidneys, and muscles
- Arrhythmias can result in sudden death
- Renal and electrolyte complications may include hypokalemia and depletion of magnesium and phosphate
- Hematological complications include anemia, leukopenia, and thrombocytopenia
- Neurological complications include cerebral atrophy with a reduction in gray and white matter volume, peripheral neuropathy, seizures, and cognitive impairment
- Anorexia nervosa has one of the highest mortality rates of any mental illness

Posttest self-assessment question and answer

Which of the following is not a complication of anorexia nervosa?

A. Osteopenia
B. Leukocytosis
C. Hypophosphatemia
D. Cerebral atrophy
E. Arrhythmias

Answer: B

Anorexia nervosa causes bone loss, so osteopenia and osteoporosis are both complications. Renal and electrolyte complications may include hypokalemia and depletion of magnesium and phosphate. Complications of anorexia nervosa include cerebral atrophy and potentially fatal arrhythmias. Leukopenia is one of the hematological complications of anorexia nervosa. This leukopenia is not associated with an increased risk for infections.

References

1. American Psychiatric Association. (2013). Eating and feeding disorders. In: *Diagnostic and Statistical Manual of Mental Disorders*, 5th edn. Arlington, VA: American Psychiatric Association, 2013. Available from: https://doi.org/10.1176/appi.books.9780890425596.dsm10

2. Arcelus J, Mitchell AJ, Wales J, Nielsen S. Mortality rates in patients with anorexia nervosa and other eating disorders. A meta-analysis of 36 studies. *Arch Gen Psychiatry* 2011; 68:724–31. https://doi.org/10.1001/archgenpsychiatry.2011.74

3. Attia E, Steinglass JE, Walsh BT, et al. Olanzapine versus placebo in adult outpatients with anorexia nervosa: a randomized clinical trial. *Am J Psychiatry* 2019; 176:449–56. https://doi.org/10.1176/appi.ajp.2018.18101125

4. Baker JH, Schaumberg K, Munn-Chernoff MA. Genetics of anorexia nervosa. *Curr Psychiatry Rep* 2017; 19:84. https://doi.org/10.1007/s11920-017-0842-2

5. Bulik CM, Tozzi F, Anderson C, et al. The relation between eating disorder and components of perfectionism. *Am J Psychiatry* 2003; 160:366–8. https://doi.org/10.1176/appi.ajp.160.2.366

6. Duncan L, Yilmaz Z, Gaspar H, et al. Significant locus and metabolic genetic correlations revealed in genome-wide association study of anorexia nervosa. *Am J Psychiatry* 2017; 174:850–8. https://doi.org/10.1176/appi.ajp.2017.16121402

7. Frank G, DeGuzman M, Shott M, et al. Association of brain reward learning response with harm avoidance, weight gain, and hypothalamic effective connectivity in adolescent anorexia nervosa. *JAMA Psychiatry* 2018; 75:1071–80. https://doi.org/10.1001/jamapsychiatry.2018.2151

8. Frank G, Shott M, Hagman J Mittal V. Alteration in brain structures related to taste reward circuitry in ill and recovered anorexia nervosa and in bulimia nervosa. *Am J Psychiatry* 2013; 170:1152–60. https://doi.org/10.1176/appi.ajp.2013.12101294

9. Frostad, S, Danielsen, YS, Rekkedal, GÅ, et al. Implementation of enhanced cognitive behaviour therapy (CBT-E) for adults with anorexia nervosa in an outpatient eating-disorder unit at a public hospital. *J Eat Disord* 2018; 6:12. https://doi.org/10.1186/s40337-018-0198-y

10. Hussain AA, Hübel C, Hindborg M, et al. Increased lipid and lipoprotein concentrations in anorexia nervosa: a systematic review and meta-analysis. *Int J Eat Disord* 2019; 52:611–29. https://doi.org/10.1002/eat.23051

11. Kaye WH, Wierenga CE, Bischoff-Grethe A, et al. Neural insensitivity to the effects of hunger in women remitted from anorexia nervosa. *Am J Psychiatry* 2020; 17:601–10. https://doi.org/10.1176/appi.ajp.2019.19030261

12. Lebow J, Sim LA, Erwin PJ, Murad MH. The effect of atypical antipsychotic medications in individuals with anorexia nervosa: a systematic review and meta-analysis. *Int J Eat Disord* 2013; 46:332–9. https://doi.org/10.1002/eat.22059

13. Lock, J. *Pocket Guide for the Assessment and Treatment of Eating Disorders*. Washington, DC: American Psychiatric Association Publishing, 2019.

14. Luz Neto LMD, Vasconcelos FMN, Silva JED, et al. Differences in cortisol concentrations in adolescents with eating disorders: a systematic review. *J Pediatr (Rio J)* 2019; 95:18–26. https://doi.org/10.1016/j.jped.2018.02.007

15. Mahon PB, Hildebrandt TB, Burdick KE. New genetic discoveries in anorexia nervosa: implications for the field. *Am J Psychiatry* 2017; 174:821–2. https://doi.org/10.1176/appi.ajp.2017.17050574

16. March M, Wildes J. Evidence-based psychological treatment for eating disorders. In: Gabbard GO, ed. *Gabbard's Treatments of Psychiatric Disorders*, 5th edn. Washington, DC: American Psychiatric Publishing, 2014. Available from: https://psychiatryonline.org/doi/full/10.1176/appi.books.9781585625048.gg30

17. Mehles P. Anorexia nervosa in adults and adolescents: medical complications and their management. In: Yager J, Solomon D, eds. *UpToDate*, 2019. Available from: https://www.uptodate.com/contents/anorexia-nervosa-in-adults-and-adolescents-medical-complications-and-their-management (accessed March 26, 2021).

18. Norris ML, Spettigue W, Buchholz A, et al. Olanzapine use for the adjunctive treatment of adolescents with anorexia nervosa. *J Child Adolesc Psychopharmacol* 2011; 21:213–20. https://doi.org/10.1089/cap.2010.0131

19. Stahl S. Olanzapine. In: *Stahl's Essential Psychopharmacology: Prescriber's Guide*, 6th edn. Cambridge, UK: Cambridge University Press, 2017; pp. 527–36.

20. Walter K, Bulik C, Plotnicov K, et al. The genetics of anorexia nervosa collaborative study: methods and sample description. *Int J Eat Disord* 2013; 41:289–300. https://doi.org/10.1002/eat.20509

21. Watson HJ, Yilmaz Z, Thornton LM et al. Genome-wide association study identifies eight risk loci and implicates metabo-psychiatric origins for anorexia nervosa. *Nat Genet* 2019; 51:1207–14. https://doi.org/10.1038/s41588-019-0439-2.

22. Yager J, Devlin MJ, Halmi KA, et al. *Treatment of Patients with Eating Disorders*, 3rd edn. In: *American Psychiatric Association Guideline Watch*. Available from: https://psychiatryonline.org/pb/assets/raw/sitewide/practice_guidelines/guidelines/eatingdisorders-watch.pdf

Case 27: Could it be both? Comorbid psychiatric diagnoses

The Question: How do you distinguish between poor academic performance due to attention-deficit/hyperactivity disorder (ADHD) versus a specific learning disorder versus both?

The Psychopharmacological Dilemma: Utilizing the biopsychosocial model to provide holistic treatment and improve patient quality of life

Ruqayyah Malik, Margaret Yau, and Dennis Alters

Pretest self-assessment question (answer at the end of the case)

Which of the follow medications is considered the first-line treatment for attention-deficit/hyperactivity disorder (ADHD) in adolescents?

A. α_2-adrenergic receptor agonists
B. Serotonin-norepinephrine reuptake inhibitors (SNRIs)
C. Stimulants

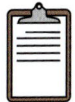

Patient evaluation on intake

- A 15-year-old male with the chief complaints of mood symptoms and inattention
- He was accompanied by his parents who felt he had reached a plateau with his previous psychiatrist and psychotherapist and wanted a fresh start to see whether further improvements could be attained

Psychiatric history

- The patient has had mood lability since the age of 8
- He was diagnosed with ADHD, inattentive type, at age 11 after having difficulty paying attention both at school and at home
- He has had initial and terminal insomnia since the age of 12
- He was diagnosed with major depressive disorder at age 13 due to symptoms of sadness and amotivation

Family history

- Mother with ADHD and depression
- Father with history of alcohol use disorder
- Younger brother with ADHD
- Elder sister with ADHD and depression
- Maternal great grandmother with suicide attempts

Medication history

- Lisdexamfetamine (Vyvanse) 30 mg daily since the age of 11 with mixed results for ADHD treatment
- Fluoxetine (Prozac) 10 mg daily since the age of 13 for depression with no improvement

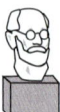

Psychotherapy history

- He sees a psychotherapist twice a month; it is unclear whether this is helpful

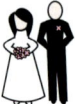

Social and personal history

- He denies alcohol, tobacco, and illicit drug use
- He attends a STEM high school, is good at math and likes science, but his grades suffer because he does not turn in assignments on time
- He does not have many friends at school and keeps to himself
- His hobbies include architecture, lacrosse, and the Boy Scouts
- He lives with his parents and younger brother; his older sister is away at college
- He frequently clashes with his mother over completing his schoolwork and house chores
- He has a history of severe temper tantrums, which have resulted in property damage

Medical history

- The patient achieved his developmental milestones appropriately
- Physiological cupping of optic disks
- His body mass index (BMI) is 16.22 kg/m^2
- His blood pressure is 89/53 mmHg
- His low BMI and blood pressure lead to concern of decreased appetite secondary to a stimulant or undiagnosed eating disorder; however, the patient denies both
- He has normal fasting glucose and triglycerides

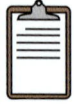

Patient evaluation on initial visit

- The patient admitted to weekly mood shifts (pleasant to irritable) lasting about 4 hours, and apathy, boredom, and anergia
- His mother is concerned about his poor performance in school
- He appeared anxious, inattentive, and depressed

PATIENT FILE

Question

Based on the information presented so far, do you agree with the patient's current psychiatric diagnoses?

- Yes
- No

Attending physician's mental notes: initial evaluation

- The patient's initial evaluation supports his current diagnoses of ADHD, inattentive type, and depression; however, there are some other diagnoses that should be considered:
  - Autism spectrum disorder given the patient's withdrawn nature and lack of a peer social circle at school
  - Disruptive mood dysregulation disorder given the patient's history of irritability, mood lability, and severe temper tantrums
- The patient's history of initial and terminal insomnia may have been an early symptom of his depression rather than a separate diagnosis
- Family therapy was recommended with an emphasis on interpersonal communication skills to help mitigate the patient's conflicts with his mother
- Lisdexamfetamine (Vyvanse) 30 mg and fluoxetine (Prozac) 10 mg were continued

Further investigation

Is there anything else you would especially like to know about this patient?

- The patient has a strong family history of ADHD and depression. What medications have his mother and siblings been on and how effective were they for them?
  - There is no available information on the siblings' psychiatric treatments; however, the mother does volunteer that she has had a good treatment response to lisdexamfetamine (Vyvanse) and desvenlafaxine (Pristiq) for her ADHD and depression, respectively

Question

The patient is on the same stimulant that his mother found to be effective but is still having difficulty at school and is receiving poor grades. Should serum drug levels be obtained to ensure the patient is in the therapeutic range?

- Yes, it is helpful to do so
- Yes, but obtaining serum drug levels is not a standard clinical practice
- No

Attending physician's mental notes: initial evaluation (continued)

- Obtaining serum drug levels is not a standard clinical practice. Serum drug levels can be difficult to obtain for medications such as lisdexamfetamine (Vyvanse) as only a few stimulants are available for testing. It is also difficult to get insurance coverage for these tests. Pharmacogenetic testing, however, is more routinely covered by insurance and can provide the patient's unique metabolism profile for various drugs. This information can help guide medication dosing and titration

Case outcome: first interim follow-up visit at week 4

- The patient had a depressive episode 2 weeks prior, with symptoms of amotivation, anergia, hopelessness, helplessness, irritability, and low self-esteem. He also admitted to initial insomnia and trouble processing information. He denied suicidal ideation and hallucinations
- He had a similar depressive episode 4 months ago that lasted 1 week during his final examinations
- He is responsible for taking his own medications and often misses doses

Question

How would you adjust the patient's medication?

- Increase his dosage of fluoxetine (Prozac), but leave the lisdexamfetamine (Vyvanse) dosage unchanged
- Increase his dosages of both fluoxetine and lisdexamfetamine
- Leave both the fluoxetine and lisdexamfetamine dosages unchanged
- Add another adjunctive medication

Attending physician's mental notes: first interim follow-up visit at week 4

- The patient likely had subtherapeutic drug levels as he often forgot to take his medications
- The decision was made to leave both the fluoxetine (Prozac) and lisdexamfetamine (Vyvanse) dosages unchanged and instead emphasize daily medication compliance with parental supervision
- Adding another new medication when the patient is already struggling with compliance on his current regimen is likely to be unsuccessful and may be overwhelming to the patient
- The parents were not interested in pursuing family therapy

Case outcome: second interim follow-up visit at week 6

- The patient reported better compliance with his medication regimen and feeling less fatigued and irritable
- However, he was still having difficulty retaining reading materials and taking notes

Question

Are the patient's learning difficulties consistent with his already established diagnosis of ADHD? Should you consider another etiology?

- The learning difficulties are consistent with ADHD, inattentive type
- The learning difficulties may be due to a learning disorder
- The learning difficulties may be due to the patient's mood disorder
- The learning difficulties may be due to an anxiety disorder

Attending physician's mental notes: second interim follow-up visit at week 6

- Although the patient's difficulty with reading and writing may be due to his inattention-predominant ADHD, his ability to excel in STEM subjects may be indicative of an underlying language-specific learning disability
- A referral to a neuropsychologist was provided to evaluate for learning disabilities
- An order for pharmacogenomic testing was also provided per parental request and to ensure that he was on the appropriate medication regimen for his metabolic profile

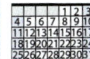

Case outcome: fourth interim follow-up visit at week 10

- The patient reported that lisdexamfetamine (Vyvanse) was effective for about 11 hours (7 a.m.–6 p.m.); however, his academic performance was declining, and he had begun lying to his parents about completing his assignments
- Pharmacogenetic testing revealed a slow metabolism, and hence a higher average serum level, for fluoxetine (Prozac). The patient also had a polymorphism of the serotonin transport gene that resulted in decreased to intermediate response to selective serotonin reuptake inhibitors (SSRIs) such as fluoxetine. Stimulant pharmacogenomic data were unavailable

Question

Should the patient's stimulant dosage be increased, given his increased difficulty at school?

- Yes, his increased academic difficulty indicates that his medication dosage is not sufficient
- No, increased academic difficulty may be attributed to other factors that cannot be addressed by medications
- No, the patient's stimulant dosage is appropriate at this point

Attending physician's mental notes: fourth interim follow-up visit at week 10

- It is important to consider each aspect of the biopsychosocial model in providing effective holistic treatment for your patients. While the biological aspect of the patient's presentation has been well investigated, the psychological and social aspects are needed to complete the picture
  - The patient's psychotherapist was contacted for more information about social stressors that may be contributing to his worsening academic struggles
  - The psychotherapist recommended that the parents stop pressuring the patient about excelling in school
  - The parents were also encouraged to communicate directly with his school and teacher about his pending neuropsychological testing
- As the patient self-reports appropriate efficacy (11 hours) for his current lisdexamfetamine (Vyvanse) dosage, uptitration is not necessary at this time
- A medication effectiveness and duration chart was provided so the patient and his parents could quantitatively chart his ADHD symptoms throughout the day

Case outcome: fifth interim follow-up visit at week 12

- The patient was very depressed, hopeless, and tearful during the visit
- The effectiveness and duration chart indicated that lisdexamfetamine (Vyvanse) was actually only effective for approximately 6 hours for the patient
- The patient's worsening depression and academic struggles warranted uptitration of both medications: lisdexamfetamine from 30 mg to 40 mg daily and fluoxetine (Prozac) from 10 mg to 20 mg daily

PATIENT FILE

Case outcome: sixth interim follow-up visit at week 14

- The patient continued to struggle in school and lie about completing his assignments. He exhibited regressive behavior (e.g. crying in fetal position) when confronted by his parents
- On interview, he did not necessarily demonstrate remorse or guilt, however, and appeared more resigned to his situation with no motivation to improve his life. The patient denied suicidal ideation
- The patient also complained of initial and terminal insomnia
- There was no suicidal ideation or plan

Question

What adjunct therapies can be added to target the patient's persistently depressed mood and insomnia?

- Doxepin (Sinequan)
- Triazolam (Halcion)
- Quetiapine (Seroquel)
- Zaleplon (Sonata)
- Zolpidem (Ambien)

Attending physician's mental notes: sixth interim follow-up visit at week 14

- Atypical antipsychotics can be used as an adjunctive treatment for persistent depressive symptoms unresponsive to monotherapy with an SSRI
- The patient was advised to start quetiapine (Seroquel) 25 mg every night as its sedating side effects could also be useful in alleviating his insomnia
- The patient's continued academic struggles despite the recent increase in his stimulant dosage reinforced the need for neuropsychological testing

Case outcome: tenth interim follow-up visit at week 26

- The patient reported improvement in his mood and focus with the quetiapine (Seroquel), and he was better able to get his homework done. He eventually had to be switched to aripiprazole (Abilify) 2 mg titrated to 5 mg daily due to the medication side effect of headaches on quetiapine
- The patient revealed to his psychotherapist that he was bullied at school and transferred to another school where he was no longer bullied. His academic performance improved significantly at the new school. He also joined the lacrosse team and made friends

- Neuropsychological testing revealed that the patient, while intellectually gifted (IQ 99th percentile), had a significant reading and writing disability that was over 1 standard deviation below his IQ. Referral was provided to an educational therapist to help develop an Individualized Education Plan (IEP)
- Lisdexamfetamine (Vyvanse) was ultimately discontinued due to insufficient efficacy. Amphetamine-dextroamphetamine 10 mg daily was started and titrated to 30 mg with better efficacy and improved focus
- The patient was ultimately stabilized on a daily regimen of amphetamine-dextroamphetamine 30 mg, aripiprazole 5 mg, and fluoxetine (Prozac) 20 mg, with significant improvements in mood and focus

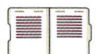

Case debrief

- The patient initially presented with mood lability, inattention, and poor school performance. Various treatment methods were trialed as his depressive symptoms worsened and his school performance continued to decline
- Skillful interviewing and careful observation over the course of many visits led to the discovery of the patient's learning disability and major social stressor of being bullied at school
- The patient showed significant improvement once he switched schools and was no longer bullied
- He also had moderately treatment-resistant depression that was unresponsive to SSRI monotherapy but improved significantly with the addition of an adjunctive atypical antipsychotic
- The patient's insomnia was a symptom of his depression and usually worsened whenever his depression worsened
- The biopsychosocial model of holistic patient care was central to this case, as well as interprofessional communication between the psychiatrist, psychotherapist, and neuropsychologist

Take-home points

- Patients with ADHD often have comorbid diagnoses that may require careful interviewing and observation to elucidate, as was the case with this patient's specific learning disorder (SLD)
- The most common types of SLD are reading disorders, written language disorder, and mathematics disorder, and these are not well documented to be responsive to stimulant treatment
- ADHD is estimated to co-occur at a rate of 25–40% with reading disorders, 55–64% with written language disorder, and 11–30% with mathematics disorder

- ADHD and SLD have shared neuropsychological factors including response inhibition, decreased processing speed, impaired working memory, and inattention
- To adequately assess and treat comorbidity between ADHD and SLD, a comprehensive multidisciplinary approach involving practitioners from both mental health and education is recommended

Performance in practice: confessions of a psychopharmacologist

What could have been done better here?

- Should family therapy have been encouraged more at the beginning of the treatment? Would this have created an environment where the patient could have confided in his parents about being bullied at school earlier?
- Should the adjunctive atypical antipsychotic have been considered and pushed far sooner, after the patient's first depressive episode?
- Should the SSRI have been uptitrated more aggressively or switched instead of adding another medication?

What are possible action items for improvement in practice?

- Communicate early and often with other allied mental health professionals
- Emphasize the importance of therapy in conjunction with medications in the patient's treatment plan
- In the case of poor treatment response, consider maximizing the dosage on one class of medications before adding another

Posttest self-assessment question and answer

Which of the follow medications is considered the first-line treatment for ADHD in adolescents?

A. α_2-adrenergic receptor agonists
B. SNRIs
C. Stimulants
Answer: C
Stimulants are considered first-line medications for ADHD in adolescents. The FDA has approved two stimulants for treating ADHD: methylphenidate (Concerta) and amphetamine. The effect size [(treatment mean – control mean)/(control standard deviation)] for stimulants as treatment for ADHD is around 1.0.

Three non-stimulants have been approved by the FDA as second-line treatments to treat ADHD in adolescents: atomoxetine (Strattera) (an SNRI) and the α_2-adrenergic receptor agonists guanfacine extended-release (Intuniv) and clonidine extended-release (Kapvay). For these three medications, the demonstrated efficacy in treating ADHD in adolescents is lower than that of stimulants, with effect sizes around 0.7 for all three.

Table 27.1 shows FDA-approved treatments for ADHD in children and adolescents:

Table 27.1 FDA-approved treatments for ADHD

Drug/device, class, and mechanism of action	Trade names	Age range (years)
Amphetamine-*d,l* A. Stimulant B. Dopamine, norepinephrine reuptake inhibitor and releaser (DN-RIRe)	Adderall, Evekeo	3 and older
	Dyanavel XR	6–17
	Adderall XR, Evekeo, Adzenys XR-ODT, Adzenys ER	6 and older
	Mydayis	13 and older
Amphetamine-*d* A. Stimulant B. Dopamine, norepinephrine reuptake inhibitor and releaser (DN-RIRe)	Zenzedi	3–16
	ProCentra	3–16
	Dexedrine Spansule	6–16
Atomoxetine A. Selective norepinephrine reuptake inhibitor (NRI) B. Norepinephrine reuptake inhibitor (NRI)	Strattera	6 and older
Clonidine A. Centrally acting α_{2A} agonist B. Norepinephrine receptor agonist (N-RA)	Kapvay	6–17
Guanfacine A. Centrally acting α_{2A}-agonist B. Norepinephrine receptor agonist (N-RA)	Intuniv	6–17
Lisdexamfetamine A. Stimulant (pro-drug of dextroamphetamine) B. Dopamine, norepinephrine reuptake inhibitor and releaser (DN-RIRe)	Vyvanse	6 and older
Methylphenidate-*d* A. Stimulant B. dopamine, norepinephrine reuptake inhibitor and releaser (DN-RIRe)	Focalin	6–17
	Focalin XR	6 and older
Methylphenidate-*d,l* A. Stimulant B. Dopamine, norepinephrine reuptake inhibitor and releaser (DN-RIRe)	Ritalin, Methylin	6–12
	Ritalin LA	6–12, adults
	Metadate CD, Daytrana, Cotempla XR-ODT	6–17
	Ritalin SR, Methylin ER, Metadate ER, Concerta, QuilliChew ER, Aptensio XR, Quillivant XR	6 and older

Table 27.2 Treatment guidelines for ADHD in children and adolescents

Age	First-line treatments	Other treatment options
Preschool-aged children (4 years to the sixth birthday)	*Psychosocial:* Evidence-based behavioral PTBM and/or behavioral classroom interventions	*Pharmacological:* Methylphenidate may be considered if these behavioral interventions do not provide significant improvement and there is moderate-to-severe continued disturbance in the 4–5-year-old child's functioning (the rate of metabolizing methylphenidate is slower in children 4–5 years of age, so they should be given a low dose to start, which can be increased in smaller increments)
Elementary and middle school-aged children (6 years to the 12th birthday)	• *Pharmacological:* stimulants (methylphenidate, amphetamine) • *Psychosocial:* PTBM and/or behavioral classroom intervention (e.g. school environment, class placement, instructional placement, behavioral supports, IEP or a rehabilitation plan)	*Pharmacological (in order):* • Atomoxetine • Guanfacine extended-release • Clonidine extended-release
Adolescents (12 years to the 18th birthday)	*Pharmacological:* stimulants *Psychosocial:* evidence-based training interventions and/or behavioral interventions, planning for the transition to adult care (during high school years)	

PTBM, parent training in behavior management.

Current evidence-based treatment guidelines

In 2019, the American Academy of Pediatrics (AAP) provided the evidence-based treatment guidelines for ADHD in children and adolescents shown in Table 27.2.

The AAP recommends screening for comorbid conditions in children and adolescents with ADHD including emotional or behavioral conditions (e.g. anxiety, depression, oppositional defiant disorder, conduct disorders, substance use), developmental conditions (e.g. learning and language disorders, autism spectrum disorders), and physical conditions (e.g. tics, sleep apnea).

References

1. Caye A, Swanson JM, Coghill D, Rohde LA. Treatment strategies for ADHD: an evidence-based guide to select optimal treatment. *Mol Psychiatry* 2019; 24:390–408. https://doi.org/10.1038/s41380-018-0116-3
2. Chan E, Fogler JM, Hammerness PG. Treatment of attention-deficit/hyperactivity disorder in adolescents: a systematic review. *JAMA* 2016; 315:1997–2008. https://doi.org/10.1001/jama.2016.5453
3. Hong DS. Here/in this issue and there/abstract thinking: learning disorders and ADHD: are LDs getting the attention they deserve?

J Am Acad Child Adolesc Psychiatry 2014; 53:933–4. https://doi.org/10.1016/j.jaac.2014.06.006

4. Masi G, Milone A, Veltri S, et al. Use of quetiapine in children and adolescents. *Pediatr Drugs* 2015; 17:125–40. https://doi.org/10.1007/s40272-015-0119-3

5. Mulder R, Hamilton A, Irwin L, et al. Treating depression with adjunctive antipsychotics. *Bipolar Disord* 2018; 20:17–24. https://doi.org/10.1111/bdi.12701

6. Pham AV, Riviere A. Specific learning disorders and ADHD: current issues in diagnosis across clinical and educational settings. *Curr Psychiatry Rep* 2015; 17:38. https://doi.org/10.1007/s11920-015-0584-y

7. Pritchard AE, Nigro CA, Jacobson LA, Mahone EM. The role of neuropsychological assessment in the functional outcomes of children with ADHD. *Neuropsychol Rev* 2012; 22:54–68. https://doi.org/10.1007/s11065-011-9185-7

8. Reale L, Bartoli B, Cartabia M, et al. Comorbidity prevalence and treatment outcome in children and adolescents with ADHD. *Eur Child Adolesc Psychiatry* 2017; 26:1443–57. https://doi.org/10.1007/s00787-017-1005-z

9. Stahl SM. *Stahl's Essential Psychopharmacology: Prescriber's Guide: Children and Adolescents*. New York, NY: Cambridge University Press, 2019.

10. Stevens JR, Wilens TE, Stern TA. Using stimulants for attention-deficit/hyperactivity disorder: clinical approaches and challenges. *Prim Care Companion CNS Disord* 2013; 15:PCC.12f01472. https://doi.org/10.4088/PCC.12f01472

11. Thapar A, Cooper M. Attention deficit hyperactivity disorder. *Lancet.* 2016; 387:1240–50. https://doi.org/10.1016/S0140-6736(15)00238-X

12. Wolraich ML, Hagan JF, Allan C, et al. Clinical practice guideline for the diagnosis, evaluation, and treatment of attention-deficit/hyperactivity disorder in children and adolescents. *Pediatrics* 2019; 144:e20192528. https://doi.org/10.1542/peds.2019-2528.

Case 28: Treatment-emergent mania/hypomania in a depressed patient

The Question: Can you observe manic/hypomanic side effects in a unipolar depression case after starting antidepressants?

The Psychopharmacological Dilemma: How careful should you be with antidepressants if you suspect unipolar depression versus bipolar depression when starting treatment?

Kevin Truong and Lawrence Yu

Pretest self-assessment questions (answers at the end of the case)

Can you experience treatment-emergent mania/hypomania in a suspected unipolar patient?

A. Yes
B. No

Which class of antidepressants most consistently carries the highest risk for treatment-emergent mania/hypomania mood switching?

A. Selective serotonin reuptake inhibitors (SSRIs)
B. Selective norepinephrine reuptake inhibitors (SNRIs)
C. Tricyclic antidepressants (TCAs)
D. Monoamine oxidase inhibitors (MAOIs)
E. Norepinephrine-dopamine reuptake inhibitors (NDRIs)

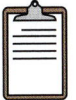

Patient evaluation on intake

- A 36-year-old male with the chief complaints of sadness and anxiety
- He is seeking mental health evaluation now because of worsening symptoms

Psychiatric history

- The patient has had no prior psychiatric evaluations
- He has had daily anxiety about worst-case scenarios since his teens
- He has had depressive episodes since his teens described by sadness, insomnia, lethargy, poor concentration, and poor appetite
- There have been no manic/hypomanic episodes
- He has no history of suicidal thoughts
- He has not had any auditory or visual hallucinations
- He does not have paranoid or delusional thoughts
- He suffered prior emotional abuse from his father during his young childhood from which he has nightmares monthly

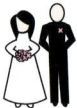

Social and personal history

- The patient graduated high school with mostly As and Bs with no goal to complete further education
- He is now working in on-demand food delivery services using his car to deliver ordered meals to peoples' homes, which he feels is becoming more difficult as his anxiety makes it more difficult to interact with strangers
- He currently lives with his mother and father who are overall supportive, but he feels they are constantly pressuring him to get a better-paying job and move out of their home
- He is single, has never married, and is not interested in romantic relationships
- He describes himself as not social and does not consider himself as having many friends

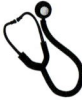

Medical history

- Asthma

Family history

- None

Patient evaluation on initial visit

- The patient hesitantly shakes the provider's hand with a loose grip and sweaty palms
- He decides to sit in the patient chair to the side of the room
- He is notably anxious, sweating, avoiding eye contact, stuttering, and often correcting himself
- He lacks insight into his symptoms and requires prompting for further elaboration on his responses; he requests medications to "make me feel better"
- He is hesitant and uncomfortable in discussing prior traumas and summarizes the emotional abuse from his father as "He made me feel worthless"
- He feels that his worsening sadness and anxiety are not due to his prior trauma
- He appears motivated to cooperate with treatment
- He asks if his mother is allowed to accompany him to future appointments

Attending physician's mental notes: initial evaluation

- His overall demeanor, paralanguage, and request to have his mother accompany him to future appointments possibly indicate low self-esteem, which may be a result of depression, anxiety, or prior traumas
- He appears guarded in discussing his symptoms

Question

As this is the first visit with the patient and his first encounter with a psychiatrist, what would your approach be to discussing his prior traumas and incorporating them into your differential?

- Ignore them
- Offer him more time to discuss his traumas
- Ask him if he would be comfortable speaking with a male or female provider
- Inform him that he should only talk about what is comfortable for him
- Ask about traumas at different points in the interview

Attending physician's mental notes: initial evaluation (continued)

- The patient prefers not to discuss his prior trauma in detail and while he feels his symptoms are not due to his prior trauma, it is important to consider it as a contributor to his diagnosis
- He has not tried any prior psychotropic medications or psychotherapy and likely does not have much knowledge on what to expect
- Given his symptoms and social history, there are multiple potential diagnoses for this patient including, but not limited to:
  - Major depressive disorder (MDD)
  - Generalized anxiety disorder (GAD)
  - Posttraumatic stress disorder (PTSD)
- The literature indicates that multimodality treatment including pharmacotherapy and psychotherapy can improve the effectiveness and rate of treatment, and as a result he should be offered psychotropic medication and psychotherapy in order to improve his self-awareness and insight
- Given his prior traumas, guardedness, and complicated relationship with his family, multiple forms of psychotherapy may be applicable including interpersonal psychotherapy (IPT) and cognitive behavioral therapy (CBT)
- IPT builds on two major principles:

- Depression is a medical illness, is not the patient's fault, and is treatable
- There is a practical link between mood and disturbing life events that either trigger or follow from the onset of the mood disorder
- A focus of treatment for IPT addresses interpersonal difficulties broken into particular problem areas that are identified and addressed, composed of unresolved grief, role disputes, role transitions, and interpersonal deficits
- IPT can be individual or group work, completed within 16 weeks, that involves phases including initial exploration of the social and relationship history, implementing and practicing healthy coping skills, and then planning for maintenance after stopping therapy
- There is an emphasis on support and being an ally to the patient, with focuses on the patient's outside environment, not on the therapy itself, whereby the therapist works with the patient to identify challenging interpersonal situations and either congratulates or provides sympathy and discusses alternative skills that can be utilized in future situations
- Applications of IPT have expanded past depression and can now be implemented as part of treatment for anxiety, eating disorders, substance use disorders, bipolar disorder, postpartum depression, and PTSD
- As this is his first encounter with mental health, the patient should be actively included in the formation of his treatment plan

Question

Which of the following would you do?
- Start sertraline (Zoloft)
- Start venlafaxine (Effexor)
- Start bupropion (Wellbutrin)
- Start methylphenidate (Concerta)
- Recommend psychotherapy

Case outcome: initial evaluation

- The patient decides that he would like to address his symptoms with both medication and psychotherapy
- He is started on sertraline (Zoloft) 25 mg daily for 2 weeks and then told to increase the dose to 50 mg daily
- He is also referred for IPT as he reports he heard about this form of psychotherapy online and this is considered the treatment of choice for unipolar depressive disorders

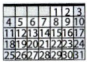

Case outcome: first interim follow-up visit at week 6

- He begins taking sertraline (Zoloft) immediately and begins IPT in the following weeks
- He calls the clinic 3 weeks after starting sertraline (Zoloft) and reports increased irritability, agitation, restlessness, racing thoughts, and anxiety
- As these symptoms may be a result of SSRI-induced hypomania, he is instructed to stop sertraline and return to the clinic for further workup
- He returns to the clinic with his mother present and reports that since stopping sertraline he feels that the irritability, agitation, impulsivity, restlessness, and racing thoughts have improved
- He states he continues to struggle with depression and anxiety
- He feels that IPT is challenging but intends to continue to follow up weekly
- His mother attends the appointment and often answers questions for the patient

Question

Which of the following would you do?
- Retry sertraline (Zoloft)
- Stop IPT
- Start bupropion (Wellbutrin)
- Start lamotrigine (Lamictal)

Attending physician's mental notes: first interim follow-up visit at week 6

- Assigning causality of emerging manic/hypomanic symptoms to an underlying bipolar disorder or treatment-induced symptoms is difficult, as a majority of patients with bipolar disorder will initially present to mental health treatment with depressive symptoms
- The literature has attempted to address this problem by defining the emergence of manic/hypomanic symptoms within 8 weeks of treatment as treatment-emergent mania/hypomania
- His symptoms including depressive and manic symptoms can be described as a mixed state, which can require similar treatment strategies as treatment of bipolar disorder
- He likely experienced treatment-emergent hypomania, which may have been caused by sertraline (Zoloft), as the hypomanic symptoms resolved after stopping sertraline; thus, this was likely treatment-emergent hypomania secondary to the SSRI

- His IPT should not be stopped as this form of psychotherapy can help with depressive symptoms, which may be caused by poor interpersonal relationships between the patient and his parents
- To minimize risk for further treatment-emergent hypomania, he was started on bupropion extended-release (XL) (Aplenzin) 75 mg PO daily
- Rather than give a monoamine reuptake blocker, he could be given an atypical antipsychotic with evidence of efficacy in mixed features, such as cariprazine (Vraylar) or lurasidone (Latuda), especially if he fails another reuptake blocker

Two-minute tutorial

Mixed affective states

- Mixed states were formerly characterized by DSM-4-TR by concurrent presence of full manic and depressive phenomena for at least 7 days, but in DSM-5 this was changed to "with mixed features" that is usable in bipolar I and II disorder and MDD, which describes the presence of only three symptoms of opposite mood polarity
- This broadening of the concept of mixed features in DSM-5 indicates that there is likely a higher percentage of patients who experience these mixed features and are therefore at greater clinical risk and who may require greater clinical attention
- Those who experience mixed episodes suffer from greater comorbid conditions including anxiety and spectrum disorders and substance misuse, and are at greater risk for completed suicide
- The existence of mixed features often indicates a more severe illness trajectory, poor treatment response, and poor outcome
- Possible causes of mood switching and exacerbation of mixed affective states include catecholamine–acetylcholine imbalances and circadian dysregulations
- The pharmacological agents employed in the treatment of mixed states are primarily atypical antipsychotics and mood stabilizers
- Treatment of mixed depression should not consist of antidepressant monotherapy, given the potential risk to destabilize mood, and consideration should be made to either taper/discontinue the antidepressant if not effective or augment with either an atypical antipsychotic or an antimanic mood stabilizer
- There are no current FDA-approved psychotropic agents for the treatment of depression with mixed features
- There is a questionable role and no clear established controlled trials of antidepressants in long-term treatment of depression with mixed features

- In severe episodes that show unsatisfactory response to pharmacological treatment, electroconvulsive therapy or transcranial magnetic stimulation is another form of therapy that can lead to resolution of intractable symptoms
- The preferred strategy for maintenance treatment is continuous rather than intermittent treatment with oral medication, given the high risk for relapse

Case outcome: second interim follow-up visit at week 12

- The patient reported improvements in his depression and anxiety after starting bupropion XL (Aplenzin)
- He denies the recurrence of irritability, agitation, and restlessness
- He has remained stable on bupropion XL for the next several months
- He reports ongoing compliance with IPT and feels it has been helping him communicate with his parents and discuss prior traumas; he states that his therapy is nearing termination but describes improved coping mechanisms
- His mother is not in attendance at this visit and he states that his mother trusts him at his appointments on his own

Case debrief

- It appears as though this patient is likely struggling with unipolar depression that was complicated with treatment-emergent hypomania after starting an SSRI, as these hypomanic symptoms started and resolved in accordance to SSRI changes
- Treatment-emergent mania/hypomania in unipolar depression is an observed phenomenon, most commonly occurring with SSRIs and TCAs, with TCAs having a consistently higher risk of mood switching than all other antidepressants combined and which has been observed in as many as 70% of recipients
- Some antidepressants have been found to induce treatment-emergent mania/hypomania in a dose-related manner
- There remains wide discussion on distinguishing bipolar depression from unipolar depression and the idea that these are diagnoses on a mood spectrum, as there are many cases of unipolar depression leading to eventual diagnostic conversion to bipolar depression, with mixed states lying on the spectrum
- Some studies have shown that treatment-emergent mania/hypomania is rare and may be a course of the illness phenomenon, rather than a treatment-induced outcome
- A family history of bipolar disorder has been considered the most reliable risk factor for bipolar depression

- The precise mechanism underlying the process of treatment-emergent mania/hypomania mood switching is not yet determined, but hypotheses are that antidepressants influence central serotonergic and catecholaminergic systems
  - This is supported by the fact that higher levels of urinary noradrenaline and dopamine are associated with mania, direct pharmacological treatment resulting in elevated catecholamine levels can mimic mania-like states, and several genetic polymorphisms linked with serotonergic and catecholaminergic systems have been proposed as risk factors for treatment-emergent mania/hypomania
- The literature has indicated that bupropion (Wellbutrin) and paroxetine (Paxil) have lower risks of treatment-emergent mania/hypomania
- If there were larger concerns of primary diagnosis of depression with mixed features instead of a treatment-emergent mania/hypomania, then there should be further consideration to switching treatment to an atypical antipsychotic and mood stabilizers with likely discontinuation of the antidepressants
- IPT is an evidence-based, targeted therapy modality focused on interpersonal relationships and social functioning that can help to reduce stress and is often used as a treatment of choice for unipolar depressive disorders; however, CBT has been shown to have equal efficacy
- The literature indicates that whether to prescribe CBT or IPT should depend on patient preference
- Meta-analyses of IPT have shown it to be effective as both an independent treatment and in combination with pharmacotherapy, indicating its ability to augment pharmacotherapy
- Pharmacotherapy may have limited benefit in some situations, and psychotherapy may relieve symptoms by different mechanisms, particularly in situational stressors including complicated grief
- In cases where there is no evidence of bipolar disorder, be cautious when starting antidepressants if the patient has other risk factors including a family history of bipolar disorder, a depressive episode with psychotic symptoms, young age at onset of depression, and antidepressant resistance

Performance in practice: confessions of a psychopharmacologist

What could have been done better here?

- For patients presenting with initial symptoms of depression and anxiety with prior trauma, suggesting a trial of psychotherapy could be considered prior to psychotropic medications
- Try to further engage the family in the treatment plan as many of the patient's symptoms may be exacerbated by interpersonal and family dynamics
- Additional forms of psychotherapy could have been encouraged such as family therapy, given the strong initial presence of the mother in treatment

Mechanism of action moment: bupropion

- Bupropion (Wellbutrin) is a NDRI
- It increases noradrenergic neurotransmission by blocking the norepinephrine reuptake pump (transporter), which results in desensitization of β-adrenergic receptors
- It increases dopamine neurotransmission by blocking the dopamine reuptake pump (dopamine transporter), and by blocking the norepinephrine reuptake as this pump usually results in dopamine deactivation in the frontal cortex
- It inhibits cytochrome P450 2D6
- Food does not affect absorption
- Plasma levels are noted to be higher in lower-weight children
- Its metabolism changes during puberty and becomes more like that of adults
- The XL formulation is largely preferred compared with the immediate-release or sustained-release formulation
- The more anxious or agitated the patient, the lower the starting dose and the slower the titration needed
- Notable side effects include: dry mouth, constipation, nausea, insomnia, dizziness, headache, anxiety, agitation, sweating, weight loss, abdominal pain, and hypertension
- Dangerous side effects include: seizures, Stevens–Johnson syndrome, rare activation of suicidal ideation and behavior, and rare induction of mania

Take-home points

- Diagnosing depressive symptoms can be difficult, as these symptoms may be a result of unipolar or bipolar depression
- The literature points to affective disorders existing on a spectrum including depression, mania, and mixed states

- Always ask for a family history of bipolar disorder as this is a key risk factor
- The treatment of depression can be complicated, as the first-line treatment with antidepressants can result in treatment-emergent mania/hypomania; this phenomenon occurs more so in patients diagnosed with bipolar disorder compared with those with unipolar depression
- Certain antidepressants carry a higher risk of treatment-emergent mania/hypomania, the highest risk being TCAs, and lowest risk including bupropion (Wellbutrin) and paroxetine (Paxil)
- Treatment of depression with mixed features as part of bipolar or unipolar affective disorder involves atypical antipsychotics and mood stabilizers, with little efficacy shown for adjunctive antidepressants
- Other modalities of treatment, including psychotherapy, should be considered in combination with or as alternative to medications, as multiple forms of psychotherapy, including CBT and IPT, have been found to be effective for both unipolar and bipolar depression

Posttest self-assessment questions and answers

Can you experience treatment-emergent mania/hypomania in a suspected unipolar patient?

A. Yes
B. No
Answer: A

What class of antidepressants most consistently carries the highest risk for treatment-emergent mania/hypomania mood switching?

A. SSRIs
B. SNRIs
C. TCAs
D. MAOIs
E. NDRIs
Answer: C

References

1. Benvenuti A, Rucci P, Miniati M, et al. Treatment-emergent mania/hypomania in unipolar patients. *Bipolar Disord* 2008; 10:726–32. https://doi.org/10.1111/j.1399-5618.2008.00613.x
2. Cuijpers, P, Geraedts, AS, van Oppen, P, et al. Interpersonal psychotherapy for depression: a meta-analysis. *Am J Psychiatry* 2011; 168: 581–92. https://doi.org/10.1176/appi.ajp.2010.10101411

3. de Almeida JRC, Phillips ML. Distinguishing between unipolar depression and bipolar depression: current and future clinical and neuroimaging perspectives. *Biol Psychiatry* 2013; 73:111–18. https://doi.org/10.1016/j.biopsych.2012.06.010

4. Dudek D, Siwek M, Zielińska D, et al. Diagnostic conversions from major depressive disorder into bipolar disorder in an outpatient setting: results of a retrospective chart review. *J Affect Disord* 2013; 144:112–15. https://doi.org/10.1016/j.jad.2012.06.014

5. Markowitz JC, Weissman MM. Interpersonal psychotherapy: principles and applications. *World Psychiatry* 2004; 3:136–9.

6. Muneer A. Mixed states in bipolar disorder: etiology, pathogenesis and treatment. *Chonnam Med J* 2017; 53:1–13. https://doi.org/10.4068/cmj.2017.53.1.1

7. Patel R, Reiss P, Shetty H, et al. Do antidepressants increase the risk of mania and bipolar disorder in people with depression? A retrospective electronic case register cohort study. *BMJ Open* 2015; 5:e008341. https://doi.org/10.1136/bmjopen-2015-008341

8. Stahl SM, Debbi A Morrissette, Gianni Faedda, et al. Guidelines for the recognition and management of mixed depression. *CNS Spectr* 2017; 22:203–19. https://doi.org/10.1017/S1092852917000165

9. Stahl SM. *Stahl's Essential Psychopharmacology: Prescriber's Guide*, 4th edn. New York, NY: Cambridge University Press, 2011.

10. Yamaguchi Y, Kimoto S, Nagahama T, Kishimoto T. Dosage-related nature of escitalopram treatment-emergent mania/hypomania: a case series. *Neuropsychiatr Dis Treat* 2018; 14:2099–104. https://doi.org/10.2147/NDT.S168078.

Case 29: The border between mood and personality

The Question: Can you differentiate between borderline personality traits (disorder) from a recurring mood disorder such as major depressive disorder (MDD)?

The Psychopharmacological Dilemma: Is it necessary to differentiate between borderline personality traits (disorder) and major depressive disorder in a teenager?

Phuong Vo and Ijeoma Ijeaku

Pretest self-assessment question (answer at the end of the case)

Which of these are considered standard of care in treating patients with borderline personality disorder?

A. Dialectical behavioral therapy
B. Mentalization-based therapies
C. Psychoeducation about condition
D. Crisis management
E. Pharmacological treatment of episodic mood and psychotic symptoms
F. All of the above

Patient evaluation on intake

- A 17-year-old girl who is in 10th grade and lives in a group home presents with an extensive history of trauma, self-injurious behaviors, and verbal aggression, and is seen for concerns of depressive symptoms and self-harming behaviors
- She was recently placed on an involuntary hold for being a danger to self after endorsing suicidal ideation with a plan

Psychiatric history

- The patient was admitted after being removed from the home and was started on psychotropic medications but it is unclear what medications. She was admitted again 6 months later. The current evaluation was done shortly after her third involuntary hold and admission
- She admits that she has struggled with anxiety attacks, poor sleep, nightmares, intermittent auditory and visual hallucinations, low self-esteem, and chronic feelings of emptiness since she was in elementary school but is unable to provide more details

Medication history

- Recently, she began escitalopram (Lexapro) 5 mg PO every morning, trazodone (Desyrel) 75 mg PO at bedtime and hydroxyzine (Vistaril) 25 mg PO at bedtime with noted grogginess and dizziness. It is unclear how long she took the medication but she was off the regimen when she came to the group home

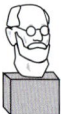

Psychotherapy history

- The patient reports being briefly in therapy starting in 8th grade following concerns for depressive symptoms and self-harming behaviors. Since being at the group home, she has been in therapy

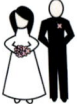

Social and personal history

- The patient has no knowledge of her biological father. Her mother and father separated after her birth, but she lived intermittently with her mother and her husband whom she considers her father. The patient has been with various caregivers over the course of her life. She has been dropped off to various friends of her parents. She reports being sexually abused and raped by one of the parents' friends, an adult male, and became pregnant. The patient admits to then being physically abused by her "father" while pregnant, sustaining a blunt injury to her abdomen (punches). She miscarried the pregnancy at 7 months' gestation
- Child Protective Services (CPS) only became involved several months ago for abuse. Since removal from her mother's home, she has been in two foster homes and is currently in a group home
- The patient denies current drug use

Medical history

- Her body mass index is over 30 kg/m^2
- She has adequately controlled asthma responsive to an albuterol inhaler as needed
- Her current caregiver reports possible *in utero* exposure to cocaine and nicotine

Family history

- The patient reports depression and anxiety in her cousins

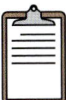

Patient evaluation on initial visit

- The patient admits to daily anxiety attacks (two per day), excessive worries and fears, social anxiety, poor sleep, nightmares, flashbacks, hypervigilance, low energy, amotivation, poor concentration, and intermittent auditory and visual hallucinations
- She lacks insight as far as the role of trauma in her current presentation, has poor coping skills, a poor sense of self, and recurrent psychiatric issues
- She is future oriented and is invested in getting better
- She denies any current suicidal ideation, homicidal ideation, or auditory and visual hallucinations

Current medications

- None

Attending physician's mental notes: initial visit

- The presentation is highly suggestive of borderline personality disorder, but given that she is only 17 years and this is the first meeting, the patient will continue to be observed very closely for the usual patterns of borderline personality disorder (e.g. significant distress associated with fear of abandonment, decreased self-image, and significant distress and hypersensitivity to rejection, all likely manifestations from previous trauma, etc.). She is also presenting with major depressive disorder (MDD) with psychotic features and posttraumatic stress disorder (PTSD) and these need to be addressed promptly
- Given her hyperarousal states noted as poor sleep, nightmares, flashbacks, and hypervigilance, as well as exaggerated startle responses, she may benefit from a centrally acting α-agonist
- Given that she had recently been on escitalopram (Lexapro) with no major side effects, this medication could be retried to address the symptoms of MDD and PTSD
- A positive response to medication and just any therapy is unlikely as this is a more chronic presentation requiring multiple modalities of treatment approach to ensure an improvement in functional capacity. Thus, she will benefit from a trauma-informed therapy approach
- She will also benefit from extensive and ongoing psychoeducation to educate her about the interaction between traumatic experiences and thoughts, feelings, and behaviors

Initial plan

- An emergency JV-220 document is filed to start psychotropic medications and prevent further decompensation
  - A JV-220 application is a document from the Juvenile Court of the Judicial Council of California. It is a document asking permission from the courts to administer psychotropic medications to a minor because the minor in the foster care or probation system is a ward of the courts. It is completed by the attending psychiatrist with statements regarding the minor who is in treatment. It could be made for an initial psychotropic medication administration (JV-220(A)) or as a request for continuation of psychotropic medications that the minor is already taking (JV 220(B)). In the outpatient setting, an approved JV-220 document is valid for 6 months
- Start escitalopram 5 mg PO at bedtime for 4 days and then increase to 10 mg PO at bedtime
- Start clonidine (Catapres) 0.05 mg PO at bedtime
- We requested a collateral history to understand the timeline of the traumatic experiences as well as the course of her psychiatric illness but we have not been able to receive any other information

Case outcome: first interim follow-up visit at 2 weeks

- The patient's weight has increased by 3 lbs since the last visit 2 weeks ago
- She is reportedly compliant on her prescribed psychotropic medication regimen; escitalopram (Lexapro) 10 mg PO at bedtime and clonidine (Catapres) 0.05 mg PO at bedtime with some improvement in sleep but ongoing daytime agitation. There are no appreciable side effects
- The patient engaged appropriately and shared some of her recent experiences from school and the group home. She was happy to be here but complained incessantly about her frustrations with school, lack of support from teachers, inadequate explanation of subject matter, and excessive work thrown at students. She reports that she is irritable due to her challenges at school and feeling unsupported
- She reports that she is sleeping really well
- She reports that her concentration is off sometimes
- Her caregiver reports that the patient has been "snappy" with peers and staff
- The patient denies suicidal ideation/homicidal ideation or auditory and visual hallucinations

Plan

- Continue escitalopram (Lexapro) 10 mg PO at bedtime
- Continue clonidine 0.05 mg PO at bedtime and start clonidine 0.05 mg PO every morning; this may be decreased to 0.025 mg PO every morning if she feels sedated on 0.05 mg PO every morning
- Recommend School Success Team/Individualized Education Plan (IEP) to address academic issues
- Recommend trauma-informed care/dialectical behavior therapy principles in therapy at the group home; this was discussed at length with the therapist at the group home
- Ongoing psychoeducation

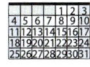

Case outcome: fourth interim follow-up visit at 3 months

- The patient is reportedly compliant on her prescribed psychotropic medication regimen: escitalopram (Lexapro) 15 mg PO at bedtime and clonidine (Catapres) 0.05 mg PO at bedtime/0.05 mg PO every morning as needed
- She was tearful during the evaluation. She cried intermittently about a recent abandonment issue with her Therapeutic Behavior Services (TBS) coach who abruptly stopped working with her about a week ago
- She reports that she has been crying a lot, having hallucinations, self-cutting, and dealing with excessive and explosive mood changes
- She reports that she has been having nightmares about her parents coming after her to hurt her
- The patient's therapist reports that she has been hysterical in the evenings at the group home with daily outbursts and the need for calls to the therapist
- The patient's licensed vocational nurse reports that various staff members have reported that the patient has been very emotionally dysregulated

Plan

- Start risperidone (Risperdal) 0.5 mg PO every morning
- Continue escitalopram (Lexapro) 15 mg PO at bedtime/continue clonidine 0.05 mg PO at bedtime and 0.05 mg PO QPM
- Order the following laboratory test: complete metabolic panel, complete blood count, thyroid-stimulating hormone, triiodothyronine/thyroxine, and lipid profile due to starting risperidone

- Continue with therapy at the group home, using trauma-informed care/dialectical behavior therapy principles as well as TBS to address her poor coping skills issues
- Continue psychoeducation

Attending physician's mental notes: fourth interim follow-up visit at 3 months

- The classic abandonment issues were re-enacted here after the patient's TBS coach left suddenly. She decompensated and started having hallucinations, self-injurious behaviors, and explosive outbursts
- The addition of risperidone (Risperdal) at this time was imperative to address the psychotic symptoms as well as explosive outbursts and mood changes. There was a huge concern for metabolic syndrome issues given that the patient is already obese and struggles with self-esteem issues. The plan will be to use this medication for as short a time period as is necessary
- Ongoing psychoeducation was done to reassure the patient that the TBS coach's behavior is not her fault and that her brain is responding to trauma as it has done in the past. She was encouraged to identify this pattern and to use new tools that she is learning in therapy to counter the effects

Case debrief

- Many patients with trauma history present in a comorbid fashion and experience symptomatology that may vary from one phase to another depending on the current stressor levels
- The use of different classes of psychotropic medications may be warranted depending on presentation and level of severity
- A multimodal approach is essential to address various issues ranging from classic axis I disorders to possible emerging personality disorders to inadequate coping skills
- Ongoing psychoeducation against the backdrop of a strong therapeutic alliance is very important to ensure that the patient remains engaged in understanding the roles of trauma, old unhealthy patterns of coping, and the use of trauma-informed therapy tools to deal with stressors
- In order to experience improvement in symptoms and a higher quality of life, this patient will need to remain adherent to her regimen and work closely with her psychiatrist to taper off medications as needed. She will likely require use of the tools that she learns from trauma-based therapy to deal with stressors in her life, bearing in mind that she may need psychotropic medications to address specific target symptoms at certain periods of her life and brief periods of therapy

Attending physician's mental notes: trauma-informed care

- Trauma-informed care is sensitive to the potential for trauma-related issues to contribute to patient conditions and behaviors; it is applied to all patients, even if patient symptoms are not clearly related to trauma at first glance
- Guiding principles include:
  - Safety: be mindful of how clinical spaces and procedures may impact feelings of physical and emotional safety
    - For example, touching without permission or entering a room without knocking may violate patient boundaries
  - Collaboration: encourage patient choice and control over treatment where possible
    - Sharing power may reduce feelings of being controlled by an authority figure, which may recapitulate the experience of trauma
  - Empowerment: use a strength-based model to reinforce a patient's positive attributes
    - If a patient interaction is only focused on discussing patient deficits, it may reinforce a message that a patient is defective and hopeless

Take-home points

Neurobiology and epigenetics of trauma

- Maltreatment in childhood, specifically chronic or sustained stress, has been correlated with brain changes that predispose the development of major depression, bipolar disorder, anxiety disorders, PTSD, substance use disorders, personality disorders, and psychosis (Figure 29.1)
- Areas of the brain in maltreated individuals have been found to have less gray matter volume and blood flow, specifically the left anterior cingulate, right occipital pole, left temporal pole, and right medial frontal gyrus with the proposed functionality:
  - The anterior cingulate regulates attention, emotions, and impulses
  - The temporal pole relates to social cognition and attribution of thoughts, intentions, and beliefs toward other people
  - The occipital poles affect visual processing and also contribute to awareness
  - The middle frontal gyrus works on memory and attention
  - The rostral portion of the middle frontal gyrus has an association with social cognition, self-knowledge, and self-perception

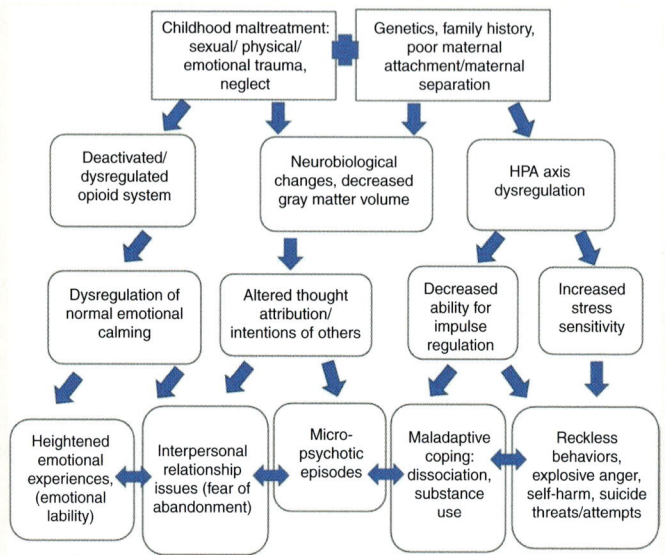

Figure 29.1 Symptom manifestation of borderline personality disorder. HPA, hypothalamic–pituitary–adrenal.

- Neuronal changes lead to decreased ability of patients to regulate impulses and accurately attribute thought/intentions of others (cognitive distortion), and create heightened emotional experiences, cravings, and self-centered mental thought processes
- Epigenetic modifications during maltreatment (sexual, physical, or emotional abuse or neglect) reprogram the brain to fire differently in response to stress, and, in developing young minds, alter the direction of brain development itself
- Sustained stress affects two systems epigenetically: the sympathetic nervous system and the hypothalamic–pituitary–adrenal (HPA) axis
  - Increases in the HPA axis increase cortisol levels, correlated with MDD or depressive symptoms and PTSD
  - Early adversity increases basal levels while decreasing cortisol responses over time via methylation and downregulation of glucocorticoid receptors, leading to chronic hyporeactivity to stress (depressive symptoms)
- Toxic traumatic stress affects epigenetics via DNA methylation and histone acetylation, modifying the expression of genes. Three regions of the brain have been correlated with the most effect from HPA axis gene dysregulation due to abundance of glucocorticoid receptors reacting to stress hormone release:

- Chronic stress impairs neuronal growth and proliferation in the hippocampus, responsible for memory and learning, thus impairing future memory function
- Toxic traumatic stress leads to amygdala remodeling (increased growth), the space that responds to stress and creates increased impulsive behavior
- The prefrontal cortex, the space for planning and impulse control, also develops fewer connections, revealing decreased impulse control in these patients
- Brain-derived neurotrophic factor (BDNF), which helps with the growth, maintenance, and survival of neurons, also decreases substantially in patients with MDD, likely due to glucocorticoid-induced neurotoxicity via HPA axis dysregulation
  - Electroconvulsive therapy, exercise, and antidepressant use has been shown to increase BDNF levels, producing antidepressant-like effects, and allows increased neuronal survival (especially in the hippocampus)
- Psychopathology development may be associated with dysregulation of genes that normally regulate serotonin, such as polymorphisms of the *5-HTTLPR* gene. Patients with shorter variants of the gene are significantly more likely to develop depression when put into a toxic traumatic stress environment

Demographics of borderline personality disorder

- The point prevalence of borderline personality disorder is 1.6% per year, with a lifetime prevalence of 5.9% in the USA
- The prevalence of borderline personality disorder is 20% in psychiatric inpatient populations, and these patients have high rates of comorbid disorders (mood disorders 80–96%, anxiety disorders 88%, substance use disorders 64%)
- Borderline personality disorder heritability is more than 50% in twin studies, showing higher heritability than major depression
- Environmental factors that contribute to the development of borderline personality disorder include childhood trauma (physical, sexual, or neglect), maternal separation or poor attachment, parental substance abuse, and inappropriate family boundaries

General treatment of borderline personality disorder

- Treatment of borderline personality disorder relies on psychotherapy. Mentalization-based therapy allows the management of emotion dysregulation to help patients feel understood and decrease assumptions made about other people's intentions (decreased splitting). Dialectical behavior therapy allows mindfulness practice to develop skills for emotion regulation and interpersonal relationship management. Transference-focused psychotherapy uses the patient–therapist relationship to develop awareness of interpersonal habits and dynamics. As mentioned above, trauma-informed care is particularly useful in borderline patients to emphasize collaboration in the patient–physician relationship and help empower them to make decisions without reinforcing the idea that the patient is "defective" or "helpless"

- There are no FDA-approved treatments for borderline personality disorder, as there has only been limited evidence of effectiveness of selective serotonin reuptake inhibitors (SSRIs), mood stabilizers, and antipsychotics (unless used for specific comorbid symptoms)

- With consistent therapy, a longitudinal study shows rates of remission of borderline personality disorder to be 35% after 2 years and 91% after 10 years. Some speculate that patients may appear to remit due to avoidance of toxic interpersonal relationships, not necessarily due to better interpersonal skills

- Patients with borderline personality disorder are more likely to attempt suicide with prescribed medications, which indicates careful follow-up when there is medication initiation

Comorbid MDD and borderline personality disorder

- Up to 80% of patients with borderline personality disorder experience one or more episodes of MDD, while 10–30% of patients with MDD have co-occurring borderline personality disorder

- Patients with borderline personality disorder have a hyperactive amygdala and may have depressive symptoms that manifest as reactions to stressful events or interpersonal challenges

- The patient's experiences of depression may be intense and exaggerated. Patients with borderline personality disorder rate their depression with substantially higher scores compared with clinician-rated scores, but clinician measures tend to match self-rates in patients with MDD without borderline personality disorder

- Features that may distinguish reactive depressive symptoms in borderline personality disorder may include feelings of loneliness, chronic emptiness, clinging dependency, intense fear of rejection or abandonment, instability or lability of negative affect, a deep sense of self-loathing, and a high prevalence of anger/hostility

- MDD that co-occurs with borderline personality disorder does not respond well to antidepressants, mood stabilizers, electroconvulsive therapy, or transcranial magnetic stimulation compared with MDD without borderline personality disorder. Dialectical behavior therapy and mentalization-based therapy have demonstrated benefits for MDD that co-occurs with borderline personality disorder, which suggests prioritizing borderline personality disorder treatment and avoiding polypharmacy

Neurobiology of borderline personality disorder and MDD

- Borderline personality disorder has a risk of intense emotional reaction and self-injurious behavior. A proposed mechanism is that it is due to reduced inhibition in the frontolimbic inhibition pathway
- Patients showed deactivation of the opioid system in brain areas and dysregulation of the normal calming function
- When thinking about self-injurious behavior, patients with borderline personality disorder show increased activity in the dorsolateral prefrontal cortex and a decrease in the mid cingulate
- Those with comorbid borderline personality disorder and MDD show altered patterns in the parietotemporal and anterior cingulate cortical regions. Impulsivity and hostility are positively correlated to increased glucose uptake in these regions in response to fenfluramine
- Dopaminergic transporter polymorphism (dopamine D_2 receptor variant alleles B1 and A1) has been correlated with borderline personality disorder in at-risk adults and has been seen as a risk factor for borderline personality disorder in depressed patients
- Besides environmental and genetic predisposition, patients with borderline personality disorder may also have serotonin dysregulation leading to reduced sensitivity of the serotonin 5-HT_{1A} receptor, corresponding to the limited efficacy of SSRIs as treatment for depression in these patients

Management of borderline personality disorder with comorbid MDD

- There is limited evidence for the use of aripiprazole (Abilify), olanzapine (Zyprexa), and ω-3 fatty acids for treatment of comorbid MDD with borderline personality disorder but no standardized data to guide clinicians
- Fluoxetine (Prozac) and olanzapine have been found to be safe and effective in blunting impulsive aggression in patients with borderline personality disorder
- Olanzapine monotherapy seemed superior with less chance of resistance for MDD management with borderline personality disorder. Olanzapine showed improvement over placebo in depression, anxiety, impulsivity, and aggressive behaviors of patients with borderline personality disorder with comorbid MDD
- Patients treated with aripiprazole showed significant changes in Hamilton Depression Rating Scale (HAM-D) and Symptom

Checklist-90-Revised (SCL-90-R) scores (MDD symptoms) and the Trait Anger inventory (borderline personality disorder impulsiveness) after about 8 weeks

- Lamotrigine (Lamictal) has promising effectiveness for treating the affect instability of borderline personality disorder

Borderline personality disorder and psychosis (other symptoms)

- Initial naming of borderline personality disorder was based on a concern that patients were "on the border" of psychosis, which has fallen out of favor. Borderline personality disorder has many comorbidities, as discussed above
- Patients with borderline personality disorder are more likely to abuse substances that may cause psychotic experiences and cause an increased severity of suicidality
- Patients with borderline personality disorder are more likely to experience micro-psychotic episodes in the setting of acute stressors; this may be associated with substance abuse but is also seen without drug effects
- Micro-psychotic episodes may warrant a short course of antipsychotics to stabilize and manage symptoms through acute stressors. Childhood trauma is more associated with psychotic symptoms in adults than trauma experienced as an adult. Child sexual abuse is strongly associated with hallucinations
- Patients with borderline personality disorder react very strongly to daily life stress with increased psychotic symptoms and hallucinations, more so than patients with psychotic disorders
- Stress reactivity may be due to dysregulation of the HPA axis, affecting processing of sensation. High PTSD comorbidity may cause flashbacks and hallucinations related to the abuse suffered (physical, sexual, or conversing with the abuser)

Posttest self-assessment question and answer

Which of these are considered standard of care in treating patients with borderline personality disorder?

A. Dialectical behavioral therapy
B. Mentalization-based therapies
C. Psychoeducation about condition
D. Crisis management
E. Pharmacological treatment of episodic mood and psychotic symptoms
F. All of the above

Answer: F

Treatment of borderline personality disorder usually involves different approaches in an attempt to deal with the myriad of issues that these individuals have to deal with. There is need for adequate education of the patient and their family about the nature of the disorder, management of crisis situations when they arise, use of psychopharmacological agents for mood and psychotic symptoms that might arise as comorbid disorders or during stressful conditions, and use of psychotherapy in both individual and group settings. Dialectical behavioral therapy and mentalization-based therapies have been useful techniques.

References

1. Barnow S, Arens EA, Sieswerda S, et al. Borderline personality disorder and psychosis: a review. *Curr Psychiatry Rep* 2010; 12:186–95. https://doi.org/10.1007/s11920-010-0107-9
2. Beatson J Rao S. Depression and borderline personality disorder. *Med J Aust* 2013; 199:S24–7. https://doi.org/10.5694/mja12.10474
3. Bellino S, Zizza M, Rinaldi C, Bogetto F. Combined treatment of major depression in patients with borderline personality disorder: a comparison with psychotherapy. *Can J Psychiatry* 2006; 51:453–60. https://doi.org/10.1177/070674370605100707
4. Chand SP, Arif H. Depression. In: *StatPearls*. Treasure Island, FL: StatPearls Publishing, 2020. Available from: https://www.ncbi.nlm.nih.gov/books/NBK430847/
5. Chapman J, Jamil RT, Fleisher C. Borderline personality disorder. In: *StatPearls*. Treasure Island, FL: StatPearls Publishing, 2020. Available from: https://www.ncbi.nlm.nih.gov/books/NBK430883/
6. Gunderson JG, Stout RL, McGlashan TH, et al. Ten-year course of borderline personality disorder: psychopathology and function from the Collaborative Longitudinal Personality Disorders study. *Arch Gen Psychiatry* 2011; 68:827–37. https://doi.org/10.1001/archgenpsychiatry.2011.37
7. Joyce P, Mulder RT, Luty SE, et al. Borderline personality disorder in major depression: symptomatology, temperament, character, differential drug response, and 6-month outcome. *Compr Psychiatry* 2003; 44:35–43. https://doi.org/10.1053/comp.2003.50001
8. McEwen BS, Nasca C, Gray JD. Stress effects on neuronal structure: hippocampus, amygdala and prefrontal cortex. *Neuropsychopharmacology* 2016; 41: 3–23. https://doi.org/10.1038/npp.2015.171

9. McLaughlin KA, Sheridan MA, Gold AL. Maltreatment exposure, brain structure and fear conditioning in children and adolescents. *Neuropsychopharmacology* 2016; 41: 1956–65. https://doi.org/10.1038/npp.2015.365

10. Mercer D, Douglass A, Links P. Meta-analyses of mood stabilizers, antidepressants, and antipsychotics in the treatment of borderline personality disorder: effectiveness for depression and anger symptoms. *J Pers Disord* 2009; 23:156–74. https://doi.org/10.1521/pedi.2009.23.2.156

11. Teicher MH, Anderson CM, Ohashi K. Childhood maltreatment: altered network centrality of cingulate precuneus, temporal pole and insula. *Biol Psychiatry* 2014; 76:297–305. https://doi.org/10.1016/j.biopsych.2013.09.016

12. Tyrka AR, Burgers DE, Philip NS. The neurobiological correlates of childhood adversity and implications for treatment. *Acta Psychiatric Scand* 2013138:434–47. https://doi.org/10.1111/acps.12143.

Case 30: The student who wanted to go to rehab

The Question: How do you manage a patient with benzodiazepine withdrawal seizure?

The Psychopharmacological Dilemma: How to delineate whether the patient has benzodiazepine withdrawal psychosis or cannabis-induced psychosis in an 18-year-old male who presented with seizure

Eduardo Javier, Louis May, and Martin Sahakyan

Pretest self-assessment question (answer at the end of the case)

Which of the following is not a symptom of both cannabis and benzodiazepine withdrawal?

A. Seizures
B. Irritability
C. Sleep disorders
D. Diaphoresis

Patient evaluation on intake

- An 18-year-old healthy male who was taken to the emergency department by his aunt for alteration in mental status, anxiety, and strange behavior
- At the emergency department, the patient had one episode of witnessed tonic–clonic seizure lasting a few minutes, controlled by intravenous (IV) lorazepam (Ativan) 1 mg. A computed tomography (CT) scan of the head was negative for any anatomic abnormality. Postseizure, the patient did not exhibit any focal neurological deficits or postictal confusion. The initial workup in the emergency department was consistent with encephalopathy, hypernatremia, rhabdomyolysis, and anion gap metabolic acidosis, which was attributed to the seizure
- The patient was admitted with lorazepam 1 mg IV every 4 hours as needed for seizures. A urine drug screen was positive for benzodiazepine and cannabis
- On day 2 of hospitalization, the patient was noted to have visual and auditory hallucinations; he was alert but oriented to self only. Diazepam (Valium) 10 mg PO three times per day was initiated. His initial laboratory derangements were improving. A sitter at the bedside was ordered. Psychiatry and addiction medicine consults were requested

Psychiatric history

- The patient had no formal psychiatric diagnosis but he had suicidal intent and a plan about 6 years ago. He has had no suicide attempts
- He was seen by a therapist for a short period of time during high school after being expelled from school for selling marijuana to other students

Substance use history

- The patient reports experimenting with alcohol but denies any use in the past couple of weeks. He also reports that he has used alcohol since middle school, around age 13, but it is not his drug of choice. His aunt reports that the patient has extensive alcohol use; she has found tequila bottles in his room many times over the previous 2 years
- Sedative hypnotics/anxiolytics: the patient admits to consuming alprazolam (Xanax) 6–8 mg every other day on average for the past 6 months, with the first use at age 14. He reports that he stopped "cold turkey" a couple of days prior to admission. The patient buys alprazolam in the street but reports that he tests all his tablets with an at-home kit for fentanyl prior to using
- The patient admit to using cannabis wax, up to 1 g per day, every day, for the last 8 months. The time of use is all day. His first use was age 13. The patient reports that he started using marijuana in middle school but did not start daily use until 8 months ago. He has a marijuana card but the qualifying illness was unknown

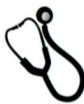

Medical history

- None

Medication history

- None

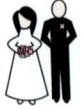

Social and personal history

- His parents are separated, but, due to an unsafe living environment, he lived with his aunt for 7 years until recently when he turned 18 and moved in with his father and grandmother. He never felt that he was welcome at his aunt's house

Family history

- Father with methamphetamine and opioid use disorder
- Mother with alcohol and methamphetamine use disorder

Current medications

- Lorazepam (Ativan) 1 mg IV every 4 hours as needed for seizure
- Ondansetron (Zofran) 4 mg IV every 8 hours as needed for vomiting
- Potassium chloride 40 mEq three times per day for hypokalemia
- Diazepam (Valium) 10 mg PO three times per day

Further investigation

Is there anything else you would specifically like to know about this patient?

- Collateral information: while an intervention was planned for the patient's father that day, the patient was observed to be acting strangely and was having delusions and hallucinations, so efforts were redirected toward the patient and he brought him to the ER instead of the father. He was seen pacing around his bedroom and having conversations with nobody in the room. The patient told his family that he needed to hide given that he owed a lot of money to "some people," but when asked about how much money, he responded that it was $100. He told his aunt that he also wanted to go to rehab; his room was searched and he stayed at his aunt's house so did not have access to alprazolam (Xanax) for 2 days during his stay. It was reported that he did not sleep at all. His aunt reported that the day before admission, he went running out of the house screaming and was very agitated. His symptoms worsened so he was brought to the emergency department and had a seizure while he was being evaluated
- During the initial consultation, the patient was noted to be calm, responsive, alert, hypervigilant, easy to startle, and oriented to self only. Very prominent mydriasis was observed. He had auditory hallucinations of people talking to him, but he knew they were not real; he thought he was at home and his father was next door. A sitter was placed at his bedside who reported that he had not slept since the night before. He was re-oriented as needed

Question

Why is the patient having auditory and visual hallucinations (hearing and seeing family members who are not there)?

- Metabolic encephalopathy
- Benzodiazepine withdrawal psychosis
- Cannabis-induced psychosis
- Undiagnosed psychotic disorder
- Severe sleep deprivation

Attending physician's mental notes: initial evaluation

- When did the symptoms start – days after he stopped alprazolam (Xanax) or was it happening prior to discontinuation of alprazolam? Benzodiazepine withdrawal delirium and psychosis should be considered if it happened hours to days after a distinct discontinuation period of the substance
- Cannabis can unmask an undiagnosed psychiatric disorder; the duration and strength of cannabis have a dose–response relationship
- Cannabis can cause psychosis if laced with phencyclidine or other psychotomimetic agents
- His current metabolic derangement can cause encephalopathy that could present with delirium
- However, the patient has persistent hallucinations, even after a few doses of lorazepam upon admission
- According to the nursing staff, the patient has not slept for 4 days and sleep deprivation can lead to symptoms that resemble psychosis. Prolonged sleep loss is both a precursor and a precipitant to psychosis
- After several doses of lorazepam (Ativan) and diazepam (Valium), the patient continued to have hallucinations
- He did not exhibit other autonomic overactivity symptoms such as increased heart rate, elevated blood pressure, diaphoresis, or tremors that are seen in benzodiazepine withdrawal
- The patient was cooperative and did not exhibit increased anxiety or irritability, and was directable

Questions

Would you continue diazepam (Valium) on the same dose?
- Yes, continue the same dose to observe for response
- No, increase the dose
- No, change it to another benzodiazepine
- No, start antipsychotics

Would you start medications for cannabis withdrawal syndrome?
- No, it should be minimal
- Yes, it might help with his sleep
- No, try to minimize psychoactive medications if possible
- Yes, it could be an adjunct to benzodiazepine

Would you start an antipsychotic?
- No, just close observation for now
- Yes, start with a very low dose
- No, they lower the seizure threshold
- Yes, it is warranted at this time

Attending physician's mental notes: initial evaluation (continued)

- The diazepam dose and frequency were continued because it may take several doses to achieve a therapeutic dose. Continue IV lorazepam (Ativan) as needed for actual seizure for rapid onset of action
- The patient was started with gabapentin (Neurontin) 300 mg three times per day for cannabis withdrawal symptoms, as it has been shown to ameliorate symptoms and decrease craving. It can also act as an adjunct to treatment of benzodiazepine withdrawal symptoms
- Quetiapine (Seroquel) 50 mg at bedtime was added to help the patient sleep and also could be used for benzodiazepine withdrawal delirium/psychosis. It also does not lower the seizure threshold, unlike other more commonly used antipsychotics

Case outcome: first interim follow-up visit at day 1

- The sitter reports that the patient slept well the night before
- The patient was more engaging and responsive with good eye contact. He answered questions more appropriately and was coherent with fair impulse control
- He denies depression and anxiety
- His hallucinations, delusions, and mydriasis have improved. His vital signs remained stable, with no recurrence of seizure

Attending physician's mental notes: second interim follow-up visit at day 1

- The patient continues his overall improvement
- Addressing withdrawal symptoms of each individual substance with the objective of augmenting the effect of the other medication has helped in his rapid recovery
- Being able to closely monitor the patient's response at the hospital has helped to titrate medications accordingly
- Sleep has also been essential to his recovery, which highlights the healing benefits of having a good night's sleep; this can often be aggravated in the inpatient setting due to frequent monitoring and interventions

Case debrief

- It is challenging to distinguish the causality of the problem when polysubstance dependence is involved, especially when most withdrawal symptoms overlap

- The patient's seizure was due to alprazolam (Xanax) discontinuation, but the hallucinations and delusion do not point to a particular substance except if you dig deeper into the temporal occurrence of the events after having collateral information from family members
- The patient's improvement was attributed to the combined administration of low doses of diazepam (Valium), quetiapine (Seroquel), and gabapentin (Neurontin) and allowing the patient to sleep by decreasing stimulation and providing a conducive environment
- The combination targets the individual withdrawal syndrome of each substance but also protects against the return of psychosis

Take-home points

- The most common symptoms associated with cannabis withdrawal are irritability, nervousness/anxiety, sleep difficulty, decreased appetite, and decreased mood (Table 30.1)
- Previous meta-analysis studies have confirmed a positive association between the extent of cannabis use and the risk for psychosis (odds ratio 3.9, 95% confidence interval 2.84–5.34)[5] (Table 30.2)
- Benzodiazepine withdrawal can happen in two stages (Table 30.3)
  - Symptoms of the early stage of benzodiazepine withdrawal are irritability, anxiety, insomnia, headache, anorexia, and perceptual disturbances
  - Later stages of benzodiazepine withdrawal present as psychosis, delirium, myoclonus, and seizure

Table 30.1 DSM-5 diagnostic criteria for cannabis withdrawal syndrome

A	Cessation of cannabis use that has been heavy and prolonged (usually daily or almost daily use over a period of at least a few months)
B	Three or more of the following signs and symptoms develop within approximately 1 week of criterion A: • Irritability, anger, or aggression • Nervousness or anxiety • Sleep difficulty (insomnia, disturbing dreams) • Decreased appetite or weight loss • Restlessness • Depressed mood • At least one of the following physical symptoms causing significant discomfort: abdominal pain, shakiness/tremors, sweating, fever, chills, or headache
C	The signs and symptoms from criterion B cause clinically significant distress or impairment in social, occupational or other important areas of functioning
D	The symptoms are not due to another medical condition and are not better explained by another mental disorder

Table 30.2 Adverse effects of short- and long-term or heavy use of cannabis

Effects of short-term use	Effects of long-term or heavy use
Impaired short-term memory, making it difficult to learn and retain information	Addiction (in about 9% of users overall, 17% of those who begin use in adolescence, and 25–50% of those who are daily users)
Impaired motor coordination, interfering with driving skills and increased risk of injuries	Altered brain development
	Poor educational outcome, with increased likelihood of dropping out of school
Altered judgment, increasing the risk of sexual behaviors that facilitate the transmission of sexually transmitted diseases	Cognitive impairment, with lower IQ among those who were frequent users during adolescence
	Diminished life satisfaction and achievement (determined on the basis of subjective and objective measures compared with such ratings in the general population)
In high doses, paranoia and psychosis	Symptoms of chronic bronchitis
	Increased risk of chronic disorders (including schizophrenia) in persons with a predisposition to such disorders

Table 30.3 Clinical symptoms and complications of benzodiazepine withdrawal

Psychopathological symptoms	Vegetative symptoms	Neurological and physical complications
Increased anxiety	Trembling	Increased risk of seizures
Sleep disorders	Sweating	Cognitive impairments
Inner restlessness	Nausea and vomiting	Pronounced perceptual impairments
Depressive symptoms	Motor agitation	Hyperacusis
Irritability	Dyspnea	Photophobia
Psychosis-like conditions, delirium	Increased heart rate	Hypersomnia
Depersonalization and derealization	Elevated blood pressure	Dysesthesia, muscle twitching, and fasciculations
Confusion	Headaches	
	Muscle tension	

- Symptoms are more abrupt and severe, and occur sooner in short-acting benzodiazepines such as alprazolam (Xanax) (start within 72 hours of the last dose)
- In our case, psychosis possibly presented earlier due to cannabis use, which was then exacerbated by benzodiazepine withdrawal
- Seizures are not documented with cannabis abuse with the exception of synthetic cannabinoids
- Taking into consideration that sleep deprivation can also be aggravated and precipitate psychotic symptoms that the patient exhibited, facilitating sleep both with pharmacological assistance and environmental adjustment was also of great importance

Performance in practice: confessions of a psychopharmacologist

What could have been done better here?

- A primary seizure workup would have been warranted if the patient did not return to baseline mental status and had neurological symptoms and postictal states. Brain magnetic resonance imaging (MRI) and an electroencephalogram (EEG) should have been done for completion of the workup
- Better coordination of care with the social worker and family to ensure the patient receives proper continuation of addiction treatment care postdischarge
- The patient has severe substance use disorder and needed more intensive treatment focusing on adolescents groups
- In-hospital initiation of psychosocial treatment would be desirable and a warm handoff to outpatient treatment to decrease the likelihood of dropout and ensure engagement with the addiction treatment program
- The patient might potentially benefit from daily delivery of inpatient motivation enhancement therapy
- Outpatient follow-up with psychiatry for a proper diagnostic workup and treatment of the underlying psychiatric disorder is advised as the risk of future psychotic events is high
- A more in-depth investigation of the family history of psychiatric disorders would be of benefit

Tips and pearls

- Benzodiazepines are relatively safe for short-term use (2–4 weeks), but their safety has not been established beyond that period, and dependence develops in approximately half of patients who use benzodiazepines for longer than 1 month
- The incidence of cannabis-induced psychosis and dependence increases as the concentration of tetrahydrocannabinol increases
- The full range of long-term consequences of high-tetrahydrocannabinol cannabis is not fully understood

Mechanism of action moment

Benzodiazepines and psychosis

- γ-Aminobutyric acid (GABA) is the chief inhibitory neurotransmitter of the central nervous system. It mediates this effect via the $GABA_A$ receptor. These receptors are present in many brain regions, including the thalamus, limbic structures, and cerebral cortex. Benzodiazepines exert their effect via modulation of the $GABA_A$

receptor. They bind at the interface of the α- and γ-subunits and lock the $GABA_A$ receptor into a conformation that increases its affinity for GABA neurotransmitters. Benzodiazepines do not alter the synthesis, release, or metabolism of GABA but rather potentiate its inhibitory actions by augmenting receptor binding. This binding increases the flow of chloride ions through the GABA ion channel, causing postsynaptic hyperpolarization and a decreased ability to initiate an action potential. This inhibition of neuropotentials causes a slowing effect within the involved pathways. Alprazolam (Xanax) is thought to have approximately 10 times the anxiolytic effect of diazepam (Valium) on a milligram-for-milligram basis, as it has a higher affinity for the benzodiazepine $GABA_A$ receptor.

- With long-term use of benzodiazepines, there is a compensatory decrease in GABA at the level of the synaptic cleft. The sudden removal of stimulation of this receptor pathway, as seen in states of withdrawal, results in less inhibition of excitatory neurotransmitters, and thus there is a pro-excitatory state. Various monoaminergic systems can be affected that include emotional, cognitive, perceptual, and autonomic pathways. Symptoms of withdrawal after long-term benzodiazepine use usually develop faster with shorter-acting agents (within 2–3 days) than with longer-acting agents (within 5–10 days). Most withdrawal symptoms are associated with a state of brain hyperexcitability and can be divided into physical, psychological, and sensory symptoms.

Gabapentin for cannabis withdrawal management

- Cannabis is the most commonly used illicit drug in the USA. Cannabis dependence is marked by compulsive use, inability to stop despite harmful consequences, and the emergence of a withdrawal syndrome upon cessation of use. Currently, there are no approved medications for the treatment of cannabis use disorder. Nevertheless, various pharmaceuticals have been studied in small ($n<80$) controlled, mostly outpatient or laboratory pilot trials: lithium, antidepressants (bupropion (Wellbutrin), nefazodone (Serzone), venlafaxine (Effexor), fluoxetine (Prozac), escitalopram (Lexapro), and mirtazapine (Remeron)), anticonvulsants (divalproex sodium (Depakote) and gabapentin (Neurontin)), norepinephrine reuptake inhibitor (atomoxetine (Strattera)), glutamate modulator and mucolytic agents (*N*-acetylcysteine), muscle relaxants (baclofen), anxiolytics (buspirone (BuSpar)), antipsychotics (quetiapine (Seroquel)), and cannabinoid receptor agonists (dronabinol and nabiximols).
- Gabapentin is an alkylated analog of GABA. It acts by blocking a specific $\alpha_2\delta$-subunit of the voltage-gated calcium channel at

selective presynaptic sites and, as a result, modulates the release of excitatory neurotransmitters that participate in epileptogenesis and nociception. Preclinical findings suggest that gabapentin normalizes the corticotropin-releasing factor-induced GABA activation in the amygdala. This activation is associated with the development of dependence on alcohol and, by extrapolation, on cannabis, because cannabis withdrawal, like alcohol withdrawal, produces both an anxiogenic-like state and increased extrahypothalamic corticotropin-releasing factor release in the central nucleus of the amygdala in rodents

Pharmacology of quetiapine

- Quetiapine is a dibenzothiazepine atypical antipsychotic. It has been proposed that this drug's antipsychotic activity is mediated through a combination of dopamine D_2 and serotonin 5-HT_2 antagonism. It is an antagonist at multiple neurotransmitter receptors in the brain: 5-HT_{1A} and 5-HT_2, D_1 and D_2, histamine H_1, and α_1- and α_2-adrenergic receptors, but appears to have no appreciable affinity at cholinergic muscarinic and benzodiazepine receptors. Norquetiapine, an active metabolite, differs from its parental molecule by exhibiting high affinity for muscarinic M_1 receptors
- Antagonism at receptors other than dopamine and 5-HT_2 with similar receptor affinities may explain some of the other effects of quetiapine. The drug's antagonism of H_1 receptors may explain the somnolence observed. The drug's antagonism of α_1-adrenergic receptors may explain the orthostatic hypotension observed

Psychosis and sleep deprivation

- Psychotic symptoms develop with increasing time awake, from simple visual/somatosensory misperceptions to hallucinations and delusions, ending in a condition resembling acute psychosis. These experiences are likely to resolve after a period of sleep, although more information is required to identify factors that can contribute to the prevention of persistent symptoms

Posttest self-assessment question and answer

Which of the following is not a symptom of both cannabis and benzodiazepine withdrawal?

A. Seizures
B. Irritability
C. Sleep disorders
D. Diaphoresis

Answer: A

Seizures happen with benzodiazepine withdrawal due to loss of GABAergic inhibition and predominance of excitatory neurotransmission. Irritability is seen following withdrawal of both substances due to dysphoria following discontinuation. Sleep disorders can manifest as hypersomnia or insomnia with cannabis use and rebound insomnia after discontinuation of benzodiazepines. Diaphoresis occurs following withdrawal of both due to autonomic hyperactivity as a result of a heightened stress response with activation of the hypothalamus by the amygdala during the withdrawal stage. Withdrawal seizure is only seen with benzodiazepine withdrawals syndrome; it could manifest in cannabis intoxication but not in cannabis withdrawals.

References

1. Bonnet U, Preuss UW. The cannabis withdrawal syndrome: current insights. *Subst Abuse Rehabil* 2017; 8:9–37. https://doi.org/10.2147/SAR.S109576
2. DeVane C, Nemeroff CB. Clinical pharmacokinetics of quetiapine: an atypical antipsychotic. *Clin Pharmacokinet* 2001; 40:509–22. https://doi.org/10.2165/00003088-200140070-00003
3. Freiberger JJ, Marsicano TH. Alprazolam withdrawal presenting as delirium after cardiac surgery. *J Cardiothorac Vasc Anesth* 1991; 5:150–2. https://doi.org/10.1016/1053-0770(91)90329-r
4. Lann MA, Molina DK. A fatal case of benzodiazepine withdrawal. *Am J Forensic Med Pathol* 2009; 3:177–9. https://doi.org/10.1097/PAF.0b013e3181875aa0
5. Marconi A, Di Forti M, Lewis CM, et al. Meta-analysis of the association between the level of cannabis use and risk of psychosis. *Schizophr Bull* 2016; 42:1262–9. https://doi.org/10.1093/schbul/sbw003
6. Mason BJ, Crean R, Goodell V, et al. A proof-of-concept randomized controlled study of gabapentin: effects on cannabis use, withdrawal and executive function deficits in cannabis-dependent adults. *Neuropsychopharmacology* 2012; 37:1689–98. https://doi.org/10.1038/npp.2012.14
7. Ortiz-Medina MB, Perea M, Torales J, et al. Cannabis consumption and psychosis or schizophrenia development. *Int J Soc Psychiatry* 2018; 64:690–704. https://doi.org/10.1177/0020764018801690
8. Pierre JM, Gandal M, Son M. Cannabis-induced psychosis associated with high potency "wax dabs". *Schizophr Res* 2016; 172:211–12. https://doi.org/10.1016/j.schres.2016.01.056

9. Sherman BJ, McRae-Clark AL. Treatment of cannabis use disorder: current science and future outlook. *Pharmacotherapy* 2016; 36:511–35. https://doi.org/10.1002/phar.1747
10. Soyka M. Treatment of benzodiazepine dependence. *N Engl J Med* 2017; 376:1147–57. https://doi.org/10.1056/NEJMra1611832
11. Waters F, Chiu V, Atkinson A, Blom JD. Severe sleep deprivation causes hallucinations and a gradual progression toward psychosis with increasing time awake. *Front Psychiatry* 2018; 9:303. https://doi.org/10.3389/fpsyt.2018.00303

Case 31: The boy who wouldn't (couldn't) listen

The Question: What do you do when nothing you try works?

The Psychopharmacological Dilemma: How to achieve diagnostic clarity and treatment simplicity through layers of reported symptoms in a child

Alex J. Mageno, Bo Ram Yoo, and Richard J. Lee

Pretest self-assessment question (answer at the end of the case)

Which of the following disorders does NOT have significant phenomenological overlap with posttraumatic stress disorder (PTSD) in children and adolescents?

A. Bipolar disorder
B. Attention-deficit/hyperactivity disorder (ADHD)
C. Conduct disorder
D. Social anxiety disorder
E. Major depressive disorder (MDD)
F. None of the above (symptoms of all can have significant overlap with PTSD symptoms)

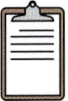

Patient evaluation on intake

- A 7-year-old male in foster care referred by his Child Protective Services social worker for management of his current psychiatric medication prescribed for bipolar disorder
- The patient has a history of physical abuse and neglect including being found with several scars of cigarette burns around his extremities. His caregiver reports the chief complaint of "he can't sit still" and reports being at her "wits' end." She has noted worsening behavior over recent months and notes the "current medications aren't working"

Psychiatric history

- The patient has been in his current foster home for over a year and has shown worsening of his behavior over the past 9 months
- He has been severely aggressive in his 2nd-grade class and recently kicked his school teacher and attempted to choke a peer. He has had multiple suspensions from school for these behaviors
- He is very impulsive and has run away from supervision at school. He has a hard time keeping his hands to himself
- His caregiver describes the patient as very hyperactive and "always on the go"
- The patient has a short attention span and is behind his peers academically in reading and math

- Additionally, he has a history of urinating and defecating around the house and has smeared feces in his bedroom and the bathroom
- He has been sexually inappropriate with peers, touching their buttocks, and frequently touches his own private parts
- The patient has a hard time making and keeping friends
- The patient describes his moods as mostly "happy." He denies any suicidal or homicidal ideation. His caregiver describes anger outbursts and irritability
- He did not admit to any psychotic thoughts on the initial visit. Overall, he was a poor historian. He responded to many questions with "I don't know"
- The patient has problems falling asleep and has complained of nightmares. He wanders the house at night
- Limited information was available about past treatments. The caregiver reported a record of atomoxetine (Strattera) making things "much worse"
- The patient has had medication trials in the past

Current medications

- Clonidine (Catapres) 0.1 mg twice per day
- Aripiprazole (Abilify) 10 mg at bedtime

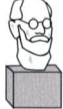

Psychotherapy history

- The patient was last receiving "wraparound services" and individual therapy at a non-profit agency serving foster children
- He had been placed 2 years ago, at the age of 5, in a residential treatment facility
- No other information was available on the first visit

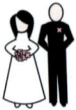

Social and personal history

- The patient was attending 2nd grade in a regular classroom. He had an active Individual Educational Plan (IEP) but details of the IEP were not available. The patient was in the process of getting referred to a non-public school due to frequent and severe behavioral problems
- The patient had been removed from his mother's custody due to neglect at age 2. The patient was placed with his grandmother for 2 years and returned to his mother where the patient had documented physical abuse
- The patient had been in eight prior foster homes and one prior residential treatment placement
- He only has occasional visits with a maternal aunt. He does not have regular visits with his mother or grandmother
- The patient has an interest in baseball and playing outside

PATIENT FILE

Medical history

- No medical problems at present
- The patient has a history of physical abuse, with documented burn scars and report of a prior "head injury"
- He is up to date with vaccinations and has no standing medications
- Blood pressure 98/61 mmHg, pulse 82 bpm, height 50", weight 59 lbs, with a body mass index of BMI 20 kg/m²

Family history

- Mother with a history of bipolar disorder and cocaine/methamphetamine use. No information available on the father
- Maternal grandmother with a history of depression

Patient evaluation on initial visit

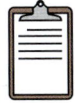

- The patient was friendly and made good eye contact
- He appeared to be respectful of and attached to his caregiver
- He spoke in short sentences, mostly responding "I don't know"
- He was restless and fidgety at times but was able to remain seated throughout the initial session
- He reported feeling "happy"
- His range of affect was constricted and neutral
- He had no current suicidal ideation, delusions, hallucinations, or thought disorder
- He reported no bad side effects to his medication

Questions

Based only on what you have been told so far about this patient's history and current symptoms, would you consider him to fall within the bipolar spectrum?

- Yes
- No

Would you continue his "mood-stabilizing" medications?
- Yes, continue aripiprazole (Abilify)
- No, discontinue aripiprazole

Attending physician's mental notes: initial evaluation

- Rather than bipolar disorder, is there more of a unifying diagnosis in this case?
- A response to medication alone may be particularly unlikely for a patient with such significant trauma history and disruptive behaviors

- Clearly, there is a history of significant trauma, likely including sexual abuse
- The presenting chief complaint is around ADHD symptoms (hyperactivity, poor focus, impulsivity)
- Many of the reported behaviors are also consistent with trauma-related disorders (sexual behaviors, sleep difficulty, fecal/urinary behaviors, social difficulties, inattention)

Question

Despite taking several psychotropic medications, the patient does not appear to have robust efficacy, nor does he report bad side effects. Which of the following would be your next step?

- Change medication strategies
- Continue the current medications and augment further
- Recommend restarting cognitive behavioral therapy (CBT) with a new therapist
- Recommend other interventions

Attending physician's mental notes: initial evaluation (continued)

- As mentioned, some form of treatment in addition to medication is likely to be necessary for this patient; however, it may also be beneficial to adjust his current medication regimen
- The patient is taking aripiprazole (Abilify) without a clear response toward current target symptoms. This could be because the dosages are inadequate, or the medication could be targeting the wrong symptoms and wrong diagnosis
- The current complaints describe significant ADHD and conduct disorder symptoms. Clonidine (Catapres) immediate-release 0.1 mg twice per day is likely not an effective level of medication for his current ADHD symptoms
- The initial plan was to treat the ADHD symptoms with a stimulant, lisdexamfetamine (Vyvanse), and to change clonidine to guanfacine (Tenex) (longer half-life); however, public insurance would not cover first-line clonidine extended-release or guanfacine

Question

Is there anything else you would especially like to know about this patient?

- The caregiver in this case was not the parent or guardian and did not have all records of past treatment. In cases like these, it is imperative to obtain all past psychiatric records, past educational records, prior psychological testing, and past medical records, including pediatric neurological records

- At age 4, the patient was hospitalized for ongoing dysregulated behavior, acting out, and aggression toward self and others. He was discharged on guanfacine 1 mg twice per day and prazosin (Minipress) 1 mg at bedtime. The patient had complained of a "ghost monster" at night and also had a history of urinating and defecating throughout the house. He would kick, scream, and hit others
- The patient had recent psychological testing. The Wechsler Intelligence Scale for Children (WISC) IV revealed his Full-Scale IQ was 97. He had been evaluated for special education and did not qualify under learning disability but did qualify under emotional and behavioral disturbances due to ADHD and PTSD
- The patient had been evaluated by pediatric neurology. He demonstrated age-appropriate social cues with no neurological deficits. Further workup for any historical head trauma was not indicated
- The patient had a history of poor sleep and possibly sleepwalking. A sleep study may be helpful

Case outcome: first interim follow-up visit at week 4

- The patient appears not to be tolerating lisdexamfetamine (Vyvanse) well; he complains of feeling twitchy and achy. He has been picking at his skin. He remains hyperactive overall
- His caregiver has seen his behavior as bizarre, and reports he is talking to himself as well
- Because stimulants can sometimes cause picking, tics, and restlessness, the decision was made to discontinue lisdexamfetamine
- There was some concern, given that aripiprazole (Abilify) had been discontinued, about whether the above symptoms were psychotic in nature or related to PTSD

Questions

Would you continue his ADHD treatments?

- Yes, continue both lisdexamfetamine (Vyvanse) and guanfacine (Tenex)
- Continue guanfacine but discontinue lisdexamfetamine
- Continue lisdexamfetamine but discontinue guanfacine

Would you restart an antipsychotic at this point?

- Yes
- No

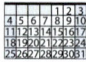

Case outcome: first interim follow-up visit at week 4 (continued)

- Lisdexamfetamine (Vyvanse) was discontinued
- The dose of guanfacine (Tenex) was increased to 2 mg twice per day
- There was no clear indication for an antipsychotic as the patient was calm and did not admit to any psychotic symptoms

Question

In addition to the adjustments to medications, which of the following would you be most likely to recommend to this patient?

- CBT
- Wraparound services
- Behavioral therapy
- Both CBT and behavioral therapy
- Both CBT and wraparound services
- All of the above

Case outcome: second interim follow-up visit at week 6

- The patient has regressed again behaviorally. He has been very hyperactive and more defiant. He has been inappropriate with other household members. He remains unable to sleep and wanders the house at night
- His caregiver complains that guanfacine (Tenex) is "not working"
- He was started on dexmethylphenidate extended-release (XR) (Focalin XR) 10 mg in the morning and recommended a trial of diphenhydramine (Benadryl) as needed for sleep

Attending physician's mental notes

- Most likely, these symptoms are not psychotic, but, in fact, related to the patient's past trauma. Children with a history of trauma commonly demonstrate fecal/urinary behaviors related to past abuse or neglect

Case outcome: third interim follow-up visit at week 10

- His caregiver continued to complain that medications are not working
- The patient did not sleep with diphenhydramine (Benadryl)
- His caregiver complains that since starting dexmethylphenidate XR (Focalin-XR) he has not had tics, but he has also been more hyperactive than before

- He remains out of control at home, acting bizarrely, urinating on the carpet, and staying up all night; he is at high risk of loss of placement
- Quetiapine (Seroquel) 100 mg at bedtime was started in an attempt to address possible psychosis and help the patient sleep
- Dexmethylphenidate and diphenhydramine were discontinued
- Guanfacine (Tenex) was restarted

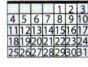

Case outcome: fourth interim follow-up visit at week 13

- Quetiapine (Seroquel) did not improve the patient's sleep and there was no improvement in behaviors, so quetiapine was discontinued
- The patient was still hyperactive but more manageable each day
- Guanfacine (Tenex) was increased back to 2 mg twice per day
- The patient is now on only guanfacine

Case outcome: fifth interim follow-up visit at week 14

- A sleep study was normal and sleep was gradually improving on guanfacine (Tenex) monotherapy
- Intensive behavioral services was added and a wraparound team was established
- The school setting was changed to a non-public behavioral school
- The target symptoms of hyperactivity were reduced
- His conduct problems related to past trauma are likely to take many more months/years to fully resolve, but may resolve with continued therapies and behavioral services

Case debrief

- The patient was referred primarily so that a psychiatrist could continue his currently prescribed medications. He had had multiple trials of medication without any clear benefit
- The target symptoms were primarily related to hyperactivity, distractibility, and conduct disorder-type behaviors, with his working diagnosis as bipolar disorder and his current pharmacotherapy an antipsychotic
- Initially, aripiprazole (Abilify) was stopped, and guanfacine (Tenex) replaced the current clonidine (Catapres) because of its longer half-life; lisdexamfetamine (Vyvanse) was started in an attempt to better control his ADHD symptoms
- Lisdexamfetamine was not well tolerated, with severe side effects and no improvement in hyperactivity or attention. Dexmethylphenidate XR (Focalin-XR) was also tried, but there was similarly no improvement in ADHD symptoms on this medication

- The patient had always had poor sleep and would wander the house at night. A trial of diphenhydramine (Benadryl) did not help his sleep and a brief trial of quetiapine (Seroquel) was attempted to try and control his symptoms of insomnia and to address possible psychotic behaviors
- After months of medication changes, the patient ended up on guanfacine 4 mg per day as monotherapy and benefited primarily from social services, therapy, and a more therapeutic school environment

Take-home points

- It is important to realize that children in the foster care setting are prescribed psychotropic medications at rates that are two to five times higher than in other children, including children in families of low economic status
  - One-third of low-income children and half of children in foster care are prescribed two or more antipsychotics
  - Commercially insured children with an autism diagnosis also have high rates of polypharmacy with one-third receiving two or more antipsychotics and 15% receiving three or more
  - One-third of children with autism under the age of 1 year are already receiving psychotropic medication(s)
- It is also true that foster children are at risk of underidentification and undertreatment of mental health issues and that there is likely a higher-than-average rate of disorders in this population. Therefore, while some higher rate of psychotropic use is likely indicated, special thought and care should be taken when diagnosing and treating foster care children. Remember that because they are a vulnerable population, they are rarely studied directly, and most treatment recommendations are actually based on adult studies or children in very different populations
- Foster homes differ in their level of experience and aptitude in dealing with the behaviors common among traumatized children. Education prior to placement about any and all possible expressions of past trauma is important. Foster families should be aware that hyperactivity, distractibility, poor ability to form relationships, and behavioral outbursts are common. If it appears they may need more education, consider providing them with resources such as The National Child Traumatic Stress Network (www.NCTSN.org), which provides education and training on trauma with the goal of raising the standard of care and improving access to services for traumatized children, their families, and communities

- Symptoms of hyperactivity and distractibility can easily be interpreted as ADHD; however, when a trauma history is present, remember that these may also be symptoms of underlying PTSD. Consider what it might be like trying to focus on reading or remembering chores when your mental framework has taught you the world is not safe and you are constantly "on edge"
- Some behaviors that are often seen as psychotic in adults, such as urinating and defecating in the bedroom or home, as well as quasi-psychotic phenomena such as talking to oneself or blurring the lines between reality and imagination, may also be behavioral problems based in the patient's severely interrupted development
- "Nothing facilitates the right answer like asking the right question," or rather, "nothing facilitates the best treatment like the correct diagnosis." The patient's primary symptoms were likely not due to bipolar disorder or ADHD, as treatments that are typically beneficial in such cases had many side effects and little efficacy. More likely, such behaviors in this patient were rooted in the early derailment of attachment and development and were better addressed by a multidisciplinary, trauma-informed care team

Tips and pearls

- Children need to feel safe in order to focus on learning/attention. Therefore, consider the following interventions, which may be more effective than medications:
  - Improving the living and/or educational environment
  - Reducing repetitive stress, poverty, abuse, and neglect
  - Reducing exposure to community violence and extreme poverty whenever possible
- Initiating trauma-informed care can be especially helpful in these children and adolescents, and will probably lead to better outcomes
- Be vigilant to irrational polypharmacy and simplify medication regimens whenever possible rather than just adding more medications

Mechanism of action moment

- Guanfacine (Tenex), a non-stimulant, is currently approved by the FDA for the treatment of ADHD in children and adolescents. It is also used off label to treat conduct disorder, motor tics, oppositional defiant disorder, and developmental disorders
- Guanfacine is a selective agonist of the central α-adrenergic receptors in the prefrontal cortex, which is responsible for planning, impulse control, working memory, and decision-making

Unlike clonidine (Catapres), which broadly acts on α_1, α_2, and β-adrenergic receptors, guanfacine binds to α_{2A} receptors (mostly localized in the brain) with the highest affinity. This increases the efficacy of guanfacine and reduces its side effects, making it a more favorable drug for treatment

- ADHD is characterized by dysfunctional dopamine pathways, which are associated with impulsivity and short reward duration. The norepinephrine pathways, which are associated with emotions, sleep, and the ability to adapt to stress, come from the locus coeruleus. Normally, the phasic release of norepinephrine by the locus coeruleus allows for focused attention. However, in ADHD, norepinephrine is released in a tonic fashion, increasing background noise and making it difficult to focus attention

- When guanfacine stimulates α_{2A} receptors, cyclic AMP levels increase and hyperpolarization-activated cyclic nucleotide channels close. This enhances prefrontal cortex function and allows better regulation of attention and behaviors

- Studies suggest that those who are traumatized or show PTSD symptoms have increased noradrenergic activity, which is associated with anxiety and hyperarousal symptoms. In children, this may manifest as sleep disturbance, irritability, and aggression. Guanfacine may improve these symptoms by mimicking the action of norepinephrine at the postsynaptic α_{2A} receptors and strengthening the norepinephrine connectivity

- Common side effects of guanfacine are dry mouth, drowsiness, sedation, and headache, but the drug has overall been well tolerated. Increasing the dose has not been associated with greater severity or an increased number of side effects

Posttest self-assessment question and answer

Which of the following disorders does NOT have significant phenomenological overlap with PTSD?

A. Bipolar disorder
B. ADHD
C. Conduct disorder
D. Social anxiety disorder
E. MDD
F. None of the above (symptoms of all can have significant overlap with PTSD symptoms)

Answer: F

All of the above can have symptoms that overlap with PTSD. Trauma affects the psyche and body in many ways, some of which can be confused with symptoms of other disorders, such as an inability to focus due to constant flashbacks being confused with ADHD; or pronounced irritability and decreased mood, which may be confused with MDD. In severe trauma or neglect, there can be accompanying social anxiety better explained by the trauma disorder than a straightforward social anxiety disorder. Rapid mood changes and poor affect regulation might sometimes be considered bipolar symptoms but could perhaps be better explained by a trauma-related disorder if trauma is also present. Finally, defiance or frequent acting out, and even violence or deceit, can be behaviors present in a traumatized child who doesn't meet all criteria for conduct disorder. Of course, all diagnoses should be considered, and an individual child may indeed have PTSD and MDD, or PTSD and ADHD. But one should always be aware of the impact of trauma and at least consider if it may unify multiple diagnoses and lead to a more complete treatment plan.

References

1. Alamo C, Lopez-Munoz F, Sanchez-Garcia J. Mechanism of action of guanfacine: a postsynaptic differential approach to the treatment of attention deficit hyperactivity disorder (ADHD). *Actas Esp Psiquiatr* 2016; 44:107–12.

2. American Academy of Child and Adolescent Psychiatry. Appropriate use of antipsychotic medication for children in foster care. 2018. Available from: https://www.aacap.org/AACAP/Policy_Statements/2018/Appropriate_Use_of_Psychiatric_Medication_for_Youth_in_Foster_Care.aspx (accessed March 26, 2021).

3. Cohen JA, Bukstein O, Walter H, et al. Practice parameter for the assessment and treatment of children and adolescents with posttraumatic stress disorder. *J Am Acad Child Adolesc Psychiatry* 2010; 49:414–30.

4. Connor DF, Grasso DJ, Slivinsky MD, et al., An open-label study of guanfacine extended release for traumatic stress related symptoms in children and adolescents. *J Child Adolesc Psychopharmacol* 2013; 23: 244–51. https://doi.org/10.1089/cap.2012.0119

5. Dosreis S, Yoon Y, Rubin DM, et al. Antipsychotic treatment among youth in foster care. *Pediatrics*. 2011; 128:e1459–66. https://doi.org/10.1542/peds.2010-2970

6. Lieberman A, van Horn P. *Psychotherapy of Infants and Young Children: Repairing the Effects of Stress and Trauma on Early Attachment*. New York, NY: Guilford Press, 2008.

7. Stahl SM. Guanfacine. In: *Stahl's Essential Psychopharmacology: Prescriber's Guide*, 6th edn. Cambridge, UK: Cambridge University Press, 2017; pp. 319–22.

8. Stein REK, Hurlburt MS, Heneghan AM, et al. For better or worse? Change in service use by children investigated by child welfare over a decade. *Acad Pediatr* 2016; 16:240–6. https://doi.org/10.1016/j.acap.2016.01.019

Case 32: The patient who went streaking

The Question: Is the patient having delirium tremens or is something else going on?

The Psychopharmacological Dilemma: Agitation: methamphetamine withdrawal delirium versus benzodiazepine disinhibition syndrome

Louis May, Martin Sahakyan, and Eduardo Javier

Pretest self-assessment question (answer at the end of the case)

Which medication would be recommended for both amphetamine withdrawal delirium and benzodiazepine disinhibition syndrome in a patient with prolonged corrected QT interval (QTc) on an electrocardiogram (ECG)?

A. Thioridazine (Mellaril)
B. Olanzapine (Zyprexa)
C. Quetiapine (Seroquel)
D. Risperidone (Risperdal)

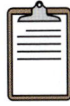

Patient evaluation on intake

- A 59-year-old male with initial complaints of chest pain and dyspnea, who became delirious on day 2 of hospitalization
- The patient went to the emergency room with the chief complaints of chest pain and shortness of breath. He was found to have atrial fibrillation with a rapid ventricular response, hypertension, and hypoxic respiratory failure with an O_2 saturation of 88% on ambient air
- On initial evaluation by the admitting team, he was alert, oriented with baseline mental status, cooperative, and able to provide a history; however on physical examination, he was also noted to have horizontal nystagmus, a computed tomography (CT) scan of the head showed possible subacute infarcts and follow-up magnetic resonance imaging (MRI) of the brain showed multifocal remote infarcts. He was given intravenous (IV) thiamine as well as morphine 4 mg IV single dose for chest pain and shortness of breath. A urine drug screen (UDS) done after morphine administration was positive for amphetamines and opiates

Case outcome: days 2–4 of hospitalization

- On day 2 of hospitalization, the patient was gradually becoming more restless and agitated. At some point during the course of the afternoon, he ran out of his room without a gown, appearing confused, disoriented, and unable to follow commands. The patient was also noted to become more tachycardic (heart rate >140 bpm) and hypertensive (systolic blood pressure 190 mmHg). An ECG showed atrial fibrillation with prolonged QTc

- Due to his history of alcohol use and it being the second day since his last alleged alcoholic drink, the patient was placed on a Clinical Institute Withdrawal Assessment of Alcohol, Revised (CIWA-Ar) protocol with an initial consideration of alcohol withdrawal delirium. His initial CIWA-Ar score was 14, accounting mostly for the agitation and anxiety; the patient was administered multiple doses of lorazepam (Ativan) as per the protocol and had to be placed in restraints. A bedside sitter was requested
- On day 3 of hospitalization, the patient became even more restless and agitated throughout the night, fighting his restraints, and was non-verbal and combative. He was given a total of lorazepam 5 mg IV. On physical examination, it was noted that he moved all extremities, had no focal findings, his pupils were normal and reactive, and nystagmus was absent
- On day 4 of hospitalization, the patient continued to deteriorate clinically. He remained on the CIWA-Ar protocol and was given a total of 14 mg IV lorazepam. The patient would calm down for a few minutes and then resume the behavior; he did not follow commands and was unable to drink or eat. At this point, addiction medicine was consulted for evaluation of withdrawal delirium

Psychiatric history

- He was diagnosed with depression 10 years ago and took fluoxetine (Prozac) for a short period of time. He was not on any medications on admission
- He denies suicidal ideations, intent, or plans
- He has had no prior psychiatric hospitalizations

Substance use history

- The patient smokes methamphetamine and cannabis daily
- He drinks three to four standard drinks according to his emergency department history, but this was not validated by the admitting team

Medical history

- Coronary artery disease
- Left ventricular systolic dysfunction with ejection fraction of 35%
- Hypertension
- Asthma
- Prior ischemic cerebral vascular accident

Medication history

- Apixaban 5 mg twice per day for secondary stroke prevention in the setting of atrial fibrillation
- Carvedilol (Coreg) 6.25 mg twice per day for rate control
- Diltiazem (Cardizem) 30 mg twice per day for rate control
- Furosemide (Lasix) 40 mg PO daily for heart failure with reduced ejection fraction
- Potassium chloride 20 mEq daily for anticipated potassium loss
- Lorazepam (Ativan) 1 mg daily

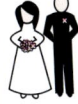

Social and personal history

- The patient has been homeless for the past 12 years following the financial crisis of 2008. His brother occasionally pays for hotel accommodation
- He is divorced from his wife and left his kids in her custody in 2008
- He has one friend who is close to him

Family history

- There are no known health problems or substance use disorder history

Question

Considering the worsening of or lack of improvement with the current management, what alternative diagnosis would you consider?

- Benzodiazepine paradoxical central nervous system (CNS) stimulation/benzodiazepine disinhibition
- Methamphetamine withdrawal delirium
- Hospital-acquired delirium
- Alcohol withdrawal delirium
- All of the above

Attending physician's mental notes: days 2–4 of hospitalization

- Due to the patient's mental status, it was a challenge to obtain a full detailed history, physical examination, and mental status examination, and therefore to come up with differential diagnoses and recommendations
- The patient was agitated, unable to give a reliable history, non-verbal, and on four-point restraints and actively fighting it, after lorazepam (Ativan) 14 mg IV. His heart rate was in the 140s, irregularly irregular, and his O_2 saturation was 96% at 2 l/minute with a nasal cannula

- What was the inciting event that caused the patient to run screaming out of the room naked? He was apparently at baseline mental status until 2 days after admission
- Why is the patient not sedated at this point? Is this resistant alcohol withdrawal? Is this a paradoxical benzodiazepine reaction? Is lorazepam helping at this point or making it worse?
- Are there any other causes of encephalopathy? What about viral encephalitis, or an evolving stroke? MRI showed multiple chronic infarcts and the patient was just started on anticoagulation for atrial fibrillation
- What about Wernicke–Korsakoff syndrome? The patient has a questionable alcohol history with the presence of nystagmus on admission; he was started on thiamine 500 mg IV every 8 hours and was decreased to 100 mg IV daily on hospital day 3
- How do I calm this patient down without compromising his respiratory and mental status?
- The UDS on admission was positive for opiates, but the patient is not exhibiting opioid withdrawal syndromes at this point – no pupillary dilatation, no nausea/vomiting, no diarrhea, and no diaphoresis, although he has tachycardia, which could be related to his agitation
- A seizure could also be a consideration; however, the possibility is remote because of high-dose lorazepam administration. Withdrawal seizure is a possibility within 7 days of the last drink

Further investigation

Is there anything else you would especially like to know about this patient?

- Further details regarding his social history and substance use during initial intake would have been helpful
- Medication history: the patient might be taking other GABAergic medications contributing to the difficult withdrawal process?
- Collateral information obtained from the brother and close friend: the patient has been smoking methamphetamine daily since becoming homeless in 2008. According to his friend, he only smokes methamphetamine and does not consume other drugs or alcohol
- His γ-glutamyltransferase level, obtained as a marker for recent large alcohol consumption, was noted to be 78 U/l, which is only slightly elevated
- A repeat ECG was obtained with a noted QTc of 517 ms

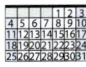

Case outcome: first interim follow-up visit at day 4

- Olanzapine (Zyprexa) 2.5 mg IM every 8 hours as needed was ordered for agitation and the CIWA-Ar was continued with instructions to score the patient as long as he is able to participate in the interview
- Olanzapine was ordered because it can be used for methamphetamine-induced psychosis, methamphetamine withdrawal delirium, and benzodiazepine withdrawal delirium, to spare the patient more lorazepam administration. It was chosen instead of other available antipsychotics due to a better safety profile regarding the patient's prolonged QTc on ECG and telemetry monitoring
- The patient rested for 3 hours after olanzapine was given and was less agitated in between doses, but at some point overnight he had to be restrained again and received lorazepam (Ativan) 6 mg IV total

Question

Would you continue the olanzapine (Zyprexa) and lorazepam (Ativan)?

- Continue with olanzapine at the lowest possible dose as needed for recurrence of agitation
- Discontinue lorazepam because he has been given substantial amounts already and prior doses could still be in his system, and also to minimize the risk of respiratory depression; watch the patient closely if mentation clears

Case outcome: second interim follow-up visit on day 5 of hospitalization

- On day 5, the patient remained confused and disoriented, but some clinical improvement was noted. The patient was less agitated and opened his eyes on verbal command. He tolerated some PO intake (liquids)
- His electrolytes were corrected. He still had atrial fibrillation (AF) and a rapid ventricular response (RVR); the diltiazem (Cardizem) IV drip was continued
- The patient had no fever, no episodes of hypotension, and no abnormal involuntary movements, or nystagmus. A neurological examination and workup showed no focal neurological signs
- The primary team was advised to remove his restraints, because this could aggravate his agitation, discontinue benzodiazepines, continue a sitter for safety, continue frequent reorientation, and consider a neurology consult if there was no improvement

- Lorazepam (Ativan) was stopped and olanzapine (Zyprexa) as needed was continued for which three doses in total were administered that day

Attending physician's mental notes

- There are subtle signs that the patient is improving, although he is still unable to verbalize his needs, which offers a glimpse that the intervention of withholding the benzodiazepine and adding olanzapine (Zyprexa) was of benefit
- Other causes of encephalopathy still needed to be ruled out. Follow-up with neurology is recommended
- New-onset seizure, acute stroke, or an infectious process seems less likely at this time. The patient's physical examination is within normal limits although he is still unable to follow commands

Further investigation

What other testing/procedures would you consider if there is no significant change in mental status?

- Lumbar puncture
- Repeat MRI
- EEG

Case outcome: third interim follow-up visit on day 6 of hospitalization

- On day 6 of hospitalization, the patient became more alert and responsive to name-calling, answered simple questions, and followed basic commands
- He was able to ambulate with physical therapy, he tolerated a regular diet, and he was completely off restraints
- Thiamine supplementation were continued
- His vital signs showed no fever, laboratory tests did not show any signs of infection, the neck was supple, and he was able to move his extremities. There were no focal neurological deficits, no abnormal limb movement, and no tremors appreciated
- Neurology added possible multi-infarct dementia due to multiple lacunar infarcts and chronic drug use, and possible cerebral hypoperfusion due to AF with RVR that decreased an already compromised left ventricular function aggravated by benzodiazepine administration

Case outcome: fourth interim follow-up visit on day 7 of hospitalization

- On day 7 of hospitalization, olanzapine (Zyprexa) was discontinued, and the patient returned to his baseline mental status; he tolerated a regular diet and participated in physical and occupational therapies

- He had no recollection of what had happened during the previous days of hospitalization. A mini mental state examination was normal and did not show impairment
- The sitter was discontinued

Case debrief

- This was a very challenging case of a patient without having the benefit of a good history and physical examination. It was difficult to obtain collateral information due to the patient being homeless and estranged from his family. The substance use history was also very difficult to assess. The patient was non-communicative, was on four-point restraints, and did not follow any command
- The mental examination was very limited and not helpful
- Immediate decisions had to be taken to offer comfort and relief, taking into consideration not to further compromise his mental and respiratory status
- Evaluation was required of the potential side effects of psychotropic medications to the cardiac rhythm and function
- Regarding his alcohol use, we learned that he had had a previous admission (about 10 years ago) to a local hospital for alcohol withdrawal. He admitted to drinking alcohol only occasionally, which was corroborated by his brother and his friend and supported by liver enzyme levels, γ-glutamyltransferase, mean corpuscular volume, and UDS
- However, the patient reported that his last use of methamphetamines was 3 hours prior to admission

Take-home points

- We cannot overstress the importance of a well-conducted initial history and physical examination that includes detailed substance use history. Most clinicians are not comfortable in broaching the subject due to the fear that they might offend the patient
- Good knowledge of withdrawal syndromes of different substances of abuse as well as experience and confidence in giving neuroleptics to patients in acute care settings are crucial in times of crisis
- Rapid and accurate recognition of the crisis and prompt referral is paramount in decreasing morbidity and length of hospital stay

Performance in practice: confessions of a psychopharmacologist

What could have been done better here?

- Early intervention and referral: the patient was already agitated and on restraint for 2 days prior to referral

- Nursing education regarding the proper use of the CIWA-Ar protocol, rather than relying on the assessment when the patient cannot answer the questions
- The family should have been involved sooner and collateral information investigated further
- Perhaps olanzapine (Zyprexa) should have been used earlier

What are possible action items for improvement in practice?

- Development of a hospital-associated delirium protocol
- Use of other validated scoring system for delirium
- Use of PAWSS (Prediction of Alcohol Withdrawal Severity Scale) on initial assessment for early identification of patients with a potential complicated alcohol withdrawal course
- Not using CIWA-Ar as a reliable scoring system once the patient is already having delirium due to falsely elevated scores and hence the potential for malignant administration of benzodiazepines, which is associated with increased mortality and prolonged hospital stay

Tips and pearls

- Clinicians should be familiar with the different neuroleptics, doses, preparation, and side effects
- Recognition of proper timing of administration of sedatives and/or antipsychotics is important to minimize complications
- All antipsychotics may cause prolongation of QTc on an ECG. QTc prolongation, resulting from blockade of ion channels, is medically significant because it can be associated with an increased risk for potentially fatal ventricular arrhythmias (torsades de pointes). These changes are particularly frequent with first-generation antipsychotics of the phenothiazine class and some second- and third-generation antipsychotics. The risk is lower for haloperidol (Haldol) and olanzapine (Zyprexa)

Mechanism of action moment
Methamphetamine withdrawal

- Methamphetamine withdrawal has been studied on a very limited basis in humans. DSM-5 defines the criteria for cocaine and amphetamine withdrawal syndromes (Table 32.1), and 87–97% of recently abstinent amphetamine users are thought to experience withdrawal
- The duration of amphetamine withdrawal is generally considered to be much longer than cocaine withdrawal, reportedly lasting from 5 days to more than 2 weeks
- Acute withdrawal from chronic amphetamine use in humans has been associated with depression, fatigue, sleepiness, aggression,

Table 32.1 Stimulant withdrawal: DSM-5 diagnostic criteria

A	Cessation of (or reduction in) prolonged amphetamine-type substance, cocaine, or other stimulant use
B	Dysphoric mood or two (or more) of the following physiological changes, developing within a few hours to several days after criterion A: 1. Fatigue 2. Vivid, unpleasant dreams 3. Insomnia or hypersomnia 4. Increased appetite 5. Psychomotor retardation or agitation
C	The signs or symptoms in criterion B cause clinically significant distress or impairment in social, occupational, or other important areas of functioning
D	The signs or symptoms are not attributable to another medical condition and are not better explained by another mental disorder, including intoxication or withdrawal from another substance *Specify* the specific substances that cause the withdrawal syndrome (i.e. amphetamine-type substance, cocaine, or other stimulant)

agitation, anxiety, hyperphagia, hypersomnia, and psychomotor retardation

Benzodiazepine paradoxical CNS stimulation: benzodiazepine disinhibition

- Although rare, disinhibitory reactions characterized by acute excitement and altered mental states have been described following the use of benzodiazepines. These reactions have been termed paradoxical and may be dangerous if interpreted as being due to pain or anxiety and treated incorrectly. The inhibitory action of benzodiazepines typically causes relaxation and decreases anxiety, and can cause anterograde amnesia. It is estimated that less than 1% of patients experience atypical responses to benzodiazepines. The majority of case reports of paradoxical reactions are in patients treated with high doses of high-potency benzodiazepines, such as alprazolam (Xanax), clonazepam (Klonopin), flunitrazepam (Rohypnol) and triazolam (Halcion), particularly when they are administered IV. There is also an increased risk from drugs with a short half-life as very high and/or rapidly fluctuating plasma levels may be responsible
- The clinical action of benzodiazepines is mediated by γ-aminobutyric acid type A (GABA$_A$) chloride channels. Benzodiazepines cause increased transmission of chloride ions by increasing the cycling rate of GABA channels. The mechanism by which paradoxical reactions occur is not completely understood, but the most likely explanation is that the anxiolytic and amnesic effects of benzodiazepines lead to a loss of the restraint that governs normal social behavior and a reduced ability to concentrate on the external social cues that guide appropriate behavior. Benzodiazepine-induced inhibition of neurotransmission may result in a decrease in the

restraining influence of the cortex, leading to excitement, agitated toxic psychosis, increased anxiety, hostility, and rage. Ingestion of alcohol, which also binds to GABA$_A$ receptors, would be expected to, and indeed can, increase the severity of this reaction

- Treatment of a paradoxical response to benzodiazepines may include supportive administration of physostigmine (Antilirium), flumazenil (Romazicon), and antipsychotics. Physostigmine is an acetylcholinesterase inhibitor that crosses the blood–brain barrier and acts to reverse the CNS depression. Physostigmine is thought to improve the paradoxical response to benzodiazepines via an antiepileptic effect. Flumazenil (Romazicon) antagonizes the benzodiazepine receptor and has clinical use in reversing benzodiazepine overdose. Antipsychotics are thought to improve atypical responses to benzodiazepines via action at dopamine receptors. This action has a calming effect on atypical responders to benzodiazepines

CIWA in patients with delirium

- The CIWA-Ar is a validated 10-item assessment tool used to quantify the severity of alcohol withdrawal syndrome (AWS) and provide clinician guidance for benzodiazepine treatment of AWS. In practice, nurses often perform the assessment hourly and may administer symptom-triggered benzodiazepine therapy dependent on the total CIWA-Ar score; the protocol may be ordered at any point during hospitalization. There are many potential limits to the safe use of CIWA-Ar. Six of the 10 items take into consideration a patient's verbal response to questions about withdrawal symptoms, and therefore patients lacking adequate cognitive status or communicative abilities due to delirium are not appropriate CIWA-Ar candidates

- The PAWSS screening tool was developed to identify patients at risk of complicated AWS. PAWSS criteria do not include all possible risk factors for AWS; however, the tool may serve to inform which patients may be appropriate candidates for the CIWA-Ar protocol. A PAWSS score of ≥4 suggests a high risk of moderate-to-AWS and that prophylaxis or treatment for alcohol withdrawal may be reasonable

Posttest self-assessment question and answer

Which medication can be used for both amphetamine-induced psychosis and alcohol withdrawal delirium?

A. Thioridazine (Mellaril)

B. Olanzapine (Zyprexa)

C. Quetiapine (Seroquel)

D. Risperidone (Risperdal)

Answer: B

Olanzapine has a safer profile, with less risk of QTc prolongation, and can be administered intramuscularly. Thioridazine has the highest risk for QTc prolongation. Quetiapine and risperidone cannot be administered parenterally or intramuscularly.

References

1. American Psychiatric Association. *Diagnostic and Statistical Manual of Mental Disorders*, 5th edn. Arlington, VA: American Psychiatric Association, 2013

2. Bramness, JG; Rognli, EB. Psychosis induced by amphetamines. *Curr Opin Psychiatry* 2016; 29:236–41. https://doi.org/10.1097/YCO.0000000000000254

3. Eloma AS, Tucciarone JM, Hayes EM, Bronson BD. Evaluation of the appropriate use of a CIWA-Ar alcohol withdrawal protocol in the general hospital setting. *Am J Drug Alcohol Abuse* 2018; 44:418–25. https://doi.org/10.1080/00952990.2017.1362418

4. Gerlach M, Mehler-Wex C, Schimmelmann BG. Antipsychotics. In: Gerlach M, Andreas W, Greenhill L, eds. *Psychiatric Drugs in Children and Adolescents: Basic Pharmacology and Practical Applications*. Vienna: Springer, 2014; pp. 157–218

5. Grover S, Kumar V, Chakrabarti S. Comparative efficacy study of haloperidol, olanzapine and risperidone in delirium. *J Psychosom Res* 2011; 71:277–81. https://doi.org/10.1016/j.jpsychores.2011.01.019

6. Kirkpatrick, D, Smith, T, Kerfeld, M, et al. Paradoxical reaction to alprazolam in an elderly woman with a history of anxiety, mood disorders, and hypothyroidism. *Case Rep Psychiatry* 2016; 2016: 6748947. https://doi.org/10.1155/2016/6748947

7. Maldonado JR, Sher Y, Das S, et al. Prospective validation study of the prediction of alcohol withdrawal severity scale (PAWSS) in medically ill inpatients: a new scale for the prediction of complicated alcohol withdrawal syndrome. *Alcohol Alcohol* 2015; 50:509–18. https://doi.org/10.1093/alcalc/agv043

8. Mancino MJ, Gentry BW, Feldman Z, et al. Characterizing methamphetamine withdrawal in recently abstinent methamphetamine users: a pilot field study. *Am J Drug Alcohol Abuse* 2011; 37:131–6. https://doi.org/10.3109/00952990.2010.543998

9. Mayo-Smith MF, Beecher LH, Fischer TL, et al. Management of alcohol withdrawal delirium. An evidence-based practice guideline.

Arch Intern Med. 2004; 164:1405–12. https://doi.org/10.1001/archinte.164.13.1405

10. Paton, C. Benzodiazepines and disinhibition: a review. *Psychiatr Bull* 2002, 26:460–2. https://doi.org/10.1192/pb.26.12.460

11. Rivière J, van der Mast RC, Vandenberghe J, van Den Eede F. Efficacy and tolerability of atypical antipsychotics in the treatment of delirium: a systematic review of the literature. *Psychosomatics* 2019; 60:18–26. https://doi.org/10.1016/j.psym.2018.05.011

12. Van der Bijl P, Roelofse JA. Disinhibitory reactions to benzodiazepines: a review. *J Oral Maxillofac Surg* 1991; 49:519–23. https://doi.org/10.1016/0278-2391(91)90180-t

Case 33: "Perseverance"

The Question: The patient with a history of anxiety, mood lability, hypomanic symptoms, psychotic symptoms, history of substance abuse, medical issues, and multiple failed trials of medications due to side effects from medication. What is the diagnosis and how should it be managed? What medications should be used to treat bipolar disorder with mixed episodes?

The Psychopharmacological Dilemma: How to manage multiple failed trials of medications from different classes, with initial benefit but then loss of effect

Kathleen Lopez, Courtney DiNicola, and Niraj Gupta

Pretest self-assessment question (answer at the end of the case)

What medications should be used to treat bipolar disorder with mixed episodes?

A. Selective serotonin reuptake inhibitors (SSRIs) or selective norepinephrine reuptake inhibitors (SNRIs)
B. Monoamine oxidase inhibitors
C. Tricyclic antidepressants
D. Dopamine antagonists
E. Serotonin-dopamine antagonist/partial agonist

Patient evaluation on intake

- A 29-year-old-woman with the chief complaint of anxiety. The patient describes her anxiety as "chest really hurts, stomach upset, heart races" that usually lasts a few hours. She has suffered from anxiety since she was 11, but 5 months ago she started taking lorazepam (Ativan) when her anxiety became severe after her grandfather's death
- She admits to elevated, expansive moods lasting 3–4 days, most recently a few weeks ago, described by the patient as "a rollercoaster of emotions, spending lots of money, talking a lot, staying up and not being tired, sleeping 3 or 4 hours, watching TV, cleaning the room, on the phone, organizing." She reports difficulty falling asleep. Her sleep patterns are not consistent; some nights she gets 8–14 hours of sleep and other nights she will not sleep at all. The patient also admitted to having a few days of feeling sad, lacking motivation, hopelessness, having no energy, and having suicidal thoughts
- Her primary stressor is her uncle, who has alcohol dependence and moved in with her and her grandmother. The patient believes her

uncle is taking advantage of her grandmother. She spends a lot of her time in her bedroom to avoid her uncle; her coping skills have included distraction, prayer, and positive self-talk

- Her solution to her current issues is "Focusing on myself, getting on the right medication, seeing a therapist every 2 weeks, and learning more cognitive behavioral therapy and dialectical behavioral therapy skills." She was two classes away from completing her Associate of Arts degree when she had her nervous breakdown 5 years ago. She wants to go to school and learn to become a social worker

Psychiatric history

- The patient started using mental health services after her parents divorced at age 5, and she has been consistently using them since the age of 11
- She has a previous history of one involuntary psychiatric hospitalization for 72 hours
- She has a history of five voluntary psychiatric hospitalizations
  - Her last hospitalization was 4 years ago for suicidal ideations, domestic violence, and a nervous breakdown
  - She has been in two crisis houses
- The last time she saw her psychiatrist and therapist was 2 years ago. Her reason for stopping these visits was as stated as "I did not like my therapist. I thought Alcoholics Anonymous was helping more than my therapist. I was going to the clinic. I got depressed and I didn't want to go. I didn't want to go because I was tired, and my kidneys were not feeling good."
- She has a history of suicidal ideations. Two years ago, she had intentions and a plan to commit suicide but did not go through with it and sought help. She stated that her plan was vague and that she did not have the intention to go through with it
- Prior to her initial visit to the clinic, she was previously treated at a partial hospitalization program for 2 weeks followed by the intensive outpatient program for bipolar and suicidal ideations after she lost her grandfather, who was her father figure
- She reports suicidal ideations, severe panic attacks for several months, and depression. She describes her moods as "a roller coaster, in the middle of a breakdown"
- She is grieving because her mother "almost died" last year, her grandfather died, and she has chronic kidney disease
- She reports feeling hopeless and helpless: "I feel like I had one horrible thing in my life happen after the other but I keep backsliding. I get better and then something happens, and it gets worse"

- She reports a tendency of stopping bipolar medications due to sexual side effects (unable to/weak climax) and feeling like she is getting better, but she subsequently becomes symptomatic after stopping medications

Attending physician's mental notes: 1 month prior to initial visit

- The patient is attending an intensive outpatient program and has been diagnosed with bipolar disorder. She meets the criteria for bipolar I disorder with psychotic features based on her frequent hospitalizations and self-reports
- She denied most symptoms of a personality disorder; she has a history of cutting behaviors and has made a few suicide attempts
- She has numerous physical health problems and when she had her last physical health exacerbation, she became suicidal again and was admitted to the hospital
- She openly discussed inconsistent behaviors with current and past treatment. She stopped seeing a therapist recently and is not 100% compliant with her current treatment
- She has a significant history of alcohol and cannabis abuse in her early teens and reports being sober since the age of 14
- She may benefit from a higher level of care due to her history of being inconsistent with treatment programs
- Assessment: bipolar I disorder, current or most recent episode depressed with psychotic features; generalized anxiety disorder
- Recommendations
  - Increase hydroxyzine (Vistaril) from 25 to 50 mg three times per day as needed for anxiety
  - Continue vilazodone (Viibryd) 20 mg daily and quetiapine (Seroquel) 75 mg daily for now
  - Taper lorazepam (Ativan); the patient agreed to attempt with the current supply
  - Consider raising the dose of quetiapine to 200 mg, the minimally effective dose approved for treating bipolar depression
  - The patient's predominant symptoms were anxiety and a history of poor compliance and substance abuse. Hydroxyzine was prescribed for anxiety. The patient does not want to change quetiapine because she reports that at 100 mg, she "gets the mouth thing" and at 125 mg she has "restless legs." The patient agreed to continue vilazodone

Question

What additional history would you like to know?

- A more extensive social history including her life during her formative years, past and current relationships, and education
- A more in-depth review of her substance use history
- Medical history
- Family history, in particular psychiatric history
- Current medications and previous medication trials
- All the above

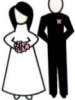

Social and personal history

- The patient was raised by her mother and grandparents and currently lives with her elderly grandmother. Her biological father did not play an important role in her life. She does not have siblings. Her father remarried and had two children. Her mother remarried and her stepfather has four children. Her half siblings were not a part of her upbringing. "It was good, but it was rough. I feel like I was raised by really good people. I have a lot of good memories with my family. My family wanted the best for me."
- She has an uncle with alcohol dependence, who recently moved in a month ago with the patient and her grandmother
- She has a history of two previous domestically violent relationships. She has had a boyfriend for the past 3 months. She has never been married and does not have children
- She graduated high school and is two credits short of an Associate of Arts degree. She was teased and bullied in high school due to early pubertal development and reports a learning disability
- Abuse:
  - Sexual abuse started around 7–9 years old and continued throughout her adult life. She was raped at age 11/12 and experienced sexual attacks throughout teen and early adult years
  - She has an emotionally abusive stepfather but has experienced no physical abuse from him
- She has been in recovery from alcohol for 15 years; she attends Alcoholics Anonymous and has a sponsor
- She has been on Social Security Disability Insurance for 4 years
- She lists the following strengths:
  - Accomplishments: "I think the fact that I got sober and stayed sober was a big deal"
  - Interests: "Art, music, nature, family, and friends"
  - Hopes: "I want to get a Bachelor's degree, get married, and have children. I want to travel. I want to be stable."

Substance use history
- She first used alcohol at age 6. She used for "probably 4 years, drinking heavily for two of those years", drinking either every day or every other day; she last used alcohol at age 14
- She first used cannabis at age 11 and smoked daily for 3 years; she last used at age 14
- Opioid, pain pills were first used at age 12/13 by either snorting or swallowing and used for 1 year; last use was at age 14
- She unintentionally smoked a joint laced with phencyclidine once at age 14
- She is currently in Alcoholics Anonymous. She completed various outpatient programs at age 15, and has never participated in a residential treatment program

Medical history
- Bipolar I disorder, current/most recent episode depressed, with psychotic features
- Generalized anxiety disorder
- Thalassemia
- Migraines
- Fibromyalgia
- Chronic kidney disease stage III
- Nephrocalcinosis
- Arthritis/joint pain
- Asthma
- Constipation/pain of bowel movements
- High blood pressure
- Urinary problems
- Tonsil removal

Family history
- Her father is not present in her life, but her mother believes that her father has bipolar disorder, diabetes, and high blood pressure
- Her mother has depression, lupus, myasthenia gravis, Sjogren's syndrome, and fibromyalgia
- Her uncle has depression
- There is a family history of heart disease and Alzheimer's disease

Current medications
- Vilazodone (Viibryd) 20 mg daily for depression
- Quetiapine (Seroquel) 75 mg daily for sleep, depression, mood stabilization

- Hydroxyzine (Vistaril) 25 mg three times per day as needed for anxiety
- Lorazepam (Ativan) 1 mg every 8 hours as needed (uses every couple of days)
- Potassium citrate 15 mEq three times per day
- Chlorthalidone (Hygroton) 12.5 mg QOD
- Ropinirole (Requip) 0.5 mg at bedtime
- Fish oil
- Folic acid
- Oral contraceptive pill

Reported medication trials

- Escitalopram (Lexapro) 10 mg daily (discontinued due to sexual side effects and headaches on 20 mg daily)
- Lithium
- Lamotrigine (Lamictal)
- Divalproex sodium (Depakote)
- Lurasidone (Latuda)
- Venlafaxine (Effexor)
- Citalopram (Celexa)
- Fluoxetine (Prozac)
- Bupropion (Wellbutrin)
- Sertraline (Zoloft)
- Mirtazapine (Remeron)
- Brexpiprazole (Rexulti)
- Quetiapine (Seroquel)

Question

Should we use antidepressants for anxiety if diagnosed with bipolar disorder?

Attending physician's mental notes: initial visit

- Take into consideration the possibility of an underlying borderline personality disorder and thus consider if the patient would benefit from dialectical behavioral therapy
- Medical causes for the patient's symptoms should also be considered, such as a possible endocrine disorder such as hyperthyroidism
- Given her history of chronic kidney disease, evaluate her medications to ensure safety and prevent risk of toxicity, consider adverse drug interactions, and consider whether any medications could be having a negative effect on her kidney function

- It is important to consider the patient's history of substance use disorder and determine, with good clinical judgment, whether controlled substances should or should not be prescribed

Further investigation

Is there anything else you would especially like to know about this patient?

- What is the status of her kidney function?
- Would it be helpful to get collateral information from her primary care provider on her other medical issues to get a comprehensive view of her health and rule out any medical causes of her symptoms such as hyperthyroidism?

Case outcome: first interim follow-up visit at 1 month

- The patient reports benefit from the recent hydroxyzine (Vistaril) increase: "It helped a lot, kicked in faster and my anxiety went away faster. I've had no anxiety problems the past few weeks or should I say panic attacks like before – now normal anxiety"
- She is no longer taking lorazepam (Ativan)
- She is sleeping 6–11 hours per night (goes to sleep between 3 a.m. and 5 a.m., sleeps until 11 a.m. or 2 p.m.), which has been a consistent pattern for 2 months. She has had sleep difficulties her entire life and describes herself as a "night owl"
- She does not take quetiapine (Seroquel) until 3 a.m. because she likes staying up late
- She wants more help with her mood: "I normally base it off my boyfriend and my relationship. I see it as unstable the most when I'm with him on the weekend. I have anger and irritability – I hold in my frustration at home during the week." The patient was recommended to discuss this with her therapist, with whom she has had one appointment with and has biweekly follow-ups
- The patient says home life continues to be difficult, but she keeps busy with medical appointments with her reported eight specialists. The patient was also directed to obtain a clinic group schedule to begin participating in group therapy
- The patient reports "slacking off at Alcoholics Anonymous meetings" but returned yesterday
- Recommendations
  - The patient requests an increase in quetiapine; increase from 75 to 100 mg daily
  - Continue vilazodone (Viibryd) 20 mg daily with meals and hydroxyzine 50 mg three times per day as needed for anxiety

- Ordered laboratory tests and encourage sleep hygiene
- Continue psychotherapy, provided psychoeducation, recommended psychotherapy/groups, provided supportive therapy, advised on healthy diet/exercise/weight loss, discussed sobriety, and discussed a safety plan
- Continue with primary care provider follow-up

Attending physician's mental notes: first interim follow-up visit at 1 month

- The patient has had symptom relief from medication but wants more help with her mood. She continued reporting mood reactivity, irregular sleep cycle and life patterns, and unstable and reactive interpersonal skills. Are these mood symptoms or personality traits?

Questions

How do we address her continued unstable and labile mood?
Does she have any personality traits that could be contributing to her symptoms?
Is she really receiving adequate treatment of either bipolar mania or bipolar depression or mixed state?

Case outcome: second interim follow-up visit at 2 months

- The patient describes herself as worse overall, despite stating that "nothing's changed from what I was doing well right after I left [the facility]"
- She reports that her "mood is a little more stable" since increasing quetiapine (Seroquel). She has been "angry, depressed, and hopeless" for 3 weeks without identifiable triggers or recent stressors. She denies any suicidal or homicidal ideation. She says, "I wonder if I'm on the right meds. I've been on them for a while, since November"
- The patient reports bad daily headaches (in the context of chronic migraines at baseline) from a higher ("doubled" = 40 mg) vilazodone (Viibryd) dose in the past; she is agreeable to retrial at a lower dose (30 mg)
- The patient is concerned about a 15 lbs weight gain since starting quetiapine. She reports an 80 lbs weight gain from quetiapine when previously taken "years ago". The patient agreed to consider switching to another antipsychotic
- She denies recent hydroxyzine (Vistaril) use (in the context of weight gain). Records indicated that her quetiapine and hydroxyzine expired, but the patient denies running out of medication

- The patient reports magnetic resonance imaging (MRI) findings consistent with "mild volume loss in parietal lobe" and says her neurologist attributed this to alcohol use, which she started at age 13
- Electroencephalogram (EEG), stress, and echocardiogram tests were reported as normal
- The patient is frustrated at the nephrologist for noting her weight gain in her chart

Attending physician's mental notes: second interim follow-up visit at 2 months

- The patient has failed multiple trials of medications and has stopped taking medications due to side effects. Given her history of obesity, is quetiapine (Seroquel) the right choice for her mood stabilization? Which mood stabilizer should we choose?

Questions

The patient has improved mood but will side effects from medication limit further titration?
What was the problem with the prior trial of lurasidone (Latuda)? Should we consider another trial of this?
Should we have considered switching quetiapine (Seroquel) or lowering the dose for a trial of cariprazine (Vraylar)?

Case debrief

- Patients with bipolar disorder, especially mixed episodes, are difficult to diagnose in complex clinical scenarios. This patient has a history of substance use disorder at different points in her life. There is also a lack of collateral information at the visit. Does this patient have a comorbid anxiety disorder? Is she providing an accurate history or does she exhibit recall bias?

Take-home points

- It is important to obtain a thorough history of mood to determine a diagnosis of bipolar disorder with mixed episodes (either bipolar manic/hypomanic episodes with subsyndromal depressive symptoms, or bipolar major depressive episodes with subsyndromal manic symptoms) early on to better guide treatment
- In patients with treatment-resistant depression, it is important to take a step back and gather a history about previous manic or hypomanic symptoms (especially irritability, distractibility, psychomotor agitation, racing/crowded thoughts, increased

talkativeness, emotional lability, impulsivity, risky behaviors, etc.) and to assess for any family history of bipolar disorder
- An underlying personality disorder should also be considered in patients with complex clinical scenarios

Performance in practice: confessions of a psychopharmacologist

- In retrospect, this patient did not receive adequate treatment of either bipolar mania or bipolar depression. Her quetiapine (Seroquel) dose could have been increased sooner or switched to another agent effective for bipolar mania (cariprazine (Vraylar) or olanzapine (Zyprexa)) or for bipolar depression (lamotrigine (Lamictal), lurasidone (Latuda), or cariprazine). Lurasidone and cariprazine cause little to no weight gain and might be preferred over quetiapine. Unstable mood symptoms require more aggressive "treatment from above" as well as "treatment from below"

Tips and pearls

- Bipolar disorder mixed episodes are more common in clinical practice, especially if they have comorbid symptoms of anxiety. Anxiety symptoms may actually be masquerading as symptoms of subsyndromal mania such as psychomotor agitation, distractibility, and irritability
- Adding antidepressants in bipolar disorder can present like mixed episodes. Thus, adding agents with direct evidence for efficacy in mixed states such as lurasidone (Latuda) or cariprazine (Vraylar) would be preferred

Two-minute tutorial

- Non-compliance with medication is common in mental health and often results in polypharmacy. In patients with multiple failed psychiatric medications, providers should consider underlying personality disorders and/or substance use disorders. It is also important to consider that mood disorders lie on a spectrum from depression to mania, rather than in discrete categories (Figure 33.1).
- The DSM-5 mixed features specifier includes full criteria for major depressive disorder (MDD) plus three or more of the following manic symptoms: elevated/expansive mood, inflated self-esteem or grandiosity, more talkative than usual or pressure to keep talking, flight of ideas or racing thoughts, increase in energy or goal-directed activity, increased or excessive involvement in activities

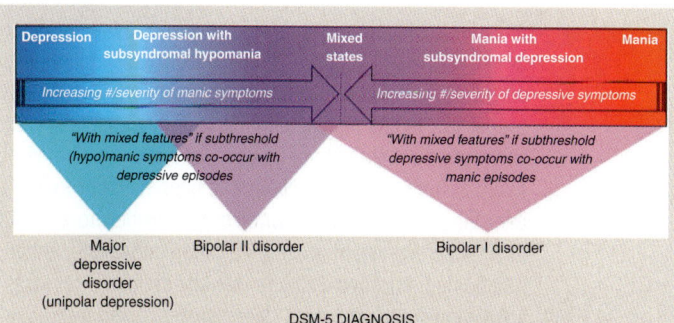

Figure 33. 1 The spectrum of mood disorders and DSM-5 diagnosis. From Stahl et al. (2017).

that have high potential for painful consequences, or decreased need for sleep.[1] However, irritability, distractibility, and psychomotor agitation are excluded from the criteria because they overlap with other disorders.[1] Making an early diagnosis of bipolar depression is difficult because patients can present with depression, but they may not notice their hypomania because it can feel pleasant and thus they do not report it. Family history is the most reliable risk factor for bipolar depression, as in our patient, whose father has suspected bipolar disorder, so it is essential to take a thorough family psychiatric history if bipolar disorder is suspected.[13] Research has shown that evolution from MDD to bipolar disorder was found in one-third of patients and was associated with treatment-resistant depression, earlier depression onset, longer treatment time, a higher number of depressive episodes, and hospitalization.[4] Mixed features are commonly seen in adults with MDD and bipolar disorder.[9] Suicide rates in patients with bipolar disorder are 20 times higher than that of the general population and two times higher than in those with MDD.[3,7]

- There is currently no mood stabilizer approved for treating depression (unipolar, mixed, or bipolar). However, there is some efficacy for lamotrigine (Lamictal) or valproate for bipolar depression, but not for lithium or carbamazepine (Equetro) as monotherapy.[2,5,6,11,14] Antidepressants should be avoided in patients with predominantly mixed states, during manic and depressive episodes with mixed features, as monotherapy in bipolar II depression with more than two concomitant manic symptoms, as an adjunct for acute bipolar I or II depressive episode with more than two concomitant manic symptoms, motor agitation or rapid cycling, and as monotherapy for bipolar I depression (Figure 33.2).[8] The new concept of treatment for major depressive episodes in unipolar depression with mixed features and bipolar disorder with or without mixed features is with a serotonin-dopamine antagonist/partial agonist with antidepressant, antimanic, and antipsychotic properties. In any patient with a hint of hypomania or mania, an antidepressant should not be used, and every patient should be asked about previous symptoms of hypomania or mania and their family history of bipolar disorder. Furthermore, addition of psychotherapy can improve medication adherence, enhance social functioning, improve ability to manage difficult stressors, encourage acceptance of the disorder, decrease denial and trauma, and decrease risk of recurrence.[10,15]

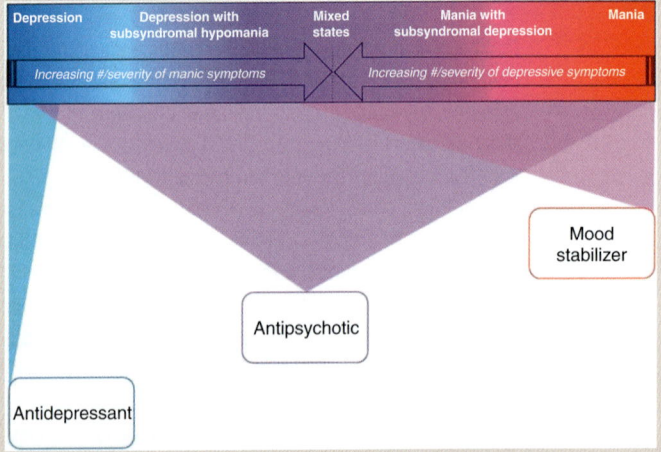

Figure 33.2. Bipolar spectrum-based first-line monotherapy treatment recommendations. From Stahl et al. (2017).

Posttest self-assessment question and answer

What medications should be used to treat bipolar disorder with mixed episodes?

A. SSRIs or SNRIs
B. Monoamine oxidase inhibitors
C. Tricyclic antidepressants
D. Dopamine antagonists
E. Serotonin-dopamine antagonist/partial agonist

Answer: E

Figure 33.3 shows a treatment algorithm for depression with mixed features.

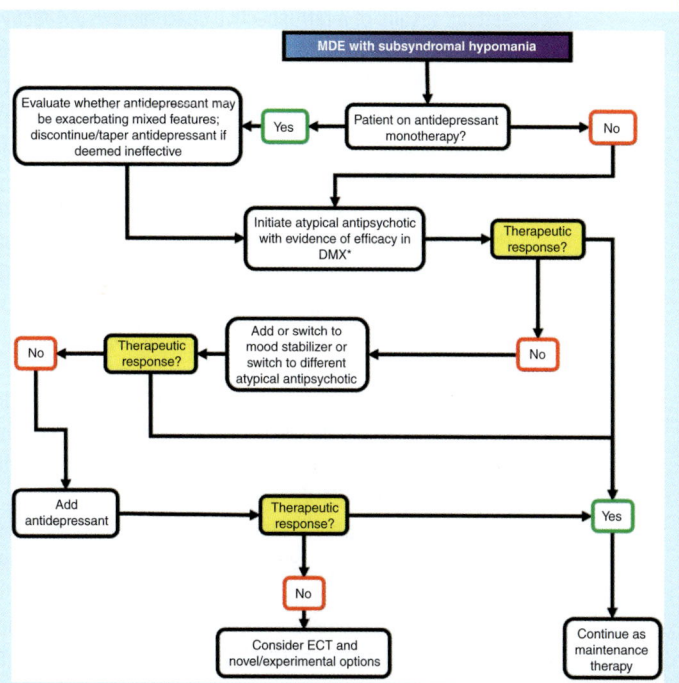

Figure 33. 3 Algorithm for treatment of a major depressive episode with mixed features Depressive Mixed States (DMX). MDE, major depressive episode; ECT, electroconvulsive therapy. *, Asenapine (Saphris), lurasidone (Latuda), olanzapine (Zyprexa), quetiapine (Seroquel), and ziprasidone (Geodon) have each shown some efficacy in treating DMX. From Stahl et al. (2017).

References

1. American Psychiatric Association. *Diagnostic and Statistical Manual of Mental Disorders*, 5th edn. Arlington, VA: American Psychiatric Association, 2013.

2. Connolly KR, Thase MD. The clinical management of bipolar disorder: a review of evidence-based guidelines. *Prim Care Companion CNS Disord* 2011; 13:PCC.10r0109. https://doi.org/10.4088/PCC.10r01097

3. Conus P, Macneil C, McGorry PD. Public health significance of bipolar disorder: implications for early intervention and prevention. *Bipolar Disord* 2014; 16:548–56. https://doi.org/10.1111/bdi.12137

4. Dudek D, Siwek M, Zielińska D, et al. Diagnostic conversions from major depressive disorder into bipolar disorder in an outpatient

setting: results of a retrospective chart review. *J Affective Disord* 2013; 144:112–15. https://doi.org/10.1016/j.jad.2012.06.014

5. Fountoulakis KN, Kasper S, Andreassen O, et al. Efficacy of pharmacotherapy in bipolar disorder: a report by the WPA section on pharmacopsychiatry. *Eur Arch Clin Neurosci* 2012; 262 (Suppl. 1):S1–48. https://doi.org/10.1007/s00406-012-0323-x

6. Goodwin GM, Consensus Group of the British Association for Psychopharmacology. Evidence-based guidelines for treating bipolar disorder: revised second edition – recommendations from the British Association for Psychopharmacology. *J Psychopharmacol* 2009; 23:346–88. https://doi.org/10.1177/0269881109102919

7. Holma KM, Haukka J, Suominen K, et al. Differences in incidence of suicide attempts between bipolar I and II disorders and major depressive disorder. *Bipolar Disord* 2014; 16:652–61. https://doi.org/10.1111/bdi.12195

8. International Society for Bipolar Disorders. Abstract 13. In: *10th International Conference on Bipolar Disorders (ICBD)*, June 13–16, 2013.

9. McIntyre RS, Soczynska JK, Cha DS, et al. The prevalence and illness characteristics of DSM-5-defined "mixed feature specifier" in adults with major depressive disorder and bipolar disorder: results from the International Mood Disorders Collaborative Project. *J Affective Disord* 2015; 172:259–64. https://doi.org/10.1016/j.jad.2014.09.026

10. McMahon K, Herr NR, Zerubavel N, et al. Psychotherapeutic treatment of bipolar depression. *Psychiatr Clin North Am* 2016; 39:35–56. https://doi.org/10.1016/j.psc.2015.09.005

11. Musetti L, Del Grande C, Marazziti D, Dell'Osso L. Treatment of bipolar depression. *CNS Spectr* 2013; 18:177–87. https://doi.org/10.1017/S1092852912001009

12. Stahl SM, Morrissette DA, Faedda G, et al. Guidelines for the recognition and management of mixed depression. *CNS Spectr* 2017; 22:203–19. https://doi.org/10.1017/s1092852917000165

13. Stahl SM. Mixed-up about how to diagnose and treat mixed features in major depressive episodes. *CNS Spectr* 2017; 22:111–15. https://doi.org/10.1017/S1092852917000207

14. Stahl SM. *Stahl's Essential Psychopharmacology: Prescriber's Guide*, 6th edn. Cambridge, UK: Cambridge University Press, 2017.

15. Swartz HA, Frank E, Kupfer DJ. Psychotherapy for bipolar disorder. In: Stein DJ, Kupfer DJ, Schatzberg AF, eds. *American Psychiatric Publishing Textbook of Mood Disorders*. Washington, DC: American Psychiatric Press Publishing, 2006; pp. 405–20.

Case 34: Clozapine (Clozaril) candidate discombobulates compassionate clinicians

The Question: How soon is too soon to consider clozapine utilization in a patient with polymorphic symptoms? The patient presents with residual symptoms of psychosis, which included delusions and hallucinations. He has been diagnosed with schizophrenia in the past and has failed multiple trials of psychotropic medication due to side effects. Does this patient need diagnostic clarification and how should this be further managed?

The Psychopharmacological Dilemma: The patient has failed trials of multiple medications in different classes, noting only transient efficacy

Darian Vernon, Nishant Prakash, and Niraj Gupta

Pretest self-assessment question (see answer at the end of the case)
Which of the following is true with regard to clozapine (Clozaril)?
A. Target range is 200–300 ng/ml
B. Efficacy is not impacted by smoking
C. It should be started after failing three antipsychotic medications
D. If dosing is interrupted for 48 hours or more, it must be reinitiated at a lower dose

Patient evaluation on intake

- A 20-year-old male with a history of paranoid schizophrenia

Psychiatric history

- The patient displays symptoms of paranoid schizophrenia, such as delusions that include "I feel that people are watching me" and states that his mother's boyfriend can read his mind. For auditory hallucinations, he states that God talks to him through radio and television. For visual hallucinations, he states that black shadowy voices "scream at me"
- The patient reports a lack of energy, and says, "I feel like a zombie" but denies other symptoms of depression. He has a history of irritable mood and anger issues, which manifest as "making mean faces, yelling, and crying," but his mother states that he does not have a history of aggressive behavior toward other people. The patient also reports having thoughts of hurting "random" people but has never acted on these thoughts. He denies suicidal ideation and homicidal ideation
- The patient also reports symptoms of anxiety and compulsive behaviors and self-harming behaviors. He engaged in self-harm 3

months ago, cutting his left arm because he "thought his mother's boyfriend was reading his mind"

- He admits to occasional use of cannabis and alcohol but does not believe the substances cause impairment in his daily life, nor does he think his current usage is a problem. On further assessment, the patient does not meet the criteria for substance use disorder

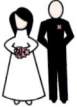

Social and personal history

- The patient lives with his biological mother, who is his main support system
- He had an Individualized Education Plan (IEP) that was done in childhood and was diagnosed with auditory processing disorder, borderline intellectual functioning, and learning disability not otherwise specified
- The patient disclosed that he had been abused at age 15, but he will not elaborate further
- The patient has been hospitalized multiple times for psychotic breaks in the past and has been diagnosed with paranoid schizophrenia
- He reported having mental health problems starting at age 14 for which he received psychotherapy only. He started receiving psychiatric medications at age 17

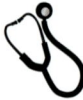

Medical history

- The patient has a history of closed head injury with loss of consciousness 6 years ago, prompting an electroencephalogram, which was found to be unremarkable

Medication history

- The patient has been on the following combination for at least a year:
  - Benztropine (Cogentin) 1 mg twice per day
  - Divalproex sodium (Depakote) 250 mg twice per day
  - Haloperidol (Haldol) 2 mg twice per day
  - Olanzapine (Zyprexa) 5 mg twice per day

Psychiatric history

- The patient has a history of one psychiatric hospitalization for 3 days, 3 years ago. He was diagnosed with schizophrenia during this time. The patient had a prior trial of quetiapine (Seroquel) 50 mg, risperidone (Risperdal) up to 4 mg and haloperidol (Haldol)

4 mg daily. An increased haloperidol dose caused extrapyramidal symptoms. The patient's previous trial of paroxetine (Paxil) and sertraline (Zoloft) made him suicidal and agitated

Attending physician's mental notes: initial evaluation

- The patient appears disheveled, with minimal speech, restless motor activity, neutral mood, blunted affect, and illogical thought processes; he admits to auditory hallucinations, and is delusional, denies any suicidal or homicidal ideations, is distracted, alert and oriented to person, place, and time; his cognition is intact, with impaired insight and fair judgment
- His medications should be simplified and the dosing optimized
- His mother is learning about schizophrenia. She is interested in the patient taking a long-acting injectable (LAI)
- The patient is currently a nearly daily user of cannabis
- Recommendations: discontinue haloperidol (Haldol) and increase olanzapine (Zyprexa) to 10 mg twice per day. Continue benztropine (Cogentin) 1 mg twice per day and divalproex sodium (Depakote) 250 mg twice per day
- The patient was given a routine laboratory slip to assess and monitor for metabolic syndrome, as olanzapine increases the risk of metabolic syndrome

Case outcome: first interim follow-up visit at 1 month

- The patient reports that he hears voices stating, "You should not live" and command auditory hallucinations telling him to kill himself. The patient reports, "My mind is controlled by someone else"
- He is restless, smiling inappropriately, and tells the provider, "There are two witches in my neighborhood"
- At this time, he denies use of any substances, including marijuana
- The patient states that daily tasks such as talking to people or brushing his hair are hard for him
- His mother states that the new medications are causing him to sleep more
- His current medications include olanzapine (Zyprexa) 10 mg twice per day; divalproex sodium (Depakote) extended-release 250 mg twice per day; benztropine (Cogentin) 1 mg twice per day
- Because he reports not using alcohol or marijuana, it is less likely to be substance induced

Questions

Does the patient have poorly controlled manic symptoms and worsening of psychosis?

Is it a predominantly bipolar disorder with psychotic symptoms?
Is the restlessness masking manic symptoms or extrapyramidal symptoms?
Is medication causing excessive sedation and hence difficulties with his activities of daily living or is this negative symptoms of schizophrenia?

Case outcome: second interim follow-up visit at 2 months

- Intervention: increase divalproex sodium (Depakote) to 500 mg twice per day and check the level
- The patient reports feeling calmer, with less pacing, and less agitation, noting that he "sees ghosts and witches periodically"
- His mother states that the increased olanzapine (Zyprexa) has caused him to be less psychotic with fewer voices telling to him to cut himself. She states that he has been more communicative but also more agitated. The patient's mother notes that he is sleeping fine and states that the voices do not distress him or appear to command him any more
- The patient is disheveled, smiling, pleasant, and cooperative, with appropriate speech, jerky movements of the arm and eye, and blinking at the beginning of the interview, but became calmer as the interview proceeded, with no further abnormal movement noted. The patient has neutral mood, restrictive affect, and normal thought processes. The patient continues to have auditory and tactile hallucinations and persecutory delusions, noting, "I can feel witches and demons pushing me in the back." The patient is oriented and alert, with adequate cognition, and fair judgment
- Medication efficacy has improved with the increase in divalproex sodium and olanzapine, but the patient continues to report episodic auditory hallucinations cursing at him and he continues feeling demons and witches pushing him
- The patient is experiencing the following symptoms: sedation, observed pacing, and subjective restlessness

Attending physician's mental notes: second interim follow-up visit at 2 months

- Is it possible the patient is experiencing extrapyramidal symptoms (EPS), such as acute dystonia or akathisia?
- Is this agitation due to uncontrolled psychosis?
- Is this schizoaffective disorder?
- Increase benztropine (Cogentin) to 2 mg twice per day
- Recommended melatonin for sleep

Case outcome: third interim follow-up visit at 3 months

- The patient's mother reports he has continued agitation, pacing, and restlessness. She notes that the patient had an episode that seemed like a panic attack
- The patient reports early insomnia and restless anxiety. He has jerky arm and leg movements that abate when he is less anxious, which is thought to be most compatible with simple motor tics

Questions

How reliable is the patient report?
Is the patient compliant with medication?

Attending physician's mental notes: third interim follow-up visit at 3 months

- The patient appears disheveled, with minimal speech, tremors and tics, anxious mood, blunted, anxious and restrictive affect, normal and goal-directed thought processes, some obsessions noted and appearing internally preoccupied, ideas of reference present, and hallucinations and delusions present; the patient seems oriented and alert with fair judgment
- The patient says his stepfather can read his mind and says he hears his stepsister's voice
- He is having panic attacks and episodic anxiety associated with obsessive and ruminative thoughts
- Ask the patient to bring his medication bottles as there is suspected poor compliance
- Add risperidone (Risperdal) 1 mg twice per day, continue divalproex sodium (Depakote) 500 mg twice per day, and continue olanzapine (Zyprexa) 10 mg twice per day and benztropine (Cogentin) 2 mg twice per day
- Consider clozapine (Clozaril) as the patient has failed trials of four antipsychotics

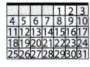

Case outcome: fourth interim follow-up visit at 4 months

- According to the mother's report, the patient is more pleasant to be around and seems mellow. The patient is not obsessively worried about other people getting hurt by witches
- He does endorse thoughts of homicide coming to mind about random people; however, these thoughts are distressing to him because he does not want to hurt them. He is also worried about father dying, as he smokes

Attending physician's mental notes: fourth interim follow-up visit at 4 months

- Increase risperidone (Risperdal) to 2 mg twice per day and monitor for EPS
- Consider the addition of a selective serotonin reuptake inhibitor (SSRI) for obsessive–compulsive disorder (OCD) as the patient has ruminative thoughts about his stepfather being hurt and thoughts of hurting random people. The patient also has fear of germs on his hands and avoids shaking hands with people
- Are these paranoid delusions true delusions or obsessive/ruminative thoughts?
- Plan: start fluoxetine (Prozac) 20 mg daily

Case outcome: fifth interim follow-up visit at 5 months

- The patient presented to urgent care with his mother because he was agitated, paranoid about individuals tampering with his food, refusing to eat or drink, not sleeping, and pacing at night. He has excessive worries about his family and the well-being of his stepfather
- His olanzapine (Zyprexa) was increased to 15 mg twice per day and risperidone was changed to the LAI formulation of risperidone (Risperdal Consta), paliperidone palmitate (Invega Sustenna), for concerns of compliance, which seemed to ameliorate his paranoid delusions regarding individuals tampering with his food

Case outcome: sixth interim follow-up visit at 6 months

- The patient is doing well on the current medication regimen
- He is less worried about the safety of his stepfather and the children in his family, and does not mention witches as frequently
- The patient admits to having unintelligible auditory hallucinations
- He seems less concerned about his food being poisoned or hands being contaminated while taking fluoxetine (Prozac)

Attending physician's mental notes: sixth interim follow-up visit at 6 months

- Plan: clozapine (Clozaril) was added and the dose was titrated to 500 mg per day in divided doses. As a result, there was a decrease in the patient's OCD and psychotic symptoms. Although clozapine was added, the patient continued to have occasional psychotic episodes. Olanzapine (Zyprexa) and divalproex sodium (Depakote) were discontinued
- His clozapine levels were titrated to approximately 550 ng/ml (normal range 350–700 ng/ml)

- Should electroconvulsive therapy (ECT) be considered? His mother did not seem agreeable to initiating ECT. Is the patient's diagnosis schizoaffective disorder with comorbid OCD?

Case debrief

- This young man has schizoaffective disorder with comorbid OCD currently in remission on clozapine (Clozaril), paliperidone (Invega), fluoxetine (Prozac), and benztropine (Cogentin)
- Providers are often hesitant to initiate clozapine, although patients are often good candidates for clozapine (if they have failed two antipsychotics at therapeutic dosage for an adequate amount of time)
- Individuals with OCD experience marked anxiety that can manifest as obsessive thoughts. The patient also had intermittent panic attacks
- There are some differences related to content of obsessions and compulsions that are dependent on age/developmental stage. For example, one might see higher rates of sexual and religious obsessions in adolescents than in children, and higher rates of harm obsessions (fears of catastrophic events such as death or illness to self or loved ones) in children and adolescents than in adults

Take-home points

- Schizoaffective disorder may have comorbid OCD symptoms that are often clinically confusing
- In individuals with schizophrenia or schizoaffective disorder, the prevalence of OCD is approximately 12%
- Up to 30% of individuals with OCD also have a lifetime tic disorder, which our patient had
- Obsessive–compulsive personality disorder and OCD sound similar in their names; however, obsessive–compulsive personality disorder is ego-syntonic (viewed as acceptable to the individual) while OCD is ego-dystonic (viewed as unacceptable) and therefore causes stress to the patient
- Patients must be compliant with clozapine (Clozaril) monitoring if clozapine is to be considered as an option for patients wanting/ needing to take clozapine
- More information on clozapine monitoring is available at https:// clozapinerems.com
- The patient adherence to laboratory tests and blood draws must be taken into account if the patient is to take clozapine. Due to this and

provider hesitancy to initiate clozapine, clozapine is underutilized in practice

- In addition to blood draws, if the patient is to initiate clozapine, the patient's bowel habits/routine must be assessed, as clozapine has a high anticholinergic burden and can precipitate necrotizing colitis and intestinal ischemia. Therefore, prophylactic bowel regimens should be considered before initiating clozapine

Performance in practice: confessions of a psychopharmacologist

- After two or more failed trials of antipsychotics, clozapine (Clozaril) should be considered as the next step. The patient might have stabilized on clozapine alone and may not have required ongoing LAI use

Two-minute tutorial

How paliperidone palmitate (Invega Sustenna) works

- It blocks dopamine D_2 receptors, reducing the positive symptoms of psychosis and stabilizing affective symptoms
- It blocks serotonin 5-HT_{2A} receptors, causing enhancement of dopamine release in certain brain regions and thus reducing motor side effects and possibly improving cognitive and affective symptoms
- Its serotonin 5-HT_7 antagonist properties may contribute to antidepressant actions
- The dosage range is 39–234 mg/month

Advantages of LAIs

- An LAI does not require simultaneous oral medication
- An LAI may work increasingly better after a few weeks of treatment in some patients
- An LAI may be very well tolerated
- An LAI may be combined with a second antipsychotic administered orally for difficult cases
- Patients with inadequate responses to atypical antipsychotics may benefit from determination of plasma drug levels and, if low, a dosage increase even beyond the usual prescribing limits

How to dose

- This is not recommended for patients who have not first demonstrated tolerability to oral paliperidone (Invega) or risperidone (Risperdal) (in clinical trials, two oral or short-acting intramuscular (IM) doses are generally used to establish tolerability)

- Conversion from oral: 234 mg delivered IM in the deltoid on day 1; 156 mg delivered IM in the deltoid on day 8; maintenance dose should start 4 weeks after the second loading injection

Oral equivalence (approximate)

Oral paliperidone (mg)	1-month Invega Sustenna (mg)
3	39–78
6	117
9	156
12	234

- The last two doses of paliperidone Invega Sustenna should ideally be the same dosage strength, so that a consistent maintenance dose is established prior to starting paliperidone Invega Trinza
- Conversion from 1-month injectable: initiate 3-month LAI when the next 1-month LAI injection is scheduled; dosing is based on the previous 1-month injection dose

1-month Invega Sustenna (mg)	3-month Invega Trinza (mg)
78	273
117	410
156	546
234	819

Dosing tips

- With LAIs, the absorption rate constant is slower than the elimination rate constant, resulting in "flip-flop" kinetics, i.e. time to steady state is a function of absorption rate, while concentration at steady state is a function of elimination rate
- The rate-limiting step for plasma drug levels for LAIs is not drug metabolism but rather slow absorption from the injection site
- Because plasma antipsychotic levels increase gradually over time, dose requirements may ultimately decrease from the initial dose; obtaining periodic plasma levels can be beneficial to prevent unnecessary plasma level creep
- The kinetics for paliperidone palmitate (Invega Sustenna) are determined by particle size: smaller particles (1-month) versus larger particles (3-month)

Posttest self-assessment question and answer

Which of the following is true with regard to clozapine (Clozaril)?

A. Target range is 200–300 ng/ml
B. Efficacy is not impacted by smoking
C. It should be started after failing three antipsychotic medications

D. If dosing is interrupted for 48 hours or more, it must be reinitiated at a lower dose

Answer: D

If the dosing is interrupted for 48 hours or more, therapy must be reinitiated at 12.5 mg once or twice per day secondary to concerns of hypotension, bradycardia, and syncope. The correct target range for clozapine is 350–700 ng/ml. Clozapine is metabolized by cytochrome P450 1A2 (CYP4501A2), as is olanzapine (Zyprexa) and asenapine (Saphris). Cigarette smoke induces the CYP4501A2 system, reducing the efficacy of these drugs. Clozapine should be initiated after failing two antipsychotics.

References

1. American Psychiatric Association. *Diagnostic and Statistical Manual of Mental Disorders*, 5th edn. Arlington, VA: American Psychiatric Association, 2013; pp.239–42.

2. Stahl SM. Paliperidone. *Stahl's Essential Psychopharmacology: Prescriber's Guide*, 6th edn. Cambridge, UK: Cambridge University Press, 2017; pp. 549–60.

Index of drug names

Index of case studies